Praise for

YOUNGER YOU

"*Younger You* challenges the long-held notion that we are helpless as it relates to the seemingly inexorable decline in our physical health as time marches on. Dr. Fitzgerald makes it clear that we can absolutely change our destiny as it relates to various parameters associated with aging and provides a straightforward program for achieving this important goal."

—DAVID PERLMUTTER, MD, *New York Times*
bestseller author of *Grain Brain*

"It is a new era—aging 'backward' is no longer a fantasy; it is now a fact proven by clinical trial. Dr. Kara Fitzgerald, lead author of this paradigm-shifting trial, now describes her approach in her new book, *Younger You*. This is the first book in the new era of 'aging reversal' medicine and health, and for all of us who are aging, this is a must read."

—DALE BREDESEN, MD, professor and author of
the *New York Times* bestseller, *The End of Alzheimer's*

"*Younger You* leads us through a compelling narrative linking food, genes, epigenetic programming of genes by life experiences and how this guides us to take control of our own lives. The book provides an engaging, clear, and understandable presentation of the complex science of epigenetics and the developmental origins of health and disease for the general audience."

—MOSHE SZYF, PhD, McGill University Medical School

"As a scientist and educator in nutritional epigenetics and longevity, I commend Kara's extraordinary ability to make science accessible and actionable to a lay audience. Her guest lecture for my course on the biology of longevity at Stanford University drew rave reviews from my students. I will recommend Kara's new book *Younger You* to my students who want to deepen their knowledge and practice of nutritional longevity."

—DR. LUCIA ARONICA, PhD

"Dr. Fitzgerald is among the first to realize that epigenetics is destined to be a game changer for twenty-first-century medicine. Now she shares her program to modify our epigenetics safely, with exercise, a natural diet, and a surprising array of other practices. Let's try it!"

—JOSH MITTELDORF, PhD, author of *Cracking the Age Code*

"Dr. Fitzgerald has published groundbreaking research that proves that we can change the aging of our body through a specific lifestyle intervention program. Now she has made this program available for all of us to benefit from in this extraordinary book. This is a 'must' for anyone interested in what they can do in slowing the aging process naturally."

—JEFFREY BLAND, PhD, president,
Personalized Lifestyle Medicine Institute

YOUNGER
YOU

YOUNGER
YOU

Reduce Your Bio Age—and Live Longer, Better

DR. KARA FITZGERALD
WITH KATE HANLEY

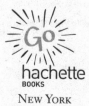

hachette
BOOKS

NEW YORK

Copyright © 2022 by Kara Fitzgerald

Cover design by Amanda Kain
Cover copyright © 2022 by Hachette Book Group, Inc.

Hachette Go, an imprint of Hachette Books
Hachette Book Group
1290 Avenue of the Americas
New York, NY 10104
HachetteGo.com
Facebook.com/HachetteGo
Instagram.com/HachetteGo

First Paperback Edition: January 2023
Hachette Books is a division of Hachette Book Group, Inc.

The Hachette Go and Hachette Books name and logos are trademarks of Hachette Book Group, Inc.

The publisher is not responsible for websites (or their content) that are not owned by the publisher.

Print book interior design by Linda Mark

Library of Congress Cataloging-in-Publication Data
Names: Fitzgerald, Kara N., author.
Title: Younger you : reduce your bio age-and live longer, better / Dr. Kara N. Fitzgerald.
Description: First edition. | New York : Hachette Go, 2022. | Includes bibliographical references and index.
Identifiers: LCCN 2021038350 | ISBN 9780306924835 (hardcover) | ISBN 9780306924859 (ebook)
Subjects: LCSH: Aging–Nutritional aspects. | Aging–Prevention. | Functional foods. | Longevity.
Classification: LCC RA776.75 .F58 2022 | DDC 613.2—dc23/eng/20211005

LC record available at https://lccn.loc.gov/2021038350

ISBNs: 9780306924835 (hardcover); 9780306924842 (trade paperback); 9780306924859 (ebook)

Printed in the United States of America

LSC-C

Printing 1, 2022

CONTENTS

Contents

*For my daughter, Isabella James, with whom I hope
to spend many more years by following this plan
as my foundational anti-aging strategy*

and for my patients, colleagues, and friends, for your faith in this work

*and for everyone who, like me, feels empowered by
the idea that we can start immediately to safely
and effectively turn back the biological hands of time.*

INTRODUCTION:
YOU CAN BECOME YOUNGER

WHAT IF I TOLD YOU, YOU COULD BE YOUNGER TOMORROW THAN you are today?

Some part of you would probably be very excited. You did, after all, pick up a book called *Younger You*. But there's probably another part of you that would be thinking something along the lines of, "Yeah, right."

But what if I followed that up by saying, it's true? And that you can do it simply by changing your diet and making some very doable modifications to your lifestyle—in other words, without expensive or high-risk drugs, or fasting for twenty-two hours a day, or any other so-called biohacking strategies?

"No way," you'd think.

I have two words for you: Yes way.

In fact, I have a two-month program that reversed the bio age of its participants by over three years.

I am the lead author on the groundbreaking, rigorous clinical pilot trial that asked participants to eat plenty of delicious food and adopt a handful of moderate practices—such as getting seven hours of sleep a night and practicing relaxation for ten minutes twice a day—for eight weeks. We measured their biological age before the study began and again when it ended. **And frankly, the results blew our doors off—our study participants lowered**

their biological age by an average of 3.23 years (compared to the control group, who received no intervention)!

This is where I need to point out that our study, while rigorous, was small. It's technically a pilot study, meaning it's designed to provide proof of concept and open the door to larger studies (which we are working on as I type). And yet, combined with our years of clinical experience using the program that we studied and that I outline in this book, it is as clear that we are headed in the right direction as it is that we need to keep researching.

In this book, as I discuss strategies to reverse biological age, you'll see that much of the research I cite is on animals or in human cells. While there is some research in humans (which I cover), there is significantly less (hence our trial being "first of its kind"). Although this is a young field, multiple lines of evidence converge on the conclusion that we might be able to control how long and how well we live through a combination of diet and lifestyle changes. In this book, I'll show you how you can follow essentially the same path that our study partipants and clinical patients have followed to become healthier and younger, too.

TURNING BACK THE BIOLOGICAL CLOCK

It's true that getting older is inevitable: no amount of wizardry can change how many years old you are. Although we all age with time, we don't all age equally. Aging is a complex process influenced by many factors, and even though two people can have the same chronological age, their life expectancy and living quality can be vastly different. That's because, in addition to your chronological age, which can only move in one direction, you also have a *biological* age—or, as I like to call it, your bio age. **And your bio age can move in reverse.**

Bio age is based on the premise that our bodies are constantly subject to damage and degradation from internal and external sources. By assessing how much damage has accumulated in your particular body, your bio age shows how old your tissues, systems, and even your genetic material are. In other words, you could be fifty chronologically but have the same amount of damage to your body as a typical fifty-eight-year-old. With our Younger You program, you could be fifty but repair your overall level of damage to that of someone in their forties. It's like turning back time.

While there have been various tools for assessing bio age for a while now, the accuracy of these tools has been mediocre at best. But recently, science has taken a massive leap forward in this arena. We can now measure bio age with exquisite accuracy by assessing how your genes are expressed in a revolutionary field of study known as epigenetics. "Epi" means "above;" epigenetics refers to the biological markers that sit on top of your genetic material and dictate which genes are turned on and which are turned off. To use a computing analogy, your DNA is the hardware—it is what it is. It can be damaged, and it can be repaired, but without software, it can't do much. So, what's the software? That is epigenetics.

So far, just a handful of human studies have shown that bio age can move in reverse. This is an extraordinary achievement, but these studies have relied on medications, and/or have taken a long time, and/or were measuring a population that started less than healthy (less healthy individuals tend to be older biologically and can therefore get younger simply by returning to health). Our study is the first to show that significant age reversal might be brought about in healthy individuals through doable diet and lifestyle changes alone, and possibly accomplished in a matter of weeks. No magic potions required. Just tweaking your normal lifestyle: food, sleep, exercise, and relaxation, but nothing beyond what most folks consider to be basic self-care.

REDUCING BIO AGE WITH DIET AND LIFESTYLE

Beyond our study participants, every one of the hundreds and hundreds of patients who have come through the doors of my clinic in the past several years have either been given, as their primary intervention, the eight-week eating plan and lifestyle prescription that our study participants followed, known as the Younger You Intensive, or been coached to incorporate some of these foods and practices—a less intensive, longer-term version known as Younger You Everyday.

At my clinic, we see patients with chronic conditions who have tried other medical avenues with limited success. They are often complex cases that represent a broad swath of the illnesses that are so common today— autoimmune diseases, chronic allergies, autism, digestive issues, diabetes, cardiovascular disease, infertility, cancer, Lyme disease, and neurodegen-erative diseases such as Alzheimer's, Parkinson's, and dementia. These are folks who have struggled with a conventional medicine model be-cause their medical realities don't necessarily fit clinical definitions, and if there are prescribed treatments, their side effects chip away at quality of life.

Regardless of their official diagnosis, the majority of our patients are at some phase of midlife, and they also want to look and feel younger. (We also have a great pediatrician on our team who uses the Younger You principles with children and young adults—because as you'll learn, they are important in all life stages.) That desire is often what gets them to book their first appointment. Yet the results my patients have experienced in search of reducing their bio age are extraordinary. We have seen their chronic, difficult-to-manage symptoms lessen, stabilize, or even go away completely.

For example, I recently started working with a woman who was dealing with a full-blown case of seasonal allergies. Ava had completely lost her sense of smell, her body was covered in hives, and every year she devel-oped a sinus infection so severe that it required antibiotics and steroids. In our first meeting, she was much more interested in developing a plan that would help reverse the signs of aging—the thickening middle, the brain fog, the loss of muscle tone—than she was in addressing her allergies. But by following the diet and lifestyle principles that I outline in this book, she lost weight, regained her ability to think clearly, built muscle, *and* her seasonal allergies fully resolved.

Ava's certainly not the only one. Across the board, our patients have reported more energy, better mood and less depression, fewer headaches, clearer skin, lost weight, and less susceptibility to succumbing to viruses. Their digestion improves—with less gas, bloating, diarrhea, and consti-pation. From a clinician's perspective, I have seen a drop in their blood sugar and insulin, reduced inflammatory markers, much lower levels of fat in the blood, higher "good" cholesterol and lower "bad" cholesterol, and even lower levels of the antibodies that are hallmarks of autoimmune conditions. Taken altogether, these results demonstrate the far reach of the Younger You program: from the epigenome to whole body balance! Essentially, it appears that we are empowering people to debug their own software.

You can use either version of the Younger You program at any age. Whether you are picking up this book because you want to feel younger or you want to address a specific condition, it doesn't matter—the Younger You program will help address both. It's a twofer, as turning back the clock should help clean up the symptoms that go along with aging.

It's so exciting to me that as we get further into what's known as the "omics revolution"—the line of study that looks at individual components of physiology such as the genome (your actual DNA), the epigenome (the material that sits on top of your genetic code and dictates which genes are turned on and which are switched off), the microbiome (the microbial population in your gut), and more, and how they interact with each other—we see that humble interventions such as nutrition, sleep, and exercise might be the most impactful and essential tools we have to improve individual health. It's a massive paradox that it took science reaching this level of sophistication to realize the power of these fundamental interventions, but it's so validating to me, a holistic physician/lab geek, to see just how exquisitely programmed for wellness we are, if we only understand how to nourish and take care of ourselves.

THE ULTIMATE GOAL: A LONGER, HEALTHIER LIFE

Our understanding of how to reduce our bio age is occurring just in the nick of time. Life expectancy in the United States has declined for three consecutive years (2015, 2016, and 2017), the longest decline since the period from 1915 to 1918, when World War 1 and the Spanish flu epidemic killed millions—and these numbers don't even take into account the COVID-19 pandemic that roared across the country starting in 2020.[1] It's not just that we're living a shorter time; it's also that we're spending a longer portion of the time we're alive with a serious disease that is a leading cause of death—according to information from the World Health Organization, we spend 20 percent of our lives sick.[2] (Although we have a life expectancy of 79.3 years, the average age for developing a serious illness is 63.1 years old, meaning we spend the last 16.2 years of our life ill.)[3]

In his incredible book *Being Mortal*, Atul Gawande included two graphs: one that showed the trajectory of a life before modern medicine, with limited years of health and then a fairly sharp decline that ended in death . . .

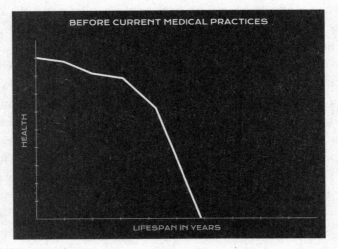

. . . and the common path of life we have now that we have learned how to survive, but not necessarily abate, disease. It shows a long, slow, gradual, and honestly, painful decline in quality of life.

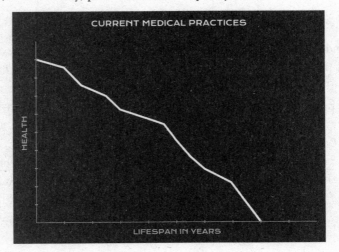

Our study and clinical work suggests a third option: that by aiming to support our epigenetics via diet and lifestyle, we might have the possibility of a new trajectory, one that combines the more consistent quality of life of Figure 1 and the overall length of life of Figure 2. Let's put an end to the sixteen-plus years of ill health we're all currently destined to endure and turn them back into years of thriving and wellness!

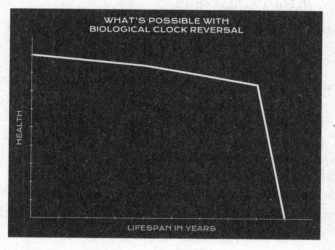

This third option isn't a new idea—it was first put forth by James Fries, a professor of medicine at Stanford University School of Medicine who published a paper on his "compression of morbidity" thesis in the *New England Journal of Medicine* in 1980. In it, Fries wrote, "Chronic illness may presumably be postponed by changes in lifestyle, and it has been shown that the physiologic and psychologic markers of aging may be modified. . . . These considerations suggest a radically different view of the life span and of society, in which life is physically, emotionally and intellectually vigorous until shortly before its close."[4]

Our Younger You program aims to postpone chronic illness—and the associated prescription drugs, surgical procedures, and poor quality of life—and improve the physiological markers of aging that Fries referenced using nutrient-rich food and time-tested lifestyle practices to empower the innate and timeless healing systems encoded within your body to slow down and even prevent chronic illness and the "aging" trajectory. By following it, you'll be aiming to influence your epigenome and genetic expression. No matter your family history, current health status, age, or weight, you can get on a path to raising your level of health, reducing your bio age, and extending your health span—maybe even your life span.

BIOHACKING FOR THE REST OF US

Doing interventions with the aim of working out the kinks in your internal health programming isn't a new idea. The biohacking trend, where health nuts are trying all manner of aggressive health interventions in an effort to live longer and healthier, is surging. Somewhere in Silicon Valley right now (so many biohackers seem to be male, tech-friendly, and wealthy), someone is injecting themself with human growth hormone, receiving an IV of a young person's blood plasma, taking an immunosuppressive drug, or even downing a cocktail of gene-editing enzymes and proteins in an effort to achieve maximum performance and longevity. While many of these methods have produced favorable health effects, and believe me, I am paying attention to (and excited about) the latest anti-aging science, for most of us, they're not available, affordable, doable, or even desirable. Some of them come with their own unpleasant—or potentially even dangerous— side effects. And because we don't know the long-term consequences of these extreme strategies, we honestly can't be sure of their safety. And only one of them (getting injections of human growth hormone for a year— something I discuss more in Chapter 1) has thus far been shown to reduce bio age in humans.

Although I love poring through research, I'm also a single mom, a business owner, and a clinician. Time is not something I have extra bits of lying around. As a fifty-three-year-old mom to a three-year-old, I am heavily invested in living as long as I can and aging as healthfully as I can.

I, like you, need any program to be *doable*. And while you can't expect to have a positive, lasting effect on your bio age without actually following the program, you could also accelerate bio aging (as you'll soon learn) if the whole program stresses you out with time and energy demands! You also won't be able to achieve your goals if the eating and lifestyle strategies take too much time and energy to figure out and activate stress responses that could adversely affect your epigenetic programs. My goal is to provide strategies that are as palatable and accessible as they are effective, based on our current clinical results. As we expand the number of people that are engaged in these interventions, as our empirical body of knowledge increases, and as we capture more and more of the "personal" variations in responses, we will be able to further optimize and personalize our plan.

There's an adage that it takes fifty years for medicine to translate new scientific discoveries into action. This number has come down some since the advent of the internet, but not by much. By writing this book, I'm seeking to dramatically reduce that timeframe.

WHAT YOU'LL FIND IN THIS BOOK

In the pages to come you'll learn how to support your body's ability to slow biological aging and increase your health span with the following:

- Lists of delicious foods that deliver the nutrients your body can then use to balance your epigenomic software
- A list of specific foods to avoid because they appear to negatively impact the epigenome and, thus, make you age more quickly
- Recipes and meal plans that have been tailored to deliver the nutrients that support healthy genetic expression
- Lifestyle practices, such as getting-to-sleep techniques and specific exercise and meditation dosages that support your body's ability to regulate its genetic expression for optimal health
- Strategies to minimize the things that can profoundly damage the epigenome and significantly throw off genetic expression, such as exposure to toxins, stress, and an overgrowth of unfriendly gut microbes

So that you understand the power of these diet and lifestyle strategies, in Part 1 you'll learn more about how your epigenome directs your genes to keep you alive and healthy—or contributes to aging and its frequent companion, illness. I'll introduce you to DNA methylation, which is a mechanism of epigenetic expression, as well as the formula to the Younger You plan.

Whether you're facing a health challenge or are very motivated to reverse the hands of time (or both!), you'll find guidance in Part 2, in which I'll share the eight-week Younger You Intensive program—the exact version that our study participants followed—as well as the more flexible Younger You Everyday, which you can adopt as your long-term eating plan after finishing the Intensive. Or if you want a more gradual transition into the Intensive rather than a full jumping in, you can start with the Younger You Everyday and then move over to the Intensive.

And in Part 3, I'll share insights on how to think about your genetic testing results if you have them, and my thoughts on how to tend to the all-important tumor-suppressor genes (the most famous one being BRCA) so that they remain hard at work for you throughout your life, keeping cancer (and aging) at bay. (As you'll see, the expression of many genes, including tumor-suppressor genes, has been shown to be favorably influenced by specific nutrients; I've started thinking of these genes as *nutrient-responsive genes*.) And you'll learn how to optimize your lifestyle at every stage of life in a way that supports your epigenome, and perhaps even pass those effects on to your children, whether you already have them, are planning for them, or even if you have adopted or fostered children. Finally, we'll take a look at what other anti-aging strategies are currently in development—their possibilities and their risks—as well as other ways DNA methylation is changing health care as we know it.

A SNEAK PEEK AT THE EATING PLAN

Both versions of the plan are designed very specifically to nourish your epigenome, and both rely heavily on whole foods—some that you may already be used to, such as eggs and dark leafy greens, as well as a few that are a little more "out there" but that I think you'll be convinced to try once you learn just how potently anti-aging they are (and you try our delicious, easy recipes for them), such as beets, shiitake mushrooms, and liver.

While the Younger You eating plan may be a different way of eating for you, it is undeniably delicious, very filling, and uberflexible: we have customized it for patients who either are constantly on the road (and don't want to pack food) or who live in food deserts and don't have access to high-quality food, and they have radically improved their health and become younger, too. Both the Younger You Intensive and Everyday programs can work with whatever therapeutic diet you are currently eating, whether that's an elimination, gluten- or grain-free, plant-based, low-glycemic, or keto diet. In fact, this is how we use the program in my clinical practice: everyone is prescribed the plan, but then we personalize it by layering it into their specific therapeutic dietary prescription.

The Everyday version is designed to help you keep the gains you'll reap with the Intensive and promote long-term health. It outlines the simple changes you can use to support your epigenome and add years to your life, like trading that extra cup of coffee or black tea for green tea (or yummy Golden Turmeric Milk), swapping your roasted potatoes for roasted beets, sprinkling rosemary on everything, and snacking on blueberries (or our delicious Matcha Coconut Crunch).

NOT A DIET—A STRATEGY FOR (LONGER) LIFE

I understand that I'm writing this book in an era where there are *so many* diets. The last thing I want to be is just another fad—particularly when the evidence is so clear that following the Younger You principles benefits all aspects of health. I also recognize that epigenetics is complicated, and that can work against even the most exciting idea being able to cut through the noise. So before I dive into the specifics of what to eat, drink, and do, I'm going to give you a layperson's tour of aging and epigenetics. Understanding *why* the Younger You Intensive is as effective as it is will help you see that it's not just some new diet—it's a science-backed guide to shaving years off your bio age by promoting a healthy epigenome.

With the Younger You program, if you're a health nut or committed biohacker in search of longevity, you won't risk taking your efforts too far, or waste effort—and time—on a less effective dietary program (even the highly respected Mediterranean diet wasn't nearly as effective as the Younger You Intensive in lowering bio age, as I'll discuss later); if you're facing health challenges and seeking relief, you'll learn how to support your ability to heal at the deepest level; if you're looking to start a family (whether through biology or adoption), you'll be able to give your offspring the best support in creating a foundation from which to thrive throughout their lives; and if you're simply seeking to look and feel your best, you'll discover a very real opportunity to delay your aging and minimize your risk of disease—in other words, to truly be a younger you.

PART 1

THE NEW SCIENCE OF AGING

1

THE EPIGENETIC EFFECT ON AGING

YOU KNOW HOW FACEBOOK SHOWS YOU MEMORIES OF OLD PHOTOS on your timeline? And you see a photo from eight, five, or even two years ago and think, "Damn, I looked good! Where have those days gone?"

It's enough to make you start Googling face creams. After all, when most of us think about anti-aging strategies, that's what we think about: various lotions and potions to rub on our skin that, in the classic language of advertisements, "minimize the appearance of fine lines and wrinkles." Or, maybe if we take it one step further, we think of taking hormones that help us feel more youthful. Because, if you're being honest, seeing that photo in your Facebook memory probably also reminds you that it's not just the way you look that's changed; you have a moment of recognizing that your memory seems to have gotten worse, your energy has flagged, and your body has lost some of its ability to do things, whether that's recover from illness, get up and down from the floor, or open a pickle jar. What you probably aren't considering is that with every passing year, the door to disease opens wider, as **age is the single biggest risk factor for every chronic disease**. And no fancy cream, no matter how expensive, is going to help you actually turn back the clock on those things.

The drive for youth is so strong in our culture (the global anti-aging industry was expected to approach \$220 billion in 2021[1]), but most of us don't connect the dots between our diet and lifestyle choices, an accelerated rate of aging, and an increase in risk for chronic disease. In fact, your bio age is *the* single biggest risk factor for all the major diseases, including diabetes, cancer, and dementia.

THE LINK BETWEEN AGING AND DISEASE

The good news about our current aging reality is that modern medicine has resulted in longer and longer life spans. We've reduced incidences of many infections—COVID-19 notwithstanding—and disabling diseases so that the average person doesn't die of flu or tuberculosis, and lives to a higher age. The bad news about longer life spans is that we have simultaneously increased the incidence of chronic, noncommunicable diseases, such as dementia, heart disease, and cancer. (As we get sicker with these chronic diseases, ironically, our risk of communicable diseases increases exponentially—as evidenced by the United States experiencing so many deaths from COVID-19.)

A whopping 80 percent of adults over sixty-five have one chronic disease. And a full 77 percent have at least two! But it's not like we turn sixty-five and—boom!—we get the disease like some kind of ghoulish birthday present. We've been on this path our whole lives—one in three Americans under sixty-five have metabolic syndrome, a collection of symptoms that includes high blood pressure, high blood sugar, high cholesterol or high triglycerides, and an apple-shaped body (accompanied by belly fat) that paves the way to full-blown chronic disease.

The scientific and medical communities have responded to this rise in disease incidence by focusing on researching and treating the diseases themselves. The problem is that once you take steps to prevent, say, heart disease, you take your eye off cancer prevention. It's what Dana Goldman, director of the Schaeffer Center for Health Policy and Economics at the University of Southern California, told PBS *Newshour*, "It's almost like Whack-a-Mole, where you push down on one disease and another one pops up."[2]

The sector that has benefited the most from this disease-centered approach is the health-care industry. In 1970, total national health-care expenditures in the United States were $74.1 billion, or $1,848 per person in 2019 dollars. By 2000, total US health-care spending was up to $1.4 trillion, and by 2019 it had more than doubled to $3.8 trillion—$11,582 per person. That's a more than sixfold increase in personal spending.[3]

Rather than treating diseases one by one, what our growing understanding of epigenetics suggests is that **we can reduce the risk of all diseases and conditions at once by seeking to either maintain or reduce bio age**. That means less suffering and more years of quality of life (increased health span and life span). Not for nothing, it also means less expense. In a 2021 paper published in *Nature Aging*, Dr. David Sinclair, professor of genetics at Harvard and author of the book *Lifespan*, and his colleagues state that "a compression of morbidity that improves health is more valuable than further increases in life expectancy, and that targeting aging offers potentially larger economic gains than eradicating individual diseases." Overall, the paper states that a slowdown in aging that results in one year of increased life span would save $38 trillion in health-care spending; a deceleration in aging that results in ten years of life span would save $367 trillion.[4]

How then do we delay aging? We focus on the thread that connects your diet and lifestyle habits, your bio age, and your risk of disease, which is epigenetics—or more specifically, an important epigenetic process called DNA methylation. If epigenetics is a collection of different types of software, as I suggested in the Introduction, then DNA methylation may be the most influential and lasting; it's certainly the best studied of all the epigenetic marks. For simplicity, we can think of DNA methylation as the operating system: it tells your hardware—your genes—what to do.

DNA methylation wields its influence by placing humble, ubiquitous molecules known as methyl groups on top of your genetic material, and those methyl groups determine which genes are turned on and which are turned off, and to what extent. (I'll delve more into how this process works later in this chapter.)

While it is true that DNA methylation has a ton of power over your health and well-being, *you* have tremendous influence over it. The choices you make every day—what you eat, when you go to bed, how stressed you are, how much you move, how much loving touch you engage in—can all negatively or positively influence how and where those methyl groups are placed, and therefore how your genes are expressed.

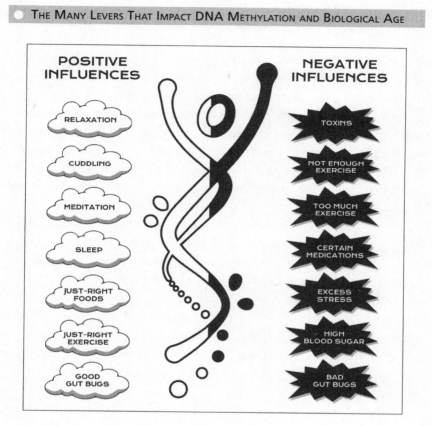

THE MANY LEVERS THAT IMPACT DNA METHYLATION AND BIOLOGICAL AGE

POSITIVE INFLUENCES

- RELAXATION
- CUDDLING
- MEDITATION
- SLEEP
- JUST-RIGHT FOODS
- JUST-RIGHT EXERCISE
- GOOD GUT BUGS

NEGATIVE INFLUENCES

- TOXINS
- NOT ENOUGH EXERCISE
- TOO MUCH EXERCISE
- CERTAIN MEDICATIONS
- EXCESS STRESS
- HIGH BLOOD SUGAR
- BAD GUT BUGS

Our study showed that when you choose to give your body more of the things that we believe promote healthy DNA methylation, and reduce your exposure to things that deregulate it, you can give yourself the DNA methylation patterns of a younger you. And that is how you can minimize your risk of developing disease in the first place, or how you might be able to mitigate or even reverse its progression if you are already ill. And, bonus, you'll also drop excess pounds, regain lost vitality, and make people wonder what you're doing to look so good for your age.

THE PATH TO THIS POINT

Before I do a deeper dive into how DNA methylation works and how it relates to aging, I just want to pause for a moment to recognize that the entire science of epigenetics and our understanding of how it works and how we might influence it is an *enormous* jump in our thinking about disease prevention. Twenty years ago, we thought that genetics held the key to reducing disease and promoting longevity. We fully expected that mapping the human genome (which was completed in 2003 by the Human Genome Project) would provide all the answers we didn't yet have—like a Rosetta Stone that would show exactly which gene, or which genetic mutation, led to which disease.

As amazing an achievement as it was, that's not what happened. What we've found since then is that most chronic diseases don't have one genetic cause. Because as much information as our genetic material contains, that information is filtered through epigenetics. On the one hand, this means that with few exceptions, there is no one smoking gun for each disease that we can eradicate with gene therapy and poof, defeat that disease. On the other hand, that means we have a ton of tools at our disposal to positively influence our DNA methylation, our genetic expression, and, thus, our health. For me, this latter approach is so much more empowering; we can *do* something about it.

Reams of research in the past ten-plus years have shown that there are a multitude of things that affect DNA methylation. And that when you change where and how DNA is methylated, you change the way you age, steering yourself away from disease and the loss of quality of life it brings with it, and toward an old age that lets you enjoy well-being throughout your final years.

THE EVOLUTION OF OUR UNDERSTANDING

Once we mapped the genome, we discovered that a mere 2 percent of our genetic material is actually the code that contains the instructions for making proteins. *Two percent!* The other 98 percent is what was at first considered "junk DNA"—a mishmash of genetic material that, because it didn't contain codes for making proteins, we at first deemed gobbledy-gook. (This assessment turned out to be wildly erroneous. We now know that the so-called junk genes actually help the DNA genes that code for proteins.)

Don't get me wrong, your DNA is vitally important. It provides a complete instruction manual for creating you and all your needed parts throughout your lifetime. It's just that DNA is inert without epigenetic inputs.

Although it communicates very complex information, a strand of DNA is structurally simple, essentially a book with twenty-three chapters written using only four letters—G (guanine), A (adenine), C (cytosine) and T (thymine). Each chapter is one long run-on sentence, printed on only two pages that sit side-by-side and are each only one character wide. Because each strand is so long—the DNA in one cell stretched all the way out is about two meters long, and all the DNA in all your cells fully extended would be approximately twice the diameter of the solar system— each gene needs to be wrapped around spools or else it gets tangled.[5] Those spools are called histones. And histones (four proteins) are further grouped in clusters of eight, called nucleosomes. Although the strands, or chapters in this example, are long, they are all written in the same language that consists of only these four characters.

Epigenetics, on the other hand, is a mess of dozens of different languages happening all over the genetic material, not just the DNA. It's as complicated as the genetic code is simple, as evidenced by a now classic cartoon that I and many of my colleagues use when presenting on the topic. It shows a woman whispering to a terrified scientist who is about to walk onstage to give a lecture, "If they ask you anything you don't know just say it's due to epigenetics."

DNA METHYLATION: A ROCK STAR OF EPIGENETICS

Methylation is an ancient and universal biochemical event that is fundamental for all life forms—we evolved to use methyl groups throughout our physiology because their building blocks were ubiquitous. A methyl group is one carbon atom surrounded by three hydrogen atoms. It's a highly stable molecule, made out of two of the most abundant elements on Earth. When a methyl group attaches to other molecules—a process that is mediated by enzymes—it is called *methylation*.

Methylation is happening in your body within every cell, all of the time. It is as ever-present and as essential as breathing. It allows you to get rid of toxins, such as mercury; to make neurotransmitters important for learning and brain health; to make white blood cells; to metabolize estrogen; and to make energy for muscles. If you have a precursor of dopamine and then you pop a methyl group on it, poof, you've got active dopamine. If you're stressed and your adrenals pump out a bunch of adrenaline, methylation is what breaks those adrenaline molecules down so that you can metabolize it. Methylation is also required to produce DNA, repair DNA, and—via DNA methylation—control DNA expression. Clearly, nature thinks methylation is one heck of a way to regulate extremely important stuff!

If you read a lot of articles about health on the internet, you've probably heard of methylation. It is a process that has garnered a lot of attention over the last decade or so as being integral to whole-body health. As it is also a process that slows down and becomes imbalanced as we age, methylation is something that functional medicine practitioners assess and address with nearly all of our patients. The primary way we've done that is to measure levels of the amino acid homocysteine, which is a byproduct of the overall methylation process; when it is elevated it indicates that methylation is impaired and is associated with an increased risk for cardiovascular disease, neurological diseases like Alzheimer's, or even anxiety and depression.

However, there is one specific type of methylation that we are realizing plays a crucial role in epigenetic expression. That is DNA *methylation*, which is when methyl groups are moved onto or off your DNA. And it is this particular form of methylation that the Younger You program is focused on.

We've known for decades that there are methyl groups that sit on top of DNA. Yet at first we thought they were extraneous. Dr. Moshe Szyf, a geneticist and professor of pharmacology and therapeutics at McGill University, founder of the journal *Epigenetics*, and one of the godfathers of the study of epigenetics, has written hundreds of studies that look at DNA methylation, the earliest of which were conducted in the 1980s. And he tells me that those methyl groups were considered irrelevant to understanding how DNA worked, pesky debris to be ignored (similar to that "junk DNA" I mentioned earlier). After all, the thinking went, how could it be possible that such a lowly, common chemical compound had such an impactful role to play?

It was only after the genome was mapped that epigenetics in general and DNA methylation specifically began to earn the respect and attention of the scientific community. You have to chuckle at how misguided our ignorance made us. Because now we know that those methyl groups that sit on top of the strands of DNA dictate which genes are turned off and which are turned on, and to what extent. Because the human body is so exquisitely complex, it's not quite as direct as it might seem, though. DNA methylation regulates both the junk DNA, which then regulates the active DNA, and the active DNA directly. But what is clear, at least at this point in our understanding, is that DNA methylation is the most influenceable link in this chain.

When I interviewed him on my *New Frontiers in Functional Medicine* podcast, Dr. Szyf said that if CTAG are the letters that form the words of DNA, then "DNA methylation is the punctuation. It makes sense out of letters, it breaks up the words and sentences, overrides and under rides, and puts exclamation marks and question marks so that the letters [of DNA] become a language."[6]

DNA methylation may be the most powerful epigenetic influencer (among other players that include acetylation, small RNAs, phosphorylation, ubiquitination, and more) because its marks can stay over a lifetime of many cell divisions and can be handed down through multiple generations. To be fair, it is also the most studied epigenetic language. There may well be other highly durable and heritable ways that genes are expressed or inhibited that we don't yet know about. But at this point in our understanding, DNA methylation is the longest lasting and most impactful of the epigenetic mechanisms and plays a key role in all the major chronic diseases of our time, including aging.

As we age, the patterns of DNA methylation predictably move in almost the exact opposite direction of where they are when we are young; this is what paves the way for disease, not necessarily the fact that we have been alive for longer. Luckily, it is possible to slow down this pattern—or even reverse it.

METHYLATION VS. DNA METHYLATION

Methylation: The addition and removal of methyl groups to molecules; this elemental biochemical process happens throughout the body.

DNA Methylation: Refers specifically to the addition and removal of methyl groups to and from strands of DNA.

• • • • •

When methyl groups are added on top of a strand of DNA—known as hypermethylation—the volume on that gene is turned down. Scientists always illustrate a methyl group attached to a strand of DNA as a little red lollipop jutting out of one of the cytosine nucleotides in your DNA strand. (In humans, the methyl group is most often placed on a cytosine nucleotide that is next to a guanine nucleotide; because nucleotides are connected by phosphates, scientific short-hand for a DNA methylation site is CpG.) The more lollipops attach to the cytosines on a gene, the more its function is diminished because the lollipops are taking up the available parking spots and no other molecules—including those that activate the gene—can get in. It takes relatively few methyl groups to silence a gene.

By the same token, **removing methyl groups—otherwise known as demethylation or hypomethylation—turns a gene on.**

Put simply, you want your DNA methylation to be working in such a way that your good genes (those that suppress tumor growth, say) are *on* and your bad genes (for inflammation, as an example) are generally *off*.

AGING FROM AN EPIGENETIC PERSPECTIVE

Imagine that you are in a gallery at the Art Institute of Chicago looking at the pointillist masterpiece *A Sunday on La Grande Jatte—1884* by Georges Seurat. When you view it from across the room, you see forty-eight people, three dogs, eight boats, one monkey on a leash, and nineteen trees, all captured in a moment of stillness. From a distance, the colors are vibrant and cohesive—a thrilling whole that immerses you in a moment of daily life in Paris in the late nineteenth century.

When you approach the painting, you begin to discern that Seurat used small dots of paint to bring the scene to life instead of the more typical brush strokes of his contemporaries. You see that what seems like one seamless painting is actually comprised of thousands of little dabs of paint.

And when you get right up to the canvas, you see that these dots of paint are even smaller than they first appeared—that each hue that you could register when you stood across the room is actually comprised of tiny dots of several different shades, and that there are *hundreds of thousands* of individual dots. You know that there must be some basic sketch underneath that guided Seurat's hand, although you can't see any evidence of it. Up close, it looks random, as if there's no way what you're seeing adds up to anything resembling anything familiar. But from a distance, every dot plays its own unique role in creating a masterpiece.

Seurat began *La Grande Jatte* by making initial drawings with a black crayon on textured white paper. These initial studies are definitive, yet they lack the details that bring the figures to life in the finished version.

Your epigenome is like a pointillist painting. Those black drawings are the equivalent of your DNA. They lay the foundation for the work of art you will become, but it's the thousands upon thousands of tiny epigenetic marks layered on top of your genes that bring the full picture of you to life. Those marks are also what determine how long you live, and how healthy you are no matter your age. In fact, they have more influence over how old you are than the calendar does.

Culturally, we're terrified of aging, but it's important to remember that aging is a natural process: We are all aging all of the time. And, if you're not aging, you're dead.

The whole process of growth and maturity when we're kids is, technically, aging. It began as soon as you were conceived—not just because the clock was ticking, but also because your epigenome began actively modifying the expression of your genes.

We've known for some time that babies who don't get loving contact become developmentally delayed (i.e., their aging is abnormally slow, and their bio age is low) and even suffer a loss in IQ points—what we've only recently come to understand is that the reason these babies don't develop fully is that their genetic expression (via epigenetics) is negatively impacted by the lack of touch.[7]

At times, DNA methylation—and therefore, aging—is moving at hyper speed, like in adolescence when you grew several inches in the span of a few months and you had to get a whole new wardrobe because nothing— not even last year's winter hat—fit. During these times, the outlines of the figures in your painting are being refined, and the colors are getting richer and more nuanced.

Once you reach adulthood, it may seem like your painting is finished, when in actuality your diet, exercise, sleep, stress, relationships, and chemical exposure are continually adding new dabs of paint/marks and removing old ones. In fact, when Dr. David Sinclair was a guest on my podcast, he shared that the epigenetic changes in adulthood are as profound as those seen in infancy.[8] And interestingly, some changes can happen quickly and last longer than you might expect—research on mice has found that a single high-glucose meal negatively impacted the epigenetic expression of DNA on vascular cells for longer than the six-day study duration, and an in vitro study of human stem cells found that a single high-sugar event produced epigenetic changes that increased the production of free radicals and downregulated antioxidant genes.[9,10] In humans, a single episode of exercise has shown favorable epigenetic changes relating to insulin sensitivity and anti-inflammation.[11] What this all means is that whether you realize it or not, you are making changes to your epigenome every day, with every choice you make about what to eat, drink, and do. By choosing to have an epigenetic-friendly meal instead of fast food, going to bed when you're tired instead of watching yet another episode of *The Great British Baking Show*, or relaxing instead of scrolling through your social media feed, those changes are favorable. And when you consistently make those choices over the long term, you can make those positive genetic changes long-lasting. And *that's* when you move the needle away from illness and disease and retain more of your youthful strength, energy, and resilience, despite how old the calendar says you are.

As I've mentioned, when left to their own devices, your epigenetic changes over time seem to reverse the exact changes that happened in your early years when you were growing. Some of this wind-down is the "normal" journey of aging. But layer into that wind-down the Western lifestyle of disease—processed foods, high stress, poor sleep, no exercise, and toxic exposures—and your epigenetic maintenance mechanisms will become even further impaired and your aging process will accelerate that much more. Both normal aging and accelerated aging share similar characteristics as far as DNA methylation goes:

- **It slows down.** Referred to as "global hypomethylation," this means more "bad" genes—which promote things like inflammation, the destruction of perfectly good cells, Alzheimer's disease, diabetes, heart disease, and cancer—can be turned on, since fewer methyl groups are essentially a green light to genetic expression.

- **It gets wonky.** The DNA methylation that does happen becomes imbalanced, which often leads to too many methyl groups getting placed on certain genes and shutting those genes off. These tend to be "good" genes, such as tumor-suppressor genes that inhibit cancer, inflammation-regulating genes, or genes that regulate detoxification and antioxidant activity or make sure our DNA itself is stable and strong.

Why would it be that genes that promote aging (and the diseases of aging) are turned on, and anti-aging genes are turned off? There are two systems of belief here. The more accepted view is that the chronic assaults from life (the bad diet, the toxins, the stress, etc.) cause random changes to DNA methylation—termed "epigenetic drift"—that ultimately accumulate in a critical mass resulting in disease and death. There is another view that is gaining acceptance among scientists that suggests all living creatures are programmed to die, and that is the theory that the length of our life span isn't determined by chance alone.[12] Meaning, aging is part of a plan where death by natural causes happens on a predictable timetable, with predictable changes to DNA methylation, just as menarche and menopause do.

One theory suggests that it's nature's way of perpetually making room and saving resources for more offspring. I see the validity of this theory, not just because there does indeed seem to be some predictability with the changes to DNA methylation over the arc of life, but because other creatures have a specific life span, too—fruit flies live only two days, while the Greenland shark lives four hundred years. The fact that there are species with profound longevity provides evidence that there is an element of genetic programming in regard to life span. (So does a 2021 paper by the best scientists across the field—it creates a DNA methylation biological clock that applies to all mammalian species that adds credence to the likelihood that our collective life spans—whether they're short, like a rodent's, or long, like a Greenland shark's—are ticking according to preprogrammed DNA methylation changes.[13]) What is important to note is that while some elements of the DNA methylation clock appear to be predetermined by evolutionary history, other DNA methylation components appear to be malleable.

If that's the case, are we trying to play God by turning back our biological clock? Well, let's just take a moment to remember those sixteen-plus years that the average American spends sick at the end of their lives that I mentioned in the Introduction. For so many of us, the quality of our final years is horrific, when we are propped up by drugs and nursing homes and hospitals. Is it wrong to want to reduce that suffering (and that profound expense, to the individual, their family, and our society)? Absolutely not. Our primary aim with the Younger You program—and what our study has shown us is achievable—is to reverse bio age, with the goal of keeping you younger longer, and not to significantly and artificially extend life span.

If you are savvy about trying to modulate DNA methylation in order to slow down bio aging—which, by reading this book, you are already becoming—you won't live forever, or transform your genetic material to be more like the Greenland shark's; but you can develop the tools to live well until you die.

Without consciously tending to your diet and lifestyle, and thus your DNA methylation—ideally, throughout all phases of life, from conception to older adulthood, although whenever you discover these principles is the perfect time to start—your aging journey will be dictated by typically imbalanced genetic expression. In addition to outward symptoms like wrinkles, thinning hair, and loss of muscle mass, you also open the door and give a warm welcome to aging's closest companion, disease. When that happens, one of the figures in your painting might end up sprouting several hats (cancer), while one of the trees might completely fade away (dementia). If you don't die immediately of the disease you develop, more and more of your canvas becomes grayed out and your quality of life declines and you lose function (represented in Figure 2 from the Introduction, page xvi). When you exert effort in adjusting your lifestyle in order to steer yourself away from the typical epigenetic drift of aging, your painting stays truer to its original form, gradually shifting to sepia tones.

THE EVIDENCE THAT YOU CAN LOWER YOUR BIOLOGICAL AGE

As I write this, there are four human studies that have shown that biological age might be lowered by dedicated interventions.

The first study was admittedly small. Run by Dr. Greg Fahy, chief scientific officer and cofounder of Intervene Immune in Los Angeles, the study followed nine healthy white men between the ages of fifty-one and sixty-five over the course of a year—seven of them from 2015 to 2016 and three of them from 2016 to 2017—during which time they took two specific medications and three supplements: recombinant human growth hormone (rhGH) injections, metformin (a drug typically prescribed for diabetes because of its ability to regulate blood sugar), the steroid hormone dehydroepiandrosterone (DHEA), vitamin D, and zinc.

Fahy wasn't even necessarily looking to improve the epigenetic clock; he was aiming to see if human growth hormone could regenerate the thymus gland, which plays an important role in immunity and which starts to shrink after puberty and slowly be replaced by fat.

What's tricky, however, is that while there were already animal studies that suggested that growth hormone stimulates the thymus gland, growth hormone is also known to increase diabetes risk. That's why Fahy also gave his participants metformin and DHEA, two antidiabetes treatments, along with the growth hormone in his study (which is known as the thymus regeneration immunorestoration and insulin mitigation [TRIIM] study).

Fahy and his team found what they were looking for—seven out of nine participants experienced thymus gland regeneration. And white blood cell counts improved in all nine participants. That was almost the end of it, until Fahy decided to analyze the biological age of his participants. He did this using the same method that we used in our study—a scientific assessment known as the DNAmAge Calculator (DNAmAge is short for DNA Methylation Age; I'll share more about exactly how this tool assesses biological age in Chapter 4).

Fahy published his results in the journal *Aging Cell* in 2019.[14] According-ing to the DNAmAge Calculator, the study participants had shaved an average of 2.5 years off their biological age over the course of a year. It was a "wow" moment—the first evidence that biological age, as measured by an epigenetic clock, could travel in reverse.

Keep in mind that this study was over the course of a year, and it re-quired self-injections of rhGH and metformin, a pharmaceutical drug that requires a prescription, and DHEA (which is available over the counter). Not only can the treatment be less than pleasant for some folks, it's not exactly accessible—after all, you can't pick up human growth hormone and metformin at the grocery store on your way home from work. It also comes with side effects that range from unpleasant (diarrhea, constipation) to potentially more menacing (increased susceptibility to infection and in-creased likelihood of developing insulin resistance, which can then pave the way to diabetes, heart disease, and cancer). While these first results of bio age reversal are very exciting, you have to wonder, is it worth it? And will these results be long lasting, or how often will the protocol need to be repeated? Stay tuned as Fahy continues to research his program.

The second study that showed that humans can turn back their biolog-ical age looked at the Mediterranean diet, the popular and well-researched approach to eating attested to by many centenarians. This 2020 pilot study included 120 individuals between the ages of sixty-five and seventy-nine from Poland and Italy. The group was supplied a Mediterranean diet and 400 IU of vitamin D_3 for one year.[15] Of the participants, only the Polish women saw a reduction in biological age, which had lowered 1.47 years at the end of the year-long study, although beneficial DNA methylation changes outside of bio age were seen across the group.[16] The authors speculated that a standard Polish diet is much different than a Mediterranean diet, and thus the switch could have been more favorable to the Poles versus the Italians, who already follow a Mediterranean diet, although they did not see the same biological age reversal in Polish men.

This study shows that the Mediterranean diet is a good, general eating plan that *can* lead to small reductions in bio age over the long term—and that probably has the biggest benefit for those who weren't already eating a diet low in red meat; high in fruits, vegetables, whole grains, and healthy fats; and with moderate intake of seafood and dairy (the hallmarks of the diet). It's excellent proof of the ability of a whole-foods-based nutrition plan plus vitamin D to favorably influence bio age, but only for certain people after a year of adherence.

The third study showed that obese or overweight African Americans, when deficient in vitamin D, can have a remarkable improvement in bio age with sufficient D supplementation. This sixteen-week study had three arms of vitamin D_3 doses: 600 IU per day, 2,000 IU per day, or 4,000 IU per day. In the group receiving 4,000 IU, bio age was significantly reduced by 1.85 years. There were no other interventions used in this study.[17] It speaks to the importance of nutrient status, and certainly vitamin D_3 supplements are easy to find and to take, although note that if you are already replete in vitamin D, starting supplementation will probably not make a difference in bio age.

And the fourth study that showed reduction in bio age is the one that I was the principal investigator on and that was published in *Aging* in 2021.

STRATEGIC FOOD AND LIFESTYLE CHANGES CAN ACHIEVE SIMILAR RESULTS—IN LESS TIME

Around the same time that Fahy's first cohort of study participants was starting their year of injections, I was developing the DNA methylation-modulating diet and lifestyle program that my practice has since prescribed in some form to the hundreds of patients we see in a year.

While we saw clinically that our program was beneficial, and we had read the research that all of the foods and lifestyle practices that our program incorporated *could* theoretically favorably influence the epigenome and maybe lower bio age, we didn't know for sure, because the tests to assess it weren't available outside of the research setting at the time we developed our program. We guessed we were doing something right based on patient response and our read on the science, but only a research study could confirm it.

In other words, we wanted proof.

So we designed a study to measure the epigenetic impact of the program. This wasn't an easy feat for a wide range of reasons—just one DNA methylation test at that time cost over $1,000, and we needed to run that test multiple times on fifty-plus subjects.

On top of that, it was a very complex study. Asking participants to change their diet for a full eight weeks, *plus* agree to take a couple of supplements, meet with a nutritionist, and modify their sleep, exercise, and relaxation habits, was a big ask. While it did take us a while, we found participants who would stick to our rather involved program (our data show impressive adherence—not often found in a nutrition and lifestyle study!).

In the end, we recruited thirty-eight healthy males aged fifty to seventy-two who came to us already eating a pretty healthy diet and exercising regularly. We targeted this particular age demographic because, as I discussed above, DNA methylation changes for the worse as we age. And we stuck to males because women of this age group have the confounding factor of fluctuating sex hormone levels of perimenopause and menopause. (Of course, I *want* to look at middle-aged women—I am one!—but we need larger study numbers to offset the sex hormone differences between middle-aged women. We are actively recruiting for this study as I type.)

Eighteen of our recruits followed the Younger You Intensive program for eight weeks; the remaining twenty participants served as a control group and received no interventions (two dropped out, as is common). Before the official protocol began, and after the eight-week study ended, we collected spit samples, sent them off to Yale's Center for Genome Analysis to be processed, and had the results analyzed by top epigenetic researchers including Dr. Josh Mitteldorf and Dr. Moshe Szyf (and his team) at McGill University. And what we found was nothing short of astonishing. As I shared in the Introduction, when we compared the biological age of the Younger You group to our controls, the Younger You group were a significant 3.23 years younger at the end of those eight weeks! Mind you, these folks (both our participants and the controls) were already pretty healthy—they ate well and most exercised regularly. While we haven't proven it (yet), it's reasonable to assume that had they been less healthy at the start of the study, their reversals would have been even greater, because those with chronic diseases, such as diabetes, are biologically older than their chronological age-matched peers.

Other benefits they enjoyed include:

- A significant *decrease* in triglycerides, the blood fats associated with cardiovascular disease, which also suggests a drop in insulin and blood sugar levels, and increased ketone production
- A significant drop in total cholesterol and LDL ("bad") cholesterol
- Nonsignificant yet still measurable trends toward improved energy and reduced anxiety, which confirms what we see in our clinical patients
- A significant increase in circulating methyl folate, a key player in DNA methylation, as compared to controls—with no folate supplements used.

These findings support what we see in our clinical practice when patients incorporate Younger You principles, including

- Weight loss in those who need to lose weight
- Lower inflammation
- Improved energy and mood
- Resolution of skin issues
- Less joint pain
- Fewer headaches
- Improved gastrointestinal health
- Improved methylation markers—measured by levels of homocysteine, B_{12}, and folate—without supplementation

What's truly remarkable is that we achieved these fast and dramatic results only with changes to diet and lifestyle—no injections or prescriptions required. This means that in order to make significant beneficial changes to your biological age, all you need access to is a grocery store.

Our study suggests that when you give your body what it needs, without beating it over the head with pharmaceuticals and synthetic hormones, you empower your body's own innate wisdom to lead the way.

This is different than the typical Western medicine approach, which is a little bit like an overbearing parent: it waits for the body to misbehave, then offers stern corrections in the form of prescriptions or procedures. What my training, clinical experience, and the results of our study have shown me is that it's far better to take a nurturing approach: give the body everything it needs to take care of itself and then let it decide, in its own inherent wisdom, how to use those ingredients to best effect. I think of it as taking an upstream approach: you sprinkle the right ingredients into the water and set them on a good path, and then let nature decide how to put them to best use.

Yes, there are cases where care needs to be more directed, but overwhelmingly, I have been humbled to witness just how wise our bodies truly are. When we give them the nutrients and the conditions they require for wellness, in the right amounts, they respond in ways that would be considered miraculous if they weren't so consistently reliable.

What's so exciting to me about our increased understanding of epigenetics, aging, DNA methylation, and biological age is that we aren't totally victims of our genetics—epigenetics offers a window of influence. It's great news, but it's a story that needs to be shouted from the rooftops again and again because it goes against what we've all thought and been taught for a long time. We'll do some dispelling of this "genes are king" myth in Chapter 2.

2

YOUR GENES DON'T DICTATE YOUR FATE

WHEN I WALKED INTO MY OFFICE, I SAW AN ATTRACTIVE WOMAN in her midforties. While she presented as very healthy, I could tell by the look in her eye that she was anxious about something. A smart, health-savvy person, Rhonda sat on the edge of her seat clutching her genetic test results. It showed that she had a single (heterozygous) mutation on one of her methylenetetrahydrofolate reductase (MTHFR) genes, which can mean (in the worst-case scenario) that it could reduce production of the MTHFR enzyme by about 25 percent, and therefore theoretically slow down her methylation cycle.

A consumer of health materials, Rhonda had read up on MTHFR and felt sure it was responsible for her brain fog, fatigue, and a few extra pounds that she could not lose. As I do with most patients, I ordered a full panel of blood work to assess many gauges of health (I share the tests I look to on page 89), including methylation status. In her case, everything related to methylation came back totally fine. It's important to note that the methylation cycle is a complex interplay of nutrients and enzymes, needs and demands, so zeroing in on one very common enzyme variant as the cause of a collection of symptoms is just too simplistic.

I did, however, see something in her lab work that concerned me—some suspicious elevated levels that are sometimes seen with multiple myeloma, which is a type of blood cancer. After a follow-up lab test did nothing to alleviate those suspicions, I referred her to a specialist.

While I understand that this was well beyond the scope of why she initially booked her appointment with me, it took a lot of conversation and education to explain that Rhonda's MTHFR status was not something she needed to worry about . . . but that her other levels warranted attention. Frustrating to me (and my colleagues in functional medicine who've encountered similar situations) is the patient who becomes absolutely convinced that their genetic report is the absolute arbiter of their health, and that "treating" their genetic imbalances with a precarious cocktail of supplements will bring about an elusive optimal health. Make no mistake: direct-to-consumer basic genetic testing can be a motivating guide to eating better, exercising, and maybe getting in touch with a long-lost cousin, but beyond that, its health insights generally aren't that remarkable and may be harmful, as they were in this case. I share Rhonda's story to show that, too often, we get hung up on our genetic testing results, when they aren't the definitive beacon that so many of us expect them to be, and that we can get fixated on our genes, to the point that we can lose sight of other aspects of health that deserve our attention.

A 2019 report by the *MIT Technology Review* found that over 26 million Americans have taken DNA tests.[1]

Why? Why do so many of us care so much?

We want to know our past—where our ancestors came from and what secrets might be hidden among the limbs of our family tree. But the main reason we get DNA testing is that we want to know our future. What diseases we are susceptible to. Our weaknesses. Our strengths. And what we might expect, health-wise, from the remaining years of our lives.

I understand the desire to ward off future threats, I truly do. But really, looking to DNA tests to give us a window into our future well-being is like looking at a newspaper published on the day we were conceived and expecting it to accurately portray today's current events. What so few of us realize is that our genes themselves by and large do not dictate our fate. The truth is, while your DNA does provide the coding for everything that makes you who you are, its influence peaks at conception. Every day of your life since that initial meeting of sperm and egg, it's not what genes you have that matter. Of greater importance is which genes are turned on and which are turned off. And this you likely have a lot of control over.

Everyday people aren't the only ones who have been eager for individual genetic testing. As I mentioned in the previous chapter, the scientific community thought mapping the genome would be the answer to all disease. I, and many of my fellow functional medicine colleagues, thought having a patient's genetic information would help us know *exactly* the collection of interventions we'd need to prescribe in order for that patient to achieve optimal wellness. We were clamoring for DNA test results for our patients—but once we got them, the turnkey solutions we were anticipating weren't there.

Genetics can sometimes offer insight into specific challenges that we need to plan for—such as a diminished ability to make antioxidants, in which case adding colorful veggies to the diet becomes even more important. And very rarely they can pinpoint a specific condition that can then be addressed—such as a mutation in an enzyme that relies on a specific B vitamin, which can result in a seizure disorder that can be remedied by supplementing with that B vitamin. But at worst—as I have seen time and again in my practice—DNA testing becomes a point of severe anxiety, and oftentimes a rationale for purchasing a raft of pricey supplements, for people who believe a certain disease or diseases are inevitable.

To be fair, DNA testing is an amazing scientific development with far-reaching ramifications. And yet, when it comes to medicine, its impact on patient care is, well, *meh*. In the mid-2000s, as genetic testing became widely available, I worked in a sophisticated clinical lab where we were looking at compounds in the body not reflected in your basic blood work. I expected that if I saw mutations in the gene responsible for creating the enzyme required to process adrenaline, for example, that I would see very elevated adrenaline levels; yet I didn't. People with that mutation *might* experience more anxiety because they didn't metabolize adrenaline that well, but it was equivocal; sometimes they did, and sometimes they didn't. And research was equivocal, too; some studies showed the mutation to be important, some showed it to be irrelevant.

It was a hard dream to give up—I looked and looked and looked for a genetic mutation that had a clear correlation to specific conditions and diseases. But only once in a great while did a patient with a significant mutation in a specific gene show a clear correlation in their lab work and symptom profile. If there were insights to be gleaned from genetic information, I and so many of my colleagues around the world realized we'd have to think about it differently.

What medical professionals and researchers have started to understand since that time is that environmental influence on gene expression—epigenetics—is the primary path of supporting and optimizing health.

As we've covered, epigenetics—and specifically DNA methylation—impacts which genes are turned on, and which are turned off. I'm not saying you can turn your brown eyes blue (with all due respect to Crystal Gayle), or reverse those age-related grays that are starting to creep into your head of hair like crabgrass. I do mean that, in addition to shaving years off your bio age, you can likely lower your chances of developing the diseases and conditions that run in your family by thoughtfully tending to your DNA methylation and, more broadly, your epigenome.

This isn't only an exciting new possibility. It's also a warning, as epigenetics don't only work in a positive direction. They can also work against you. And if you aren't consciously taking steps to support your DNA methylation, your epigenetics are most likely steering you down the path to disease. While there is still much to be learned about epigenetic interventions, we shouldn't sit idle waiting for a full understanding of these complex issues. We have already gathered some knowledge that could instruct us in choosing ways to improve our epigenetic clock.

THE AMERICAN EPIGENETIC NIGHTMARE

Let me give you an example from my own family tree to show how genetics are affected by epigenetics, and how these changes can accelerate aging and pave the road to a premature death (and how they can even be passed down to our children, grandchildren, and great-grandchildren).

Like so many other Americans, my family came to this country as immigrants. My great-grandparents came from Poland, where they grew their own food and led a physical-labor-intense life. However, Poland was not an easy place to live at the time. Russia and Germany controlled various regions of the country, and Poles were not treated well. While I don't know that my family members were technically starving, like most Poles, they didn't have money and thus food could be scarce. Their epigenetics would have adapted to this limited food availability, and their genetic expression probably became geared toward survival. Meaning, they became genetically programmed to hold on to every calorie they could, in what scientists call the "thrifty epigenotype." It worked to keep them alive back in Poland. But it also impacted their future health, and the health of their future generations. Especially after they came to America.

My great-grandparents settled in Cleveland in the early twentieth century. They bought a house in a neighborhood populated by other immigrants from other Slavic countries. True children of immigrants, my grandparents went full throttle on the American dream—and the American lifestyle. They ate a lot, drank a lot, smoked a lot, and worked a lot (in their Polish delicatessen that sold as many candies and pastries as it did pierogies and pickles). Outside of working, one thing they didn't do a lot was move their bodies, and they gave no thought to limiting their diets in order to minimize unhealthy foods. They ate high-carb, high-animal-fat Polish American foods (that, truth be told, I still love) daily, and swished them down with a cool glass of Tang by day, alcohol by night.

The American lifestyle my grandparents embraced with open arms was filtered through the calorie-saving thrifty epigenotype of previous generations, which likely explains why my grandfather dropped dead of a massive heart attack at age sixty. And why, although my grandmother outlived my grandpa, she struggled with type 2 diabetes, obesity, and severe arthritis that significantly decreased her quality of life and was a primary factor in her death. And why my dad struggles with a similar collection of issues. And why my siblings and I are basically "allergic" to the simple sugar and processed foods our grandparents loved—when we eat poorly and skip exercise, we rapidly develop high cholesterol, high blood sugar, and inflammation. (Seriously, if I even look at a slice of cake, my blood sugar jumps up.)

You might say: *But most Americans suffer with these same issues*. And of course that's true; being epigenetically vulnerable to the American diet and lifestyle certainly isn't limited to my family. You can see the evidence when you look at the stats: obesity occurs in a whopping 70 percent of adults in the United States, and cardiometabolic disease happens in almost one out of three Americans.[2]

I suspect there are two epigenetic processes happening here that increase our vulnerability: many Americans' ancestors either came from countries with food insecurity or lived through regular periods of food abundance and food insecurity (such as in an agricultural setting where there are good and bad seasons). The result of this history is that thrifty epigenotype that makes their genetics primed to hang on to every calorie. It gets passed on to subsequent generations, making them, too, vulnerable to chronic disease. Then, once they develop a chronic disease, that disease state further impairs epigenetic expression.

Of course, this explanation doesn't include indigenous Americans, whose ancestors lived in this country for millennia. Their collective epigenome was profoundly impacted by forced changes to their diet and lifestyle—marked by periods of deep famine, being compelled to become significantly more sedentary, and having a new diet imposed upon them that relied heavily on fat and bleached flour.[3] As a result, their rates of type 2 diabetes skyrocketed, suggesting that their native diet likely supported far healthier epigenetic expression.[4] This is also in addition to the harms caused by the longstanding stressors of being colonized and marginalized, as we now know that stress and trauma also have a negative impact on epigenetic expression, something I'll cover more in depth in Chapter 7.

A similar story is true for Black Americans, who have a greater risk for the chronic diseases of aging, such as diabetes, hypertension, and heart disease, which contributes to an increased risk of COVID-19, as reported in a 2020 article, "Health Inequality Actually Is a 'Black and White Issue', Research Says."[5] This hard truth is indicative of the fact that a history of trauma—particularly for those Black Americans whose ancestors were enslaved—and pervasive stress—such as that which comes from living in a racist society that often undermines the quality of health care and breeds economic inequities that then provide a stress all their own—can predispose epigenetics to disease.

While it's true that epigenetic changes are the likely mechanism that explains how trauma experienced by your ancestors gets biologically embedded into your genetic material, there is good news here: research, including our study, is starting to demonstrate that some epigenetic marks need not be forever, and new research suggests that we may also be able to unembed even the deepest traumas from the epigenome. (More on this in Chapter 7.)

WHAT IDENTICAL TWINS CAN TEACH US ABOUT EPIGENETICS

Identical twins—a pair of humans with identical DNA—offer a fascinating window into the role epigenetics play in our health. An extraordinary example of epigenetic changes that occurred within one lifetime are Scott and Mark Kelly, the identical twin astronauts. This pair of brothers share so much on both the nature and the nurture side of the coin: the same genetic code, the same upbringing, and even many of the same career experiences. They were both captains in the US Navy, both participated in several spaceflights, and both lived for a time on the International Space Station (ISS).

The major difference between them is that Scott had two missions that required him to spend an extended period of time in space—the first was 159 days aboard the ISS in 2010, and the second was 340 days on the ISS in 2015 and 2016. With its lack of gravity and oxygen, space is a hugely different environment than Earth, and environment is a big influencer of genetic expression. In fact, three years after Scott returned to Earth in 2016, scientists studying the twins found that 7 percent of Scott's genetic makeup (not the genes themselves, but how they are expressed) remained different from Mark's, and not in a good way—Scott is now biologically older than his identical twin.[6] His altered epigenetics aged him.

But it certainly doesn't take something as epic as a year in space to alter the epigenetics of identical twins. We get a glimpse of this in the story of identical twin sisters who have been involved in research by the Twin Studies Center at the California State University at Fullerton.

In 2015, when the twins were in their early thirties, one was diagnosed with stage 2 breast cancer—she had a tumor in one breast the size of a tennis ball, and the cancer had already spread to her lymph nodes. The other twin stayed healthy. Their doctors and, later, the researchers at the Twin Studies Center, asked the girls to pore over their personal histories to try to find any differences in their experiences. Because the girls grew up in the same house, ate the same foods, went to the same schools and universities, played the same sports (softball and volleyball), and even dressed the same (tank tops and flip flops, year round, like the Southern Californians they are), there weren't many differences in experience to find. Except one. The twin who did not contract breast cancer told the *Atlantic*: "My mom was so tired that she still couldn't remember who she fed, who she bathed, who she burped. She would just cry. So our grandparents came over. They put my mom to bed. They washed both of us. They fed both of us, and they painted [the twin who got breast cancer]'s toenails."[7] As a mother, I don't want to contribute to any parental (or grandparental) guilt—I had such a hard time transitioning to being the mother of one child, I can only imagine what it's like to be the mother of twins! Yet as someone who regularly reads epigenetic research, I can't help but wonder: could such an innocuous (and cute) habit have influenced that twin's epigenome in a negative way? Research has demonstrated that chemicals in nail polish, including formaldehyde, toluene, and phthalates, can all be absorbed. And formaldehyde is recognized as a potential cancer-causing agent.[8]

Of course, there could have been differences in the womb that set these sisters on different epigenetic paths—one placenta could have been smaller than the other, or one umbilical cord longer, impacting how many nutrients that baby had access to. Perhaps the twins had different sleep patterns, or ways of coping with stress, or other toxic exposures. In truth, there are so many things that influence epigenetics that there likely isn't one smoking gun. But this family's story is evidence of the power of epigenetics.

It may seem like a negative example of the power of epigenetics, but that's only looking at one side of the equation. There are *so many* things within our power that beneficially impact our epigenetic health, and knowing what those things are gives us an enormous opportunity to positively influence our own health—and the health of future generations.

This story also refutes the idea so many people have that their genes render them helpless, like when you're gathered around the Thanksgiving table and your auntie says, "I just look at that stuffing and I gain weight, it's in my genes." Not only is this notion false, it's dangerous. What you eat, how you live, what you do, whether you exercise, what you think, what your stress level is, how much you're sleeping, all have a more important influence on your health than your genetics.

When you, or your auntie, blame your tendency to gain weight on the diabetes that runs in your family, it makes you feel like there's nothing you can do, so why bother? When in fact it's just the opposite: no matter what age you are, you have the power to change how your genes express, and that means you can influence how your body processes sugar, and even whether you develop diabetes at all.

It's true that I just got through saying that if I even look at cake my blood sugar jumps. But, using the Younger You principles that I outline in this book, I have been able to keep my blood sugar dialed in to a healthy range *and* improve my epigenetic health. Even with my admittedly not always perfect habits—even during stressful times, like during a pandemic, when we had to shift our practice to telemedicine, the kitchen in my home flooded, I was on deadline for this book, and my two-year-old started having epic nightmares, I've been able to drop my bio age by almost four years by following the Younger You Intensive (even though it's called Intensive, it *is* doable, even during stressful times!). It's tremendously exciting and motivating, especially as I feel fantastic on the full program. Although we haven't thus far monitored our patients' biological ages, as the epigenetic tests until very recently have been prohibitively expensive for routine clinical use, I see the same kind of resilience in my patients as I'm experiencing. I can say for certain that the folks who have incorporated elements of the Younger You programs into their daily routines have seen their aging-related issues either lessen considerably or fully resolve, and their self-assessment scores and blood work that we use to gauge biological age dramatically improve. The eating and lifestyle strategies, when ingrained into habit, provide benefits for the long term. (Also, excitingly, these tests are becoming readily available even as I write this! See Resources, page 429.)

EPIGENETIC CHANGES ARE IMMEDIATE—AND LONG-LASTING

When it comes to DNA, it takes millennia for a meaningful change to take hold throughout a species. DNA methylation, on the other hand, can create changes to your genetic expression quickly—so quickly as to be almost instantaneous, especially when compared to the glacial pace of evolution. Remember, methylation is happening in every cell of the body all the time. Your body is constantly deciding where to lay down and where to remove methyl groups from the DNA based on what you're experiencing—getting a decent night's sleep, opting for a handful of seeds for a snack instead of chips, moving your body by doing some activity you love, or meditating can all have a beneficial effect that can show up in just a couple of hours. When you consciously make these choices again and again over the long term, you can likely regain the DNA methylation patterns of a younger you.

Conversely, if you don't pay attention to the things you eat or take steps to mitigate the toxins or stress you're exposed to, you can speed up the pace at which your DNA methylation gets disordered. One study found that short periods of exposure to air tainted with particulate matter from car traffic caused noticeable epigenetic changes on genes that govern blood leukocytes (a type of immune cell). While there were bigger impacts with longer exposures of four and seven days, there were still noticeable changes after only four *hours*.[9]

How DNA Methylation Changes Become Lasting

WHATEVER EPIGENETIC CHANGES YOU EXPERIENCE, POSITIVE OR NEGATIVE, they become lasting because some of your cells are replicating through division all the time. When they do, your DNA creates a new copy of itself, so that there's a new, daughter strand as well as the original strand. Because methyl groups bind to your DNA strand with a strong bond, known as a covalent bond, and there is an enzyme whose sole job is to accurately copy these methyl groups on identical positions at the daughter strand, at every cell division, these methyl groups can stick around. The more you make those changes to your epigenome, the more cells adopt those changes. This is how something you're exposed to today can create changes to your DNA methylation patterns and genetic expression that last inside your cells and can even be passed down to future generations of offspring. One caveat: epigeneticist Lucia Aronica, PhD, thinks that those with chronic disease (and associated accelerated aging) might need to stick with epigenetic-nourishing activities over a longer time frame to create lasting beneficial changes to the epigenome than people who don't have chronic disease do, because their epigenomes may be more resistant to change. So while we know that people with health challenges can perhaps reverse bio age more significantly than healthy peers, it might take longer. We hope to answer this question in future studies.

● ● ● ● ●

Although changes can happen quickly, it's really the choices you make every day over a sustained period of time that impact your long-term health—and even the health of your offspring—most significantly.

Much of what we understand today in terms of the heritability of epigenetic changes and the role of nutrition in what gets handed down was first illuminated by Randy L. Jirtle, PhD, a professor of epigenetics at North Carolina State University and senior scientist at the McArdle Laboratory for Cancer Research at the University of Wisconsin at Madison. A true pioneer in the field of epigenetics, Jirtle conducted an experiment on female agouti yellow mice—a strain of mouse that has an expressed (i.e., not hypermethylated and thus inhibited) agouti gene that makes the mice obese and gives them a distinctive yellow coat. Jirtle, and his postdoc Robert Waterland, supplemented their diets with vitamin B_{12}, folic acid, choline, and betaine—these are key players in the methylation process, known as methyl donors, which I'll explain in a bit—before, during, and after pregnancy. Three generations of offspring of these mothers were normal weight and their coats were either mottled with brown or fully brown, rather than the distinctive yellow. The methyl donors had in effect shut the agouti gene off. It was a true "wow" moment; his paper describing this study has gone on to be the *most* cited study in the history of science.[10]

We already knew that a mother's nutrient levels had a huge impact on the health of her child. For example, we've long known that mothers with low levels of folate have a higher rate of giving birth to babies with birth defects, which is why grains have been required to be fortified with folic acid since 1998 (and why rates of birth defects have come down, although there are perils to folic acid supplementation, too—more on this on page 51). Turns out that's because folate is an important component of the methylation process throughout the body, including DNA methylation.

But our understanding of just how impactful the nutrition of pregnant human mothers is on the health outcomes of their children was furthered by three fairly recent epidemiological studies.

The first, a 2013 study, looked at children who were born to women who were pregnant during what's known as the Dutch Hunger Winter. In September 1944, at the tail end of World War II, train workers in the Netherlands went on strike, hoping to slow the movements of Nazi troops and give the Allies a leg up. The Nazis retaliated by implementing a blockade that prevented food supplies from reaching the country, plunging the Western half of the Netherlands into famine conditions. Until the country was liberated in May 1945, most people in the affected area subsisted on somewhere between four hundred and eight hundred calories a day. More than twenty thousand Dutch people died of starvation.

Perhaps not surprisingly, scientists who evaluated the health of the people who were born during and just after the Dutch Hunger Winter found that they experienced health issues that even their own siblings (who were not in utero during the winter in question, either because they were already born or hadn't been conceived yet) didn't. What *is* a surprise is that this cohort, in adulthood, was more likely to be overweight and have higher levels of LDL cholesterol and triglycerides—all things associated with eating too *much* food, not too little. They also had obesity, diabetes, and interestingly, schizophrenia at higher rates, as well as a 10 percent higher incidence of death from any cause by the time they were sixty-eight.[11] Put simply, the early life experiences caused accelerated biological aging and early mortality.

These findings flummoxed the scientists who first observed the higher incidence of obesity. And then, in 2018, thanks to advances in science that allow lab researchers to observe the methylation marks present on over 350,000 different spots on the genome, came a big "Aha!" moment:[12] they saw evidence that those who were in utero during the Dutch Hunger

Winter were more likely to have more methyl groups on a gene known as PIM3, which is involved in metabolism, and different methylation patterns on other genes implicated in cell growth, lipid metabolism, and glucose tolerance. Perhaps the mothers' hunger caused hypermethylation on this gene and imbalancd methylation patterns on other genes, and thus their children's metabolism always ran a little slower in an effort to hang on to food a little longer (that thrifty epigenotype I referred to earlier), leading to gaining weight.[13]

Another foundational study found a similar result. The Överkalix co-hort study analyzed multiple environmental factors on the population of Överkalix, a small city in Sweden where they kept copious records, such as the size of the harvest and the price of food, for decades. The researchers were seeking to determine the effect of the amount of food readily available on epigenetic inheritance in populations born in 1890, 1905, and 1920, as well as in those populations' children and grandchildren. The researchers found that eating too much in childhood—specifically in boys in preadolescence, when sperm are actively maturing—in generation zero correlated with diabetes and diabetes-related mortality in the subsequent *three* generations! Interestingly enough, the same study shows a protective effect from eating less, suggesting that there is a sweet spot of food consumption—not too much, not too little, but just right.[14]

The third study that has shaped our understanding of the inheritance of epigenetic changes came in 2014, when Moshe Szyf, Suzanne King, and team conducted a study called Project Ice Storm. In it, they evaluated the DNA methylation of children born to mothers who lived in Montreal and were pregnant during a severe two-week 1998 ice storm that cut the power off in large swaths of Ontario, Quebec, upstate New York, and Maine. The mothers did not starve, but rather experienced profound physical and psychological stress. King's team found that these children were likely to develop a distinctive DNA methylation pattern on the genetic code in their T cells—an important immune system cell—and were more prone to displaying symptoms of asthma and autism.[15]

It may seem like bad news that if your mother was exposed to stress or trauma when she was pregnant, you're doomed to have genes that don't work as well as they could. When in truth, the opposite is true:

knowing that you can influence DNA methylation, and how to do it, can help you make mindful choices that optimize the genetic—and the circumstantial—hand you're dealt. Even genetic conditions where your fate seems carved in stone can be minimized by bolstering your DNA methylation.

THE EPIGENETIC ROOTS OF COMMON DISEASES (AKA AGE ACCELERANTS)

An overarching theme in modern medicine that has largely been missed is that disordered DNA methylation is a driver of disease, and not just an indicator. In addition, the often co-occurring diseases—including cardiovascular disease, obesity, diabetes, and dementia—are also "age accelerants."

From inheriting a thrifty epigenome from our recent ancestors who experienced food insecurity, to the challenging or even traumatic circumstances or events that we experience, to our own lifestyle choices that may further entrench unfavorable DNA methylation patterns, we have a lot of epigenetic patterns we need to rewrite. That means addressing DNA methylation is essential to prevent and treat chronic illness, which is why we prescribe some aspect of the Younger You principles with every patient we see.

Let's take a look at how the epigenome has been shown to impact various conditions and diseases.

Obesity

The truth is that weight—as measured by BMI—is associated with accelerated aging, as measured by DNA methylation.[16]

Based on what we saw in our research study with a few participants (most didn't need to lose weight as they were healthy at the start) and in our clinical practice, those who follow the Younger You Intensive, certainly, and even the Younger You Everyday, and who can benefit from weight loss do lose weight. The Younger You Intensive employs the well-established weight-loss guidelines of being a low-glycemic, keto-leaning program that incorporates mild time-restricted eating (otherwise known as intermittent fasting). It's also free of allergenic foods, such as dairy and gluten, so it's also anti-inflammatory. Taken altogether, the Younger You Intensive lowers inflammation and increases energy and satiety, which allows for weight loss, if needed.

Following the Younger You principles of avoiding toxins (more on this in Chapter 7) also reduces your exposure to endocrine-disrupting chemicals, also known as obesogens, that contribute to the epigenetic dysregulation that is associated with metabolic impairment and weight gain.

On top of these direct influences on weight loss (and this doesn't even include the weight-loss benefits of regular moderate exercise, improved sleep, and boosted relaxation), modulating your DNA methylation may also affect expression of obesity-associated genes that influence what your body does with calories.[17] If these genes are shut off due to hypermethylation, you're more than twice as likely to be obese. Because the Younger You program includes ample amounts of foods that affect the methylation-demethylation balance, the eating plan may help turn back on the genes that promote a healthy weight.

By the same mechanism, eating the DNA methylation–supportive nutrients that are a hallmark of the Younger You program may help to change the epigenetic patterns that you've inherited from parents, grandparents, and great-grandparents.[18] It gives you hope of breaking the cycle of "The chubby gene runs in our family."

Alzheimer's Disease

Having a family member with Alzheimer's can feel like receiving that diagnosis is an unavoidable part of your future. Yet, while there can be a genetic component to Alzheimer's disease, 95 percent of those who have it have the nongenetic form. That means epigenetics dictate the vast majority of cases.

As with obesity, it's known that epigenetic mechanisms play a variety of crucial roles in the development of Alzheimer's disease, to the extent that several epigenetic-based therapies are being considered now.

Most broadly, accelerated biological age is associated with Alzheimer's, and patients with Alzheimer's are biologically older than same-aged healthy folks.[19] Alzheimer's and other neurodegenerative diseases are accompanied by marked global methylation decrease overall (very often this population has elevated homocysteine, a marker of decreased methylation), along with a higher expression of genes you *don't* want to be turned on and a lower expression of genes you *do* want in the on position.

More specifically, a number of genes involved in Alzheimer's disease have been found to have aberrant methylation patterns in those with the disease as compared to those without the disease, meaning some genes are on when they should be off, or off when they should be on.[20]

The APP (amyloid precursor protein) gene gives rise to amyloid beta protein when it is in the on position, and APP is often in abundance in the brains of Alzheimer's patients. When we're young, this gene tends toward the off position; as we age, it can turn on, which likely plays a role in higher levels of beta amyloid in the brain and, thus, higher risk of Alzheimer's disease. Furthermore, the gene for the protein that breaks down beta amyloid is actually hypermethylated and turned off—a double Alzheimer's whammy. In addition, the ApoE4 gene, well known to be associated with the disease, has a complex and unusual pattern of methylation, with some areas hypomethylated and others hypermethylated. Scientists speculate that these changes may induce the pathologic alterations seen in the brains of Alzheimer's patients.[21]

From my standpoint, any program effectively addressing Alzheimer's disease requires interventions that address DNA methylation and epigenetics in general, supporting both methylation and demethylation.

The functional medicine approach to Alzheimer's disease (as developed by Dale Bredesen, MD) is a powerful intervention for both preventing and treating Alzheimer's disease—a 2021 multicenter clinical trial validated its benefit.[22] Much of the Younger You program and the Bredesen program overlap: Each focuses on healthy, low-carb/keto-leaning, good-fat and polyphenol-rich foods with time-restricted eating windows. Each prioritizes exercise, sleep, and stress reduction. And each approach minimizes toxin exposures, which is essential in protecting brain function and DNA methylation. Dr. Bredesen also recognizes hypomethylation as an issue and pays attention to homocysteine levels in his patients.

Where Younger You differs from Bredesen's approach is its wholesale focus on balancing DNA methylation.

In our clinic, we use the Bredesen approach as a foundation and then layer Younger You components onto his program. Our patients with neurodegenerative conditions routinely experience lower levels of inflammation, homocysteine, and toxins and demonstrate improved nutrient status. We see the best outcomes in cognitive scores with mild cognitive impairment (MCI), although we can see favorable changes in cognition even in those with advanced disease.

Reducing elevated levels of homocysteine, the biomarker associated with poor overall methylation, including DNA methylation, has also been shown to slow the rate of whole brain atrophy and cognitive decline in elderly people with cognitive impairment.[23] And the patients in our clinic routinely lower their homocysteine to healthy levels when following the Younger You program.

Heart Health

Cardiovascular disease is the number one cause of death worldwide. We cannot overstate the significance of heart disease in terms of quality of life and medical costs: it's absolutely enormous.

Bio age, as measured by DNA methylation patterns, is well correlated with risk of cardiovascular disease—the higher your bio or chronological age, the greater your risk of heart disease.[24]

In addition, inherited altered DNA methylation patterns—like those seen in the Dutch Hunger Winter and Överkalix studies—contribute to conditions including diabetes, hypertension, and obesity that increase your cardiovascular risk.

Disordered methylation patterns on numerous genes associated with hypertension, atherosclerosis, heart failure, and myocardial infarction have been identified in humans.[25] What I find most interesting is the connection between early and midlife stress and altered DNA methylation patterns that have been associated with later onset heart disease and cognitive decline. Of particular note is the gene NR3C1, which codes for the human glucocorticoid receptor (glucocorticoid is a class of steroid hormone that is released during stressful times and plays many roles, including curbing inflammation). Different methylation patterns of NR3C1 have been identified in a broad spectrum of stress disorders, heart disease, and cognitive decline, making it a common gene of interest in all of these conditions.[26]

Elevated homocysteine, a foundational marker of imbalanced total methylation (including DNA methylation), has long been touted as a risk factor for cardiovascular disease and stroke. Yet, the research does *not* clearly show that simply lowering homocysteine alone will prevent heart disease.[27]

So how do we interpret these seemingly conflicting findings? DNA methylation patterns, changed by broad environmental exposures ranging from previous generational experience to early and midlife stress exposures, to diet, toxins, exercise patterns, and more all influence methylation patterns that in turn influence heart disease risk. Myopic focus on correcting homocysteine—or limiting treatment to cardiology alone—isn't enough; as with all of the conditions discussed in this chapter, a full Younger You Intensive may favorably influence the occurrence of heart disease in a broad, beneficial manner, as getting biologically younger reduces risk.

Type 2 Diabetes

In the United States alone, a diabetic is diagnosed every twenty seconds. This metabolic disease burns through bio age like dry kindling on a hot day: diabetes is associated with a six- to nine-year increase in biological age![28]

It's well established that type 2 diabetes results in general dysregulation of DNA methylation with far-reaching effects, including hypermethylation of important tumor-suppressor genes and antioxidant-regulating genes,[29] as well as a particular gene that impacts insulin, PPARGC1A.[30]

The obesogenic toxins that play a role in excess weight—like PCBs and pesticides—even in low doses of exposure, are also potent drivers of diabetes, in part because they contribute to abnormal DNA methylation patterns.[31] And higher levels of exposure to obesogens are associated with a whopping thirty-eight-plus-fold increase in diabetes![32]

The good news is that type 2 diabetes is very responsive to the Younger You protocol. One patient in particular is a perfect example of the kinds of results we see in the clinic.

Linda was fifty-six when I first saw her. A smart, funny university professor, she'd been diagnosed with type 2 diabetes a decade ago, and her family history was riddled with diabetes and diabetes-associated conditions like high blood pressure and heart disease. Despite her best efforts at lifestyle change and a cocktail of medications, her blood sugar and lipids, weight, blood pressure, and food cravings were all high. Her mood was low. Linda was sick and tired of the conventional approach and was looking for a new approach to her care. At a glance, Linda's diet looked pretty good: she was eating a lot of your basic salad-and-protein meals. She also engaged in a daily meditation practice. Her real struggle came at night, when she got home from a long, intense day. Her cravings would hit, and she'd go for sweets and a glass of wine; in fact, her red wine intake was high (as you'll learn in Chapter 5, alcohol inhibits methylation).

We placed her on the full Younger You Intensive program, with an emphasis on even lower carbs, since we needed to get her glucose and insulin levels down. We had her prioritize eating specific DNA methylation–supportive nutrients that have a powerful anti-inflammatory effect, including those found in turmeric, green tea, and rosemary. I also started her on moderate doses of fish oil, magnesium, and vitamin D supplements. After her first month on the plan, her morning fasting blood sugar had dropped from 300 to 90! At four months, she was down twenty pounds and exercising most days. She was thrilled with her progress and committed to the journey. We could all see her getting younger before our eyes, and most importantly, she could see the Younger You coming through in herself!

Depression

Mental health has epigenetic roots. In adults with depression, two key genes have been found to be hypermethylated and inhibited:

- Brain-derived neurotrophic factor (BDNF), which is involved in the formation of new neurons and is vital to learning, memory, higher thinking, and mood, is often hypermethylated and switched off. In early life, adverse chemical toxin exposures can negatively impact DNA methylation and stressful events can become biologically embedded in the epigenome, changing BDNF gene methylation, which has potential long-lasting impact on behavior and memory.[33] Exercise, a fundamental part of both the Intensive and Everyday programs, helps BDNF re-expression.[34]

- Depression, along with alcoholism and obsessive-compulsive disorder, is associated with specific epigenetic changes to the serotonin transporter gene (SLC6A4), which is involved in serotonin reuptake. Interestingly, SLC6A4 is also involved in energy metabolism and its methylation status can predict obesity over the life span.

In addition to these two genes, oxytocin—known as the love hormone—also plays a role in depression. When the gene that codes for the oxytocin receptor is hypermethylated and turned off, it lowers empathy and prompts a lack of connection to others, both common experiences that can happen with depression. One study on depression in African American women involved one hundred middle-aged participants. It found that when the oxytocin receptors were hypermethylated and off, the women were more likely to have negative thinking patterns, such as pessimism and distrust, both common in depression—and this effect was seen regardless of relationship status, childhood trauma, age, and overall methylation status. The researchers concluded: "epigenetic regulation of the oxytocin system may be a mechanism whereby the negative cognitions central to depression are biologically embedded."[35] In other words, getting stuck in a negative thinking loop may further embed the experience you're thinking about in your epigenome. Doesn't that make sense? If you "indulge" in negative thinking, it can become a habit that is hard to break, even though it keeps you feeling lousy.

In our clinic, we've seen time and time again that the combination of a diet rich in DNA methylation–supportive nutrients as well as moderate exercise, meditation, and sleep all support mood and mental health, sometimes to remarkable ends (see Morgan's story at the start of Chapter 3).

Autoimmune Diseases and Allergies

Both autoimmune diseases and allergies are hallmarks of an overreactive immune system: in autoimmunity, your immune system goes on the attack of your own tissues; in allergy, it mounts an overwhelming immune response to a benign substance. Incidence of both is markedly on the rise across the globe, which means that genetics, while there is a connection, doesn't explain the increase. That leaves epigenetics.

While clear, actionable epigenetic patterns in autoimmunity and allergy are still being established, what we know so far is that epigenetic deregulation of the immune system contributes to disease onset and severity—meaning the imbalance begins long before symptoms manifest. As a specific example, the DNA methylation of genes in key insulin-producing cells is considered "potentially causal" for type 1 diabetes and may be present years before the onset of diabetes.[36] The other thing we currently know about these conditions is that lower methylation reduces immune control, allowing proinflammatory genes to be hypomethylated and turned on, something we see in other chronic diseases and in aging itself.

A 2021 study (that cited our study!) showed that women with the autoimmune disease lupus (SLE) had higher rates of hypomethylation on a specific immune cell gene when disease activity was high, and those who ate a higher methyl donor diet reported significantly lower disease activity. The authors concluded that "dietary methyl donors may influence DNA methylation levels and thereby disease activity in SLE."[37]

As I write this book, epigenetic biomarkers to test for autoimmune and allergic diseases as well as epigenetic therapeutics for treatment are being considered. While we wait for those breakthroughs to come, the Younger You program has been helping the many patients in our clinic who present with allergic or autoimmune conditions. One of our rheumatoid arthritis patients, Marian, is a prime example.

Marian came to my practice with severe pain and swelling in her fingers, wrists, and elbows. Her pain was ten out of ten, and while she was taking ibuprofen regularly, it was barely helping. According to her blood work, Marian's antinuclear antibodies and rheumatoid factor autoantibodies were off the charts.

Marian's triggering event was the loss of a very close loved one; her grief was relentless and made it hard for her to care for herself. She maintained herself on a steady intake of diet soda and take-out and didn't exercise. Marian's plan needed to be simple, but effective. I focused on all of the components of the Younger You Intensive (including removal of gluten, dairy, and legumes and lower carbohydrates overall), with supplementation of curcumin, fish oil, and vitamin D. We initiated grief counseling. And one of our nutritionists worked closely with her to help her order her food from restaurants and still stay within the guidelines of her eating plan.

Almost overnight, Marian's pain level dropped from a ten to a four. That initial relief helped her keep going—and eventually learn to cook, an important component because the epigenetic disarray starts long before the onset of a full-fledged autoimmune condition and she needed to stick with the plan for the long term.

An important part of Marian's plan was also getting off the ibuprofen, as nonsteroidal anti-inflammatory drugs (NSAIDs) damage the gut microbiome and the intestinal wall, allowing microbial debris to leak into the bloodstream and trigger a potent inflammatory response, inhibiting inflammation resolution. While they help you feel good short term—and are OK to be used occasionally—the pain-reducing benefit of NSAIDs isn't lasting, and it's likely that, long term, they help perpetuate the illness.

It's been known for decades that autoimmune and allergic diseases share underlying root causes, including genetic and epigenetic susceptibility, filtered through poor diet, imbalanced microbiome, leaky gut, hormone imbalances, toxin exposures, and in some cases, infections.[38] Each of these in turn influence DNA methylation and other epigenetic processes. Therefore it's not surprising, as our clinical experience bears out, that focusing on optimal DNA methylation using our program is generally helpful to both of these all-too-common conditions of immune dysregulation.

In addition to being designed to sweet-talk DNA methylation, the Younger You program is also potently anti-inflammatory and hypoallergenic, healing to the microbiome, and low in sugar and simple carbs with time-restricted eating—all of these features make it an ideal foundational program for those suffering from allergies and autoimmunity. You may need further individualization of the program—for example, if you have an egg allergy, clearly those should be removed from the program. But in general, our clinical experience shows the Younger You Intensive to be very useful for folks with allergies and autoimmunity. The lifestyle pieces of the Younger You program are also essential, as stress has a significant negative impact on both allergies and autoimmunity, as do toxins.

Cancer

Epigenetic aging, left to its own devices, marches us toward all of the diseases we've discussed so far. But nowhere is this march so well studied, and perhaps so scary, as it is with cancer.

Cancers of all type (brain, bladder, breast, lung, prostate, colon, skin, ovarian . . .) hijack our epigenetic machinery for their own nefarious end, like expert computer hackers can take down a country's defenses with chilling ease.[39] Also, even if we do not have cancer present, as our biological (and chronological) age creeps higher, all-important tumor-suppressor genes (including the most famous, BRCA1) and tumor repair genes can become hypermethylated and shut off. In addition, genes that promote cancer (called "oncogenes") are hypomethylated and turned on. It's just not fair: aging makes us epigenetically vulnerable to developing cancer, and cancer itself takes over our epigenetics.[40]

Because problem DNA methylation is a big piece in many conditions, scientists are working hard on developing DNA methylation tests as diagnostic tools for many, many disorders. This is most evident in cancer, where the methylation status of tumor repair and tumor-suppressor genes is used in diagnosis. Perhaps the best known example of this is the Cologuard at-home colon cancer screening test, which assesses two genes in particular that are typically hypermethylated in colon cancer (NDRG4 and BMP3).[41]

Hypermethylation of tumor-suppressor genes is such a strong factor in cancer development that there are demethylating drugs for certain cancers. They can be important players in therapy, but they are riddled with potential toxicity because they indiscriminately inhibit DNA methylation. After all, you don't want to turn genes on, or off, for that matter, willy-nilly. Better to seek the precision changes that our study suggested diet and lifestyle can produce—our participants reduced their biological age by moving methyl groups to DNA sites that are associated with youth (instead of age), and therefore health (instead of disease, including cancer).

It's starting to look like many of these cancer-associated genes are what I suspect are nutrient-responsive genes—meaning, their DNA methylation patterns change rather predictably in the presence of specific nutrients. There are certain DNA methylation–supportive nutrients (we call them DNA methylation adaptogens, which I'll cover more in depth in Chapter 3) that have some very exciting benefits for cancer prevention. For example, we've long known that EGCG (a component of green tea) and curcumin (a component of turmeric) are important interventions in integrative cancer care. Now we believe that a chief reason is that they favorably influence epigenetics, and in particular, DNA methylation.

Research is also suggesting that *combinations* of these supportive nutrients may be powerful in cancer prevention and treatment, which strongly reinforces the power of a whole foods diet that provides not only ample amounts of specific nutrients, but also creates the conditions they need to work synergistically with each other.[42] I look forward to continuing to research the impact our Younger You program has on cancer epigenetics via these nutrient-responsive genes.

In our practice, patients come to us most often to be comanaged with their oncology team. With most patients in active cancer treatment, we individualize the Younger You to them as appropriate: common customizations include longer periods of intermittent fasting in association with their chemo regimen, reducing carbs to make the eating plan more ketogenic, prescribing extra doses in diet and supplement form of the DNA methylation adaptogen nutrients I just mentioned and will share many more details about in Chapter 3, and perhaps prescribing blood sugar–supportive nutrients or medications as needed.

One final word on working with cancer patients (and anyone with a chronic illness or simply wanting to reverse biological age): the mind/body component of care cannot be overlooked. My good friend and colleague Dr. Patrick Hanaway recovered from stage 4 laryngeal cancer. While he incorporated the components I've discussed above along with radiation and chemotherapy, he said it was sloshing barefoot through the creek on his property that grounded him and was, as he says, a turning point in his healing.

ALL OF THIS points to one fact: a healthy diet and lifestyle unequivocally reduces incidence of all chronic disease.[43] This is great news. Whether you are fairly healthy or someone with a chronic condition (and perhaps wondering if it's too late to change), it's always a good time to support your DNA methylation and your bio age. And interesting research I'll share later suggests that the older you are, chronologically and biologically, the more bang for your buck you'll get with these changes. Meaning, it's never too late.

In the next chapter, we'll unpack exactly which foods and lifestyle practices we used in our research study and show evidence that they favorably influence DNA methylation and reverse bio age.

3

THE POWER OF DIET AND LIFESTYLE TO LOWER BIO AGE

WHEN MORGAN FIRST CAME TO OUR CLINIC, HE WAS CLINICALLY depressed. Although he was on Ritalin and prescription anti-anxiety meds, he started missing work and avoiding family functions. Things had gotten so bad that Morgan had become suicidal. Existing on a diet of fried chicken and greasy take-out, he was also fifty pounds overweight.

Luckily, his sister was a nutritionist doing her residency at our clinic; her support helped him seek help and implement changes.

Our approach with Morgan was twofold—to gradually improve his diet to include the vegetables, nuts, seeds, eggs, and healthy fats that support DNA methylation, and to get him to start moving his body doing something he enjoyed. His sister volunteered to cook his first week of meals as a Christmas present and convinced him to add prebiotic fiber to his morning coffee to start nurturing the friendly bacteria in his gut, as there is a well-established link between gut health and mental health. The fiber also helped curb his cravings for take-out.

When his mood lightened a bit and his energy perked up as a result of eating that nutrient-dense food, he decided to use a healthy meal delivery service for his breakfasts, and started eating canned soup and Goldfish crackers for his other meals (Morgan was, shall we say, not a cook, and it was important to him that he didn't feel totally deprived). It wasn't perfect, but it was an important start.

A few weeks later, because he was feeling better, he had the energy to take up jogging. The boost from that change inspired him to switch his midday meal to a larger mixed-vegetable salad and Goldfish crackers. After two months, he had dropped twenty pounds and started tapering his meds. Because he saw that the change in diet was giving him more relief than the meds, and even the therapy he was undergoing, he decided to invest in a meal delivery service for a few of his weekly dinners, too. As he felt better, he started spending more time with family and friends. Another turning point came when Morgan committed to a regular bedtime and started getting more and higher-quality sleep.

For Morgan, the gradual process of implementing changes was hugely important—he says, "If you had given me fifty things to do at first I never would have started."

A year later, Morgan is down fifty pounds and off of Ritalin completely. He's tapered his anti-anxiety meds and is running regularly. Although we weren't able to test his bio age at the start (this is only now just beginning to become available in a clinical setting), because obesity is an age accelerant, it's reasonable to guess that he reversed his aging very significantly. His story shows the power of diet changes, even imperfectly implemented, plus a few well-chosen lifestyle pieces—like community, sleep, and moderate exercise—to step out of the river that flows toward disease.

Up until now, you may have opted to eat a certain food because it was low-calorie and you wanted to lose weight, or done a workout because you wanted to look better in your jeans or strengthen a particular muscle, or taken a supplement because you wanted to rejuvenate your immune system. These are all honorable inspirations, but what epigenetics is revealing to us is that they are only scratching the surface of what our diet and our habits have the power to do for us. When viewed through the lens of how they impact DNA methylation you can see the awesome power of the things you eat, drink, and do to nourish your genetic expression and make you biologically younger (and, if you plan to have children, to improve their epigenetic inheritance, too).

Knowing the power of your daily decisions will give you motivation that perhaps you've never had before to make the choices that influence your health all the way down to your genes. As you'll see, it doesn't require huge sacrifices—you don't have to commit to restricting your caloric intake for the rest of your life, inject yourself with potent hormones, or experiment with off-label prescription meds that may come with their own host of side effects. You can make more mindful choices about what and when you eat, and make time for the exercise, sleep, and stress reduction—not too much, and not too little—that help you feel your best, and you can redirect the path of your health trajectory away from chronic disease and toward a longer health span. I can't wait for you to see just how moderate the plan is. We've broken it down into one formula with three simple components that, when combined, reverse bio age:

Methyl donors + DNA methylation adaptogens + lifestyle = Y2 (Younger You)

I'll delve more deeply into each of these components at the end of this chapter; for now, you need to know the following:

- **Methyl donors** are the foods that contain the nutrients the body uses to create methyl groups, which are then used in multiple processes throughout the body, including DNA methylation. These are the *ingredients* of DNA methylation.

- **DNA methylation adaptogens** are the foods that provide the molecules that have been shown to *regulate* DNA methylation. They help make sure the methyl donors get used in the right amounts and in the right places.

- **Lifestyle** refers to the practices that foster healthy DNA methylation, including getting adequate sleep and exercise, relaxation, and mild intermittent fasting, among others.

This combination of factors is what makes the Younger You program unique. No one has put these elements together this way, and certainly no one, except us, has researched it. But it's not like we came up with the formula all on our own: using diet and lifestyle to bolster genetic expression is a natural progression from the thinking of some of functional medicine's forebears and top thinkers.

THE HISTORY OF USING NUTRIENTS MEDICINALLY

Our approach of using well-chosen nutrients to influence health is part of a lineage that goes back to two of the pioneers of functional medicine: Linus Pauling, PhD (a two-time Nobel laureate), and Bruce Ames, PhD (professor emeritus of biochemistry and molecular biology at the University of California, Berkeley, and a senior scientist at Children's Hospital Oakland Research Institute).

In the 1960s, Linus Pauling coined the term *orthomolecular medicine* for the study of giving the correct (ortho) molecules in the right amounts for individual needs—an alternative to population recommendations like the Recommended Daily Intake. Pauling maintained that we can nudge physiological pathways with impaired function toward normal by giving specific supplements in specific (and typically very high) doses. In 2002, Bruce Ames, PhD, corroborated and furthered Pauling's ideas in a seminal review of 377 studies and concluded that "about 50 human genetic diseases . . . can be remediated or ameliorated by the administration of high doses of vitamin[s]."[1] In other words, in many instances, nutrients, not medications, were effective treatments for genetic mutations associated with disease.

One genetic condition in particular—maple syrup urine disease (MSUD), a genetic disease with severe neurological impairments—yielded resounding proof of the power of the right nutrient, in the right amount, to the right person. Patients with MSUD have a mutation in a gene that codes for an enzyme that needs vitamin B_1 in order to work. Ames discovered that some forms of MSUD could be wholly resolved with high-dose B_1 supplementation.

Dr. Jeff Bland and other founders of functional medicine brought forth Pauling's and Ames's papers and wove them into the fabric of functional medicine. Most functional medicine doctors have studied carefully and deeply embrace these concepts as cornerstone to our practice: that the right vitamin and minerals for an individual, prescribed in the right amounts to affect the right pathways, can nudge physiology toward optimal function, whether the individual has a genetic mutation, is a very healthy athlete who wants optimal performance, or is a "regular" person looking for best health.

It's in part these empowering ideas (along with the important concept of "treating the whole person") that inspire many doctors and practitioners from other specialties to dive back into the medical and nutritional bio-chemistry that is foundational to the practice of functional medicine. Supporting nature to lead the way with the right nutrients in the right doses is powerful, and it works. I've seen biotin successfully resolve a seizure disorder, B_6 greatly improve the behavior of a child with autism (in both cases, laboratory findings were suggestive of a mutation in enzymes requiring said nutrients), and high-dose fish oil stop painful abdominal muscle contractions in an ALS patient. The list goes on. In all of these cases, pharmaceuticals wouldn't have worked. The right nutrient(s) in the right doses were needed, just as Pauling and Ames taught us.

While there are many instances where high-dose nutrient supplementation is absolutely appropriate, as we have learned more about epigenetics, we have come to see that there may be some risks involved in this approach, too, and that sometimes less is actually more—much more.

THE POTENTIAL DOWNSIDE OF HIGH-DOSE SUPPLEMENTS

Learning about the power of high doses of nutrients offers a tempting choice: to load up on the nutrients that support DNA methylation in supplement form—*and get really young*! After all, Pauling and Ames taught us we could beneficially influence biochemistry with specific nutrients, sometimes in very high doses. But in the age of epigenetics, we're starting to be able to see that this power may be taken too far. Even Jirtle and his fellow researchers in the famous agouti mice study, which had overwhelmingly favorable findings, cautioned against excessive supplementation, concluding in their seminal paper: "These findings suggest that dietary supplementation, long presumed to be purely beneficial, may have unintended deleterious influences on the establishment of epigenetic gene regulation in humans."[2]

Why do we need to be concerned?

Some of these nutrients potently influence epigenetic expression—and that influence can be either for better or for worse. And if we're giving those nutrients in high doses, there's a possibility that we may inadvertently nudge the needle toward "for worse."

While there are certainly instances when laboratory testing or clinical experience demonstrates a need for a certain supplement in high doses, I'm much more cautious about prescribing higher-dose nutrients in supplement form. Especially now that we can see that you can influence the epigenome positively with much more moderate amounts of nutrients. In fact, we're seeing that right combinations and right amounts of nutrients delivered in a whole-food package, in what we're calling *orthomolecular nutrition*, may be our most powerful—and safest—ally yet.

A PERFECT EXAMPLE: FOLIC ACID VS. FOLATE

Folate, otherwise known as vitamin B_9, is an essential nutrient and a primary methyl donor—and therefore a crucial component of DNA methylation. Folate also helps make DNA and RNA and repairs DNA.

Folic acid, on the other hand, is a synthetic form of folate. Importantly for food and supplement manufacturers, it is shelf-stable. The body can turn folic acid into folate, but the process is time—and energy—consuming, and many people don't do it all that well.

Because it's such a key player in all things DNA and RNA, folate is needed wherever cell division is happening. As such, folate plays an important role in embryonic development; without enough of it, the neural tube (which is what will eventually become the baby's brain, spine, and nervous system) may not close properly, and whatever neural material remains exposed suffers damage that can result in birth defects.

We've known about the connection between folate levels in the mother and the risk of neural tube defects since 1991; as a result of this knowledge, the United States started fortification with folic acid in 1996, and it became mandatory in 1998.

Like most things in life, and nearly every nutrient, there is a U-shaped curve to folate's benefits. Both having too little and too much have risks.

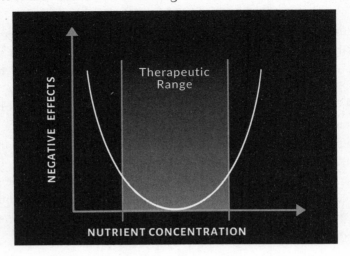

If you don't have enough folate, your DNA can become unstable, resulting in birth defects if you're an embryo or cancer if you're an adult (and loads of other conditions—from ulcerative colitis to dementia). But too much folate can also be dangerous; it has its own risks of increased cancer, especially in older people. On either leg of the U, the mechanisms behind the cancer risk are different—too little folate means the synthesis and repair of DNA is hindered, while too much means potentially increased cell proliferation and DNA methylation, which can mean tumor-suppressor genes and other good-guy genes are more likely to be inhibited.

It's only the flat portion of the U curve that's in the sweet spot of lowest risk and highest benefit—and it's eating a diet rich in naturally occurring folate that is the most no-brainer, safest way to live in that sweet spot. While it may seem like fortifying foods with folic acid supports the goal of helping more people have the right amount of folate, it's by no means clear-cut.

While fortification of folic acid has been a public health win—in the United States alone, the occurrence of neural tube defects has dropped by as much as 31 percent since we started fortifying[3]—there are two main problems with it:

1. Many people can't process folic acid into folate easily, meaning that these folks can have a lot of unmetabolized folic acid in their blood. In one study looking at older adults with low B_{12}, high levels of circulating unmetabolized folic acid was associated with reduced cognitive performance.[4]

2. For folks who can process folic acid into folate efficiently, if there is a high intake of fortified foods (especially combined with supplementing extra folate), there is a risk of having more active folate than needed and pushing DNA methylation into potentially dangerous territory—resulting in more methyl groups being added to more DNA, including on beneficial genes like tumor-suppressor and anti-inflammatory genes, and perhaps even shutting those genes off. And if cancer is already present, folate can increase the synthesis of tumor cells and promote DNA methylation in an unhelpful way. Indeed, the rate of colorectal cancer in the United States started to tick upward (some researchers called it an "abrupt reversal"[5]) in 1996 after a fifteen-year decline, peaking in 1998, the very year that all grain manufacturers were required to fortify their products with folic acid.[6] While mere timing doesn't prove causation, a 2010 study found that in individuals with high blood folate, two tumor-suppressor genes were hypermethylated and turned off.[7]

There are some countries that are exploring ending folic acid fortification because of the potential risks (I would not be surprised if the United States considers this step at some point in the future), and still other countries deciding against starting fortification programs.

To me, it's clear that while we need an ample amount of folate, we don't need to get it from folic acid–fortified foods *or* from routine supplementation. To my view, the best way to obtain our nutrient requirements is through a whole foods diet, but a healthy microbiome can play a role, too, although we're still learning about the extent of the contributions. Beneficial gut bugs actually make a lot of vitamins, and folate is just one of them (B_1, B_2, B_{12}, biotin, B_6, vitamin K, and PABA are others).[8] In our study, we increased circulating folate solely via food sources and by prescribing a probiotic that contains *Lactobacillus plantarum*, a strain that has some research to suggest that it makes folate.

To be clear there are rare times when high-dose supplementation with folate is needed. For example, there is a condition called cerebral folate deficiency—an autoimmune disease where folate can't get from the blood into the brain, which creates a host of neurological issues including memory loss, vision loss, and hearing loss—that can be completely resolved with high doses of folinic acid, a type of folate.[9] Some other conditions where I think supplemental folate is warranted (often along with B_{12} or other nutrients) include pregnancy, macrocytic anemia, certain neurological conditions, elevated homocysteine, malabsorptive conditions, and some dietary limitations.

Otherwise, generally speaking, we don't want to get our folate through high-dose supplements.

COULD HIGH-DOSE METHYL DONOR SUPPLEMENTS OPEN THE DOOR TO CANCER?

Around 2014, I saw something in the scientific literature that stopped me dead in my tracks. In a study published in that year, researchers randomized a group of over twenty-five hundred participants aged sixty-five and older with elevated homocysteine levels (remember, elevated homocysteine levels are associated with suboptimal biochemical methylation, including DNA methylation) to either take a daily folic acid (400 mcg) and vitamin B_{12} (500 mcg) supplement or a placebo for a duration of two years.[10] Study authors were seeking to measure whether supplementing with these nutrients, which are both important methyl donors, would help prevent bone fractures in older adults. While researchers did not see a significant decrease in the number of fractures (except in those who were over eighty), they were surprised to learn that those who took the supplements experienced 51 percent more incidences of colorectal cancer than the placebo group did. Mind you, these dosages were very moderate. Which suggests that even low-doses of methyl donor supplements can tilt DNA methylation toward genetic expression that favors cancer.

This study was controversial and was challenged by other researchers analyzing the same data. Some maintained that the higher likelihood of colon cancer was the result of chance. But a 2019 follow-up that re-analyzed the data and included more recent incidences of cancer in the original participants verified an increase in the risk of all cancers in those who took the real supplements, and a significantly higher risk of developing colon cancer in particular.[11]

A 2018 review stated the issue clearly in its title: "Folate and Cancer: A Tale of Dr. Jekyll and Mr. Hyde?" It examined multiple studies and found that folic acid supplementation of 1 mg per day for six years increased risk of a recurrence of colon polyps with malignant potential by a whopping 67 percent, and ten years later, there was also a significantly increased risk of prostate cancer. Another study in this review found a 70 percent increase in risk of recurring bladder cancer in those with medium to high folic acid intake (compared to those with low folic acid intake)—while natural (whole foods, not supplements) folate consumption had no similar increase in risk. Yet another study in the review found that between 26 and 77 percent of cancer survivors take multivitamins that contain folic acid. (While these studies didn't specifically assess folic acid intake through fortified foods, it's a reasonable assumption that the study participants were also getting folic acid through consumption of these foods.) **Meanwhile, two studies included looked at intake of foods rich in folate, and they showed either protection against cancer or no effect on cancer risk.**[12]

The very thought of giving patients supplements that could nudge them toward getting cancer made me break out in a cold sweat. Could it be that those all-important tumor-suppressor genes were being overly methylated and shut down, essentially told to stop doing their job in some kind of epigenetic round of layoffs?

And then I had a patient come to me who personified these fears. A woman named Sharon, in her early fifties with a strong family history of colon cancer, had recently had a large portion of her colon removed because it seemed her genetic number had been called: she had been diagnosed with colon cancer. Prior to showing up at my practice, she had developed noncancerous polyps in her colon, and so had worked with an integrative doctor who happened to notice her homocysteine level was high and started her on a common treatment of high-dose folate supplements. While her homocysteine level initially dropped, her next colonoscopy showed that the polyps had become cancerous. While we cannot know that the folate prescribed contributed to the polyps becoming malignant, there is suggestion in the literature that her precancerous cells may indeed have been fortified with high doses of folate, and her tumor-suppressor genes could have been hypermethylated and turned off.

Because I knew I had to find a way to support Sharon's ability to methylate without the unwanted risk of nudging her genetic expression toward a recurrence of cancer, I scoured the scientific literature looking for anything to suggest that eating too much of any one food that impacts DNA methylation carries risks with it. I found none. Instead, what I saw—and continue to time and again—is the power of whole foods and the combination of the nutrients they provide to regulate genetic expression in an exquisitely balanced way.

At the same time that I began working with Sharon, I treated a patient named Paul, who was dealing with multiple health challenges. His primary complaint was burning nerve pain (called neuropathy) in his thighs and his hands. He also had chronic Lyme disease that was exacerbated by the presence of mold in his home. It was as if he had aged twenty years in the past twenty-four months.

Paul's neuropathy, and his blood work, suggested that he was critically low in nutrients that support the methylation process, especially B_{12} and folate. As was standard in functional medicine at the time, I started Paul on a regimen of supplements to get his levels of these important nutrients up. Troublingly, he did not tolerate these supplements well *at all*. We tried everything—taking the supplements as pills, as shots, as drops under the tongue. But every supplement we tried—and we tried many—only made Paul's searing nerve pain worse.

This was no good for anyone; not for Paul, who had to endure worsening pain, and not for me, who took an oath as a physician to first do no harm. It just didn't add up. How could I support Paul's ability to methylate if his body wouldn't tolerate the supplements that contained the nutrients needed for methylation to work?

Although Sharon and Paul were presenting with different issues, the root cause was the same—impaired DNA methylation was likely accelerating their age and increasing their risk of illness. We had to find a way to support their ability to methylate without the high-dose supplements that could increase risk of cancer recurrence (in Sharon's case) or that only made their current symptoms worse (as was happening with Paul).

With the help of the brilliant nutritionists in my practice, especially Romilly Hodges, CNS, IFMCP, we devised an eating plan for Sharon and Paul that would deliver ample amounts of the nutrients the body needs to optimize DNA methylation using whole foods only. This was Younger You 1.0, chock-full of foods like beets, eggs, cruciferous vegetables, dark leafy greens, and nuts and seeds; foods that we chose because they deliver plenty of DNA methylation–supportive nutrients in a whole foods matrix. It also excluded the foods that either impair DNA methylation (like charred foods) or provoke an inflammatory response (like gluten and dairy) so that Sharon and Paul would have plenty of tools to help them heal and nothing that would detract from the process. I also prescribed very moderate amounts of movement and fifteen minutes a day spent on a relaxation practice (Paul chose to prioritize time spent on his favorite hobby, playing the piano).

As for Paul, he started to feel better almost immediately. His pain subsided. His mood lifted, and he started sleeping better. From a clinical perspective, his levels of folate, red blood cells, and B_{12} rose. His homocysteine lowered. And his vitality returned—the haggard look in his eyes receded and his whole face shone with relief.

When Sharon first came to me, her homocysteine level was a whopping 90 (normal levels are between 4 and 15 micromoles/liter). Within a few months of following the plan, her level dropped dramatically to 45; after about a year it was close to normal at 19, and today it's around 14. Her bowel issues from the surgical resection are much better, which dramatically improved her quality of life. And importantly, she has remained cancer-free in the three years since I first saw her, despite her personal and family history.

The two patients were proof that we were on to something—that perhaps we shouldn't be telling the body what to do by flooding it with isolated nutrients, but that we could give the body what it needed as whole-food and lifestyle interventions and it, in its own wisdom, could find its way back to balance. Seeing that we could profoundly influence methylation with food and lifestyle was a game changer.

What I have come to see is that in all but the most specific cases, when we isolate nutrients and prescribe alone, we're stepping outside of mother nature's intended design. We're losing the benefit of synergistic interactions between the myriad components in any whole food, and in so doing we're creating the possibility of unforeseen risk.

The key takeaway here is while *supplementing* with methyl donors can be risky and ineffective, *eating* a methyl donor-rich diet is not. Not only is it possible to look to diet and lifestyle to provide pretty much everything the body needs to achieve the DNA methylation of a younger person, but also it is the only prudent choice.

OTHER EATING PLANS ASSOCIATED WITH LONGEVITY

FOOD IS POWERFUL ANTI-AGING MEDICINE: AS DR. VALTER LONGO, DIREC-tor of the Longevity Institute at the University of Southern California, puts it, "Other than genes, it is hard to think of something that can be more powerful than food in determining whether someone is going to make it to 100 or die before 50 years old." There certainly have been other nutritional approaches to longevity; here are three eating strategies in particular that are well studied, both what they are, and how they are similar to, or different from, Younger You:

Caloric Restriction. This dietary approach requires limiting food intake to only 70 percent of the recommended daily caloric intake. It has been considered the gold standard strategy for longevity, shown to work in thousands of animal studies, and benefits are strongly suspected to extend to humans—although, it's important to note, similar results in humans have not been replicated. It may also carry risks to humans, who live significantly longer than most animals. When I interviewed him on my podcast, Dr. Longo expressed suspicion that severe caloric-restricting humans were likely vulnerable to developing other issues, such as increased incidence of infection.[13]

In addition, there is research that suggests that carrying a little extra weight is associated with longevity, and extra weight is hard to come by on an eating plan that restricts calories over the long term.

An Ohio State University study that came out in 2021 analyzed data that followed over five thousand people for seventy-four years and found that those who lived the longest were an average weight in their early adulthood and gained weight slowly into old age. And the cohort with the lowest BMI had a 40 percent higher risk of all-cause mortality than those who gained weight.[14] Because these new study findings fly directly in the face of an overwhelming amount of research that suggests lower body weight is ideal for longevity, I don't recommend you change your good lifestyle habits to put on pounds. But it does give me pause, and will be something important to keep on eye on as science continues to explore it.

Another factor is that consciously choosing to eat 30 percent less every day is not exactly easy to do. Especially over the long term. Eating is one of the pleasures of life, particularly when you commune with others as you do it. Truly, I want to help people expand health span, life span, *and* quality of life. Continually being hungry and counting calories, to me, does not contribute to that aim. This is an important reason why Younger You is focused more on taking in DNA methylation–supportive nutrients and *not* on counting calories. I can promise you that both the Intensive and Everyday versions are plenty filling.

Fasting Mimicking Diet. A variation of caloric restriction that is designed to be more—forgive the pun—palatable, the "fasting mimicking diet" consists of practicing caloric restriction five days a month for three or more months, depending on your health goals. On the days you aren't mimicking a fast, you follow a higher calorie, nutrient-dense program. The term "fasting mimicking" was coined by Longo, whose research suggests much of the anti-aging benefits of caloric restriction are seen with fasting mimicking, with considerably less difficulty.

I wholeheartedly agree that intermittent fasting is beneficial for genetic expression and longevity, but I also believe in keeping things simple and doable. The Younger You Intensive and Everyday versions both include a gentle daily fast between 7 p.m. and 7 a.m. (something I discuss more on page 97), so it does incorporate intermittent fasting (sometimes called time-restricted eating)—but in a way that takes little to no planning. And this twelve hours feeding/twelve hours fasting pattern is considered to be very important by Dr. Longo.[15] If you're already a proponent of intermittent fasting and use a smaller number of hours as your eating window, as long as it's doable for you, it's probably fine, too. My only caveat is that I have experienced in my own life, and seen it in my patients and colleagues alike, that excessive restrictions and multiple guidelines can nudge some folks toward an unhealthy obsession with clean eating; a phenomenon that's gotten so much more popular that it has a new scientific name: orthorexia.

Mediterranean Diet. As I discussed in Chapter 1, this popular and well-researched approach to eating has also recently been shown to reduce biological age in a specific population.[16] It's clear that the Mediterranean diet is a good, general eating plan that one study showed *can* lead to small reductions in age over the long term. Yet, compared to the Younger You Intensive, the Mediterranean diet used in that one study offers much more modest gains in aging and takes a longer time to achieve. The two plans do have some similarities—namely, plenty of healthy veggies, some fruits, good fats, and moderate amounts of healthy animal protein—but they also have plenty of differences. For the eight weeks of the Younger You Intensive, we omit legumes (except for vegetarians and vegans—more on this on page 114), grains, and wine or any alcohol, and recommend a little liver and eggs, and we greatly turn up the volume on specific DNA methylation–supportive nutrients.

· · · · ·

THE POWER OF WHOLE FOODS

Hippocrates said, "Let food be thy medicine" around 400 BC. It's taken almost twenty-five hundred years, but we're starting to prove just how effective the nutrients contained within whole foods can be.

This is the precept my team and I used when developing the Younger You program. We wanted to build on the genius of Ames and Pauling by prescribing higher-dose nutrients that are known to optimize DNA methylation, but to minimize risk delivering them by using whole, natural foods instead of isolated supplements. (Except in those unique cases where higher doses than foods can provide are warranted, and then ideally only in the short term.) To my knowledge, ours is the first practice to develop a diet based on the Pauling and Ames principles, although scientists studying epigenetics are suggesting that the "combinatorial" approach of a whole foods diet packing in many lower-dose nutrients together is probably more effective than a single nutrient.[17]

Orthomolecular nutrition provides two key differences to the high-dose approach espoused by Pauling and Ames:

- The dosages are significantly lower, but you're "taking" these nutrients multiple times per day at each meal—just as we evolved doing.

- The nutrients are housed within the complex matrix of a whole food and work synergistically with each other, improving the absorption and actions of individual nutrients.

Whole foods, which are exactly what they sound like—foods in their original form like vegetables, fruits, nuts, seeds, and quinoa—have incredible healing abilities, not just because of their superstar nutrients, but also because of their full roster of components and the interplay that happens between them that we are only beginning to understand. Honestly, we may never fully grasp all the nuances of how the components of whole foods influence physiology, because the complexity of nature's wisdom truly is mind-boggling. In fact, there is a concept known as the "dark matter of nutrition," which reminds us that, as extraordinary as the components of whole foods that we already know about are, most of what is contained within a whole food hasn't yet been defined.

Take an apple, for example. Just one bite contains an extraordinarily complex packet of information, as opposed to a drug or a supplement, which is typically only one thing. Its primary component is carbohydrates, mostly in the form of sugar—a medium apple has 25 grams of carbs, of which 19 are naturally occurring sugar. It also has a scant amount of protein (1 gram) and 3 grams of fiber, which serve to slow the release of those sugars once in your digestive tract so that your blood glucose levels don't rise and then crash quickly. Much of the fiber comes from an apple's pectin content; pectin is a source of soluble fiber, meaning it is broken down in the digestive tract and stimulates elimination. It is also fermented by your gut bugs, a process that produces short-chain fatty acids such as butyrate that researchers have shown play a role in preventing some cancers and bowel diseases.

That's not nearly all. An apple also contains many, many phytochemicals (primarily in the skin), including quercetin, a known antihistamine that can also help lower cholesterol and protect against viruses. Quercetin is a senolytic compound, too, meaning it wards off aging. And it helps optimize genetic expression.

And that's just one phytochemical component of an apple. Others include epicatechin, cholorogenic acid, and anthocyanin. These and other biologically active compounds in apples are beneficial for most chronic diseases—from cancer, dementia, and diabetes to heart disease and lung disease—via a variety of mechanisms, including helping to process the higher sugar content in apples through improved insulin sensitivity. Most of them can also regulate genetic expression (they're what's known as DNA methylation adaptogens, a concept I'll explain more in just a moment). And of course, an apple contains ascorbic acid, also known as vitamin C, which is an essential antioxidant, as well as a very important regulator of DNA methylation that helps get rid of methyl groups where they shouldn't be.

As soon as you turn that whole apple into something else, you modify these components and hamper their benefit. Removing the skin from the apple also removes much of the fiber and the majority of the quercetin and most of its other potent phytochemicals—buh bye, short-chain fatty acids, hello, blood sugar spike. Drying the apple concentrates the sugar and evaporates most of the vitamin C. Juicing an apple also concentrates the sugar, and removes the fiber and most of the phytochemicals.

Beyond the magnificence of its components, the process of eating an apple—or any whole food—kicks off a cascade of events that can't even compare to swallowing a pill.

First, just thinking about the food triggers a chain reaction in your brain that preps your entire digestive system for the incoming work to be done. Just think about applesauce—peels on!—simmering on the stove, its scent wafting through the house. Congrats, you just started activating your digestive enzymes!

Next, seeing and smelling the food cues the release of saliva, which contains the digestive enzyme amylase, which alerts your stomach to make acid, your pancreas to make digestive enzymes, and your microbiome to ready itself to further break down and transform the food. Chewing that bite begins to liberate the nutrients and further prompts the digestive chemical cascade.

As the food passes through your digestive tract, your microbiome population will take what it needs to produce neurotransmitters, fatty acids, and vitamins. In fact, one of your gut bacteria's most important roles is to take the phytochemicals in your food and ready them to do their important work, which often includes regulating gene expression. Meanwhile, your gut lining readies itself to absorb these transformed packets of information. Right on the other side of your gut, your immune system reviews what's been ingested and determines what the immune response will be, whether it's to trigger inflammation or not. Isn't it just astounding how beautifully complex our internal interaction with food is? And just take one more moment and imagine what happens when you eat a big garden salad, with apple slices and maybe some seeds on top. The potential benefit of thousands upon thousands of nutrients from this full meal interacting with each other, your microbiome, and you, is nothing short of extraordinary.

Eating whole food ensures you get a balance of synergistic nutrients in ample, but not excessive, amounts. The beauty of mother nature's design, and how it falls in lockstep with what we need to flourish, blows me away every day. And our understanding of whole foods and how they benefit all the systems of the body is only continuing to grow.

Let's look at the three components of the Younger You formula—the two categories of whole foods that comprise the bulk of the Younger You program, as well as the lifestyle practices that have been shown to positively influence DNA methylation.

Methyl donors + DNA methylation adaptogens + lifestyle = Y2 (Younger You)

YOUNGER YOU FORMULA COMPONENT #1: METHYL DONORS

Methyl donors are the nutrients that the body uses to create methyl groups. The most important methyl donors are folate—not to be confused with folic acid, as I covered starting on page 54—and vitamin B_{12}, as they are the primary components the body uses to produce S-adenosylmethionine

(SAMe), a natural and universal compound that's used in the biochemical reactions of methylation, including DNA methylation.

Other important methyl donor supporting players include betaine and choline, followed by minerals zinc, magnesium, potassium, and sulfur; B vitamins riboflavin, niacin, and pyridoxine; the amino acids methionine, cysteine, and taurine; and the omega-3 fatty acid DHA.

You simply can't have balanced DNA methylation if you don't have plenty of methyl donors on hand. We have about 20 million DNA methylation sites in each cell of the body that we are replenishing all of the time; we need these building blocks in ample supply to keep all those sites stocked.

Not only do you want the right nutrients to support DNA methylation, but you want them in the right amounts (orthomolecular nutrition!). And the best way to ensure you hit the sweet spot of methyl donor intake is to eat plenty of whole foods that are rich in methyl donors and to not get too much by over-relying on high dose supplements, *or* by inadvertently taking in too much through fortified foods.

YOUNGER YOU FORMULA COMPONENT #2: DNA METHYLATION ADAPTOGENS

You may have heard the term *adaptogen* before — it describes a compound that promotes a healthy balance in a given biochemical pathway and is used most specifically in reference to herbs that help the body modulate its physiological response to stress (to get technical, adaptogens help regulate the central nervous system, which in turn helps balance the output of stress hormones secreted by the adrenal glands). If you guess that DNA methylation adaptogens promote healthy, balanced DNA methylation, you get a gold star.

Once we have all the ingredients for robust methylation activity floating down the river in the right amounts, we want to make sure that the genes we don't want turned on get methylated (and, thus, inhibited) and the genes we do want turned on don't get methylated (and thus, expressed). We can do this in two ways: we can actively remove methyl groups from genes and we can passively inhibit methyl groups from being added to genes. This is where the DNA methylation adaptogens come in. DNA *methylation adaptogens*, as their name suggests, help DNA methylation find its sweet spot of not too much, not too little, and in just the right places.

In financial terms, DNA methylation adaptogens rebalance your portfolio. In fact, we saw a thoughtful redistribution of methyl groups in our study: methyl groups that were powering down a beneficial, youthful gene were removed, while methyl groups that were needed to shut off pro-aging genes were added. I believe it was the ample amounts of DNA methylation adaptogens that are part of the Younger You Intensive that helped this rebalancing happen.

DNA methylation adaptogens include foods that are widely hailed for their health-giving properties in traditional cultures around the globe—a fact that I believe has a lot to do with the epigenetic regulatory role—including turmeric, green tea, cruciferous vegetables, and soy.

DNA methylation adaptogens fall into two basic categories: flavonoids (which are a category of the phytochemicals known as *polyphenols*) and nutrients. Members of the flavonoid team are curcumin (found in turmeric); EGCG (green tea); rosmarinic acid (rosemary); quercetin, luteolin, lycopene, sulphoraphane (cruciferous vegetables); and genistein (soy). And for the nutrients: vitamins A, C, and D_3, and alpha ketoglutarate.

The flavonoid adaptogens appear to primarily inhibit hypermethylation of DNA, while the nutrients help actively remove unfavorable methylation marks.

Whichever type they are, together DNA methylation adaptogens work to "clean up" DNA methylation in three primary ways:
- Keeping certain "good" genes turned on by preventing new methyl groups from being laid down
- Maintaining appropriate gene expression by preventing new methyl groups from being laid down
- Adding methyl groups to where genes are expressed inappropriately so that they stay turned off

Newer research suggests that DNA methylation adaptogens might elicit a beneficial epigenetic alteration of tumor-suppressor genes, anti-inflammatory genes, and—as our study suggests—methylation sites on genes that are associated with aging. What makes them so powerful is that they appear to be selective in their influence. Whether that selectivity comes from low doses of many different flavonoids working together or some other mechanism, they seem to use the body's wisdom to remove methyl groups where they are causing harm and leave them where they are doing good. For example, luteolin—an adaptogenic flavonoid found in Mexican oregano, thyme, and celery—has been shown in a cell study to be as effective as a pharmaceutical demethylating drug.[18] That effectiveness becomes even more exciting when you consider that luteolin comes with a near-total absence of risk of side effects, as opposed to demethylating drugs, which are nonspecific in the genes that they target—which means they are known to have far-reaching unintended consequences.

SELECT METHYL DONOR AND
DNA METHYLATION ADAPTOGENIC FOODS

While there are many, many foods that contain these two types of DNA methylation–supportive nutrients—you'll find a complete list in the Nutrient Reference at the back of this book (page 407)—here are the superstars, listed in order of importance.

	NUTRIENTS	FOODS THAT CONTAIN THESE NUTRIENTS
Methyl donors	Folate (B$_9$)	Liver, chickpeas, beans (although legumes can be problematic for some, so we omit them from the Younger You Intensive unless you are vegetarian or vegan—more on page 114)
	Vitamin B$_{12}$ (cobalamin)	Clams, liver, fish
	Betaine	Beets, spinach, quinoa
	Choline	Egg yolks, liver, lentils

DNA methylation adaptogens	EGCG	Green tea
	Curcumin	Turmeric
	Romarinic acid	Rosemary
	Quercetin	Apples, onions, berries, broccoli, and capers

YOUNGER YOU FORMULA COMPONENT #3: LIFESTYLE PRACTICES

Although I do believe in letting food be thy medicine, you are a whole, multifaceted person, and, thus, the things you do when you *aren't* eating also have enormous influence on your health.

Since I first started delving into the scientific literature to uncover foods that optimize DNA methylation, I have been pleasantly surprised to find so many lifestyle practices that we already knew to be supportive of health—such as exercise, sleep, and meditation—are also known to impact genetic expression. Also, steering yourself away from toxins, both in your food and your environment, is a vital piece of the plan, so that you aren't regularly ingesting substances that can impair "normative" DNA methylation.

Seeing this research showed me that we needed to be prescribing things like exercise, relaxation, and sleep in much the same way that we prescribed an eating plan. When you combine these lifestyle pieces into a doable, regular routine, their positive benefits are increased.

DNA methylation supportive lifestyle habits include:

Sleep

OK, all you insomniacs out there. Let me attempt to *not* stress you out by haranguing you with how important sleep is to health; especially epigenetic health. (Believe me, as someone who struggles with sleep and whose child is still a toddler, sleep has not been my self-care strong suit.) Just keep in mind as you read that you don't need to get epic amounts of slumber. In fact, in our study, we advised our participants to get a very moderate seven hours of sleep a night, which is generally considered to be healthy.[19] They didn't have to completely overhaul their lives or their sleep habits in order to reap the benefits of healthy sleep and reduce their bio age. So if you've given up on ever being able to get eight hours regularly, let me just start by lowering the bar a bit.

That being said (here it comes), sleep *is* a vital piece of your health. There is an emerging body of science in humans and animals looking at changes to the epigenome that poor sleep triggers in everyone from infants to adults, and it's not pretty. For instance, sleep and accelerated aging: one fairly large study of over two thousand women showed insomnia (chronic sleep deprivation) significantly accelerated DNA methylation age.[20] A similar, smaller study showed the same thing again: a consistent sleep record of short duration and poor quality accelerated aging.[21] Changes noted include accelerated cognitive deficits, metabolic changes (think weight gain and diabetes), and changes to circadian rhythm genes.

What's interesting—and concerning—is that changes can be noted quickly. As in, after one poor night's sleep.[22] I know—painful! Rather than fixating on how a bad night's sleep can wreak epigenetic havoc (especially while you're lying there, awake), remember that what you do consistently matters more than what you do once in a while. Meaning, it's chronic deprivation that we're concerned about. I'll cover many ways to optimize sleep so that you get more of it in Chapter 7.

Exercise

You may think of exercise as a way to burn calories, build muscle, improve cardiovascular health, or clear your head. Exercise is all of these things, yet it is so much more. Because exercise is such great nourishment to your DNA methylation, it is also an anti-aging elixir.

Exercise is well known to be broadly beneficial for almost every aspect of health—regulating insulin sensitivity, decreasing inflammation, and lowering homocysteine—and has been shown to extend mean life span in animal models. Exercise triggers what's known as *hormesis*, or a biological process where a beneficial effect is triggered by a limited exposure to something harmful or challenging to the body. You probably know that lifting weights causes microtears in the muscle that the body then knits back together to make it bigger and stronger. A similar process happens on the cellular level, too: exercise causes increased free radicals in the mitochondria, which are the energy factories within your cells that you may recall learning about in high school biology class. Free radicals are destructive molecules, which might seem like a bad thing until you consider that those free radicals induce a hormetic response where your antioxidant system is turned on to put out the fires. As a result, every time you exercise, your mitochondria are drenched in the potent antioxidant elixirs that only our body can make. It's important to note that you want *just enough* exposure to free radicals, as too many can be definitively damaging. Like most things, exercise has a U curve of benefit, and exercise that is too extreme breaks the body down in greater amounts than it can recover from. A 2018 study found that Polish elite athletes, especially those involved in power sports (such as competitive weight lifting), were significantly biologically older than healthy controls of similar mean ages.[23] This suggests a sweet spot for exercise, which may be more or less than what you are currently doing.

When it comes to DNA methylation, research suggests that reasonable exercise is nearly always beneficial, with changes that can be seen almost immediately. Multiple studies have shown exercise reduces methylation of tumor-suppressor genes. This mechanism is probably a big reason why exercise is an important preventative measure for cancer, as well as an invaluable intervention if diagnosed, as was shown in a 2012 study looking at breast cancer.[24]

Just as knocking yourself out at the gym to the point that you can barely walk the next day is counter-productive, so is not moving enough. Being sedentary is as woven into the typical American experience as a diet of highly refined foods, and it is another piece of our collective way of living that we have to consciously move away from. Luckily, you don't need to attend a CrossFit class, buy a Peloton bike, or hire a trainer to ensure you're moving enough. Even cleaning house showed anti-aging DNA methylation changes (not that I recommend this one . . .)![25] Generally speaking, moderate and consistent movement is the name of the game when it comes to helping your genes be the best they can be.

In our study we had people exercise at least thirty minutes a day, five days a week, at only 60 to 80 percent of perceived exertion, doing some activity that they truly enjoyed. It was a potent part of the mix that led to their significant reduction in bio age.

Stress-Reducing Practices

Stress plays an enormous role in DNA methylation. In fact, almost 25 percent of the methylation sites in the specific epigenetic clock that we used in our study to determine biological age are related to stress. Research has shown that cumulative life stress,[26] PTSD,[27] and even how much stress your mother was exposed to when she was pregnant with you (recall the Project Ice Storm study I mentioned in Chapter 2) can all negatively impact your epigenome. And you can hand this pattern down to your offspring.

I know this probably sounds like a big fat bummer—after all, the world is a stressful place and much of the stress you've been exposed to you had no control over whatsoever (you may not even have been alive). Yet there *is* good news.

We may not be able to control the things that cause us stress, but we do have quite a lot of influence over our own response to stress. There are many practices that induce the relaxation response.

Research has found alterations in DNA methylation in long-term practitioners of tai chi[28] or meditation,[29] and even in "regular" people who started a yoga class and practiced only one hour a week.[30] A 2019 study by Italian researchers demonstrated that sixty days of relaxation practice—such as meditation or listening to peaceful music—for twenty minutes twice per day significantly reduced the biological age in their group of healthy participants (though not in their "patient" group).[31] In our study, we had the participants complete ten to twenty minutes of breath-focused meditation twice a day. (I'll share more of the specifics about that practice in Chapter 7.)

The more stress you have encountered, the more vital it is that you adopt relaxation-inducing practices. I get the paradox in that—being stressed out can make it seem mighty hard to pursue anything that isn't absolutely vital to survival. I'm arguing that doing things that reduce your stress, and doing them consistently for the long term, *are* vital to your survival. They are a huge part of how you heal from the stressors you've endured.

We absolutely have the ability to *reverse* stress-induced epigenetic programming. These favorable changes can be detected even after a single contemplative practice.[32] Yet, like anything else, the longer you practice, the longer lasting and more profound your results.

Even as a functional medicine practitioner, who is trained to see a patient as a complex being, I find it awe-inspiring to see just how many things can alter our DNA methylation—it shows just how many levers we have to improve our own health. While that could sound overwhelming, that you have more to take care of in order to be healthy, think of it this way: if any one of these levers is a little off, you have a lot of other tools you can use to shore yourself up. If your diet goes off the rails, for example, you can ramp up your relaxation practices and your sleep to keep yourself in a good place until you can get back on track. Or if you go through a spate of poor sleep, you can make sure you're eating plenty of methyl donors and DNA methylation adaptogens and keep your epigenetics in a good place.

THE RESULT: A YOUNGER YOU!

The combination of these three components appears to result in beautifully balanced DNA methylation, resilience to disease, and a lower biological age.

Following this simple formula is like buying an umbrella insurance policy for your health and resilience—whatever current health challenge you're facing, this will help. And whatever is lurking beneath the surface, waiting until a vulnerable moment to appear, this will help ward it off. Because aging is the root cause of the vast majority of diseases, by shaving years off your biological clock, you're not just getting younger, you're warding off diseases and steering your ship away from the sixteen-plus years that the average American spends ill and unhappy at the end of their life.

As with most things, the best time to get started is two years ago; the second best time is today. Before I dive into the specifics of the Younger You Intensive plan, let's take a look at how you can assess how old you are, biologically, *now*, before you start making any changes. This will help you gauge your progress and give you incentive to get started and keep going.

PART 2

THE PLAN TO REVERSE BIO AGE

HOW OLD ARE YOU, REALLY?
TESTS TO ASSESS YOUR BIO AGE

THERE HAVE BEEN MANY ATTEMPTS OVER THE YEARS TO DEFINE BI-ological age, which, as I've covered, is not how old you are in years, but how old your physiology suggests you are.

Over the past decade or so, telomeres (pronounced TEE-loh-meers) have gotten a lot of attention from the scientific and medical community as indicators of biological age, particularly thanks to the work of Elizabeth Blackburn, PhD, professor of biology and physiology at the University of California, San Francisco, who won the Nobel prize for her work on telomeres, and Elissa Epel, PhD, professor of psychiatry at the University of California, San Francisco, authors of *The Telomere Effect*. These sequences of genetic material are found at the end of the strands of our chromosomes—they protect DNA by keeping it from fraying and from fusing with other strands. They are often compared to the plastic tips that seal the end of shoelaces.

Telomeres are made out of pairs of the same nucleic acid bases that DNA is comprised of: guanine (G), adenine (A), thymine (T), and cytosine (C). Every time a cell divides, it replicates its DNA, and with each replication, the telomere loses some of its base pairs and gets a little shorter; so as we age, the length of our telomeres goes down. And the shorter our telomeres, the greater our risk of diseases.

Telomere length seems like a great way to assess how old you truly are, and it certainly is an important consideration when taking stock of how healthy your whole being is. But the length of your telomeres only has a .4 correlation with your actual age (with 1 being perfect correlation). That means they have a 60 percent chance of being wrong. Not great odds.

In 2013, Steve Horvath, a professor of human genetics and biostatistics at UCLA, published findings that he could determine biological age by analyzing the DNA methylation on hundreds of sites on the genome with only a cheek swab or a drop of blood. Extraordinarily, the results of that test had a correlation of .96 with chronological age. Even more impressive: much of that missing .04 is not a mistake—it's the difference between your calendar age and your biological age. He essentially discovered an epigenetic clock—one that has become the gold standard of determining true physiological age, which he titled the DNAmAge clock, and which is now colloquially known as the Horvath clock.

Horvath's DNAmAge epigenetic clock works by looking at methylation at hundreds of specific sites on DNA that change with age. Some get more and more methylated as you live longer, and some are the opposite—they get less and less so the older you get. By looking at the methylation status of these specific sites on the genome, the clock can calculate your bio age by assessing how old the methylation patterns on your genes are. The DNAmAge clock is what has made possible studies—like ours—that measure the impact of different strategies on bio age.

Since we began our study, many second-generation epigenetic clocks have been released, including the GrimAge clock and the PhenoAge clock, which correlate with disease and mortality risk, not chronological age. In fact, research into the world of epigenetic clocks has galloped forward since we began our study, and it's all quite exciting. There are clocks that can measure the age of skeletal muscle, the brain's cortex, and the immune system.[1] We will be using some of these second-generation clocks in our next study, which will be larger and include men and women, although we will also include the Horvath clock again, since it correlates most closely with true chronological age. We suspect that these second-generation clocks may be even more responsive to our program because they track with health and disease rather than the Horvath clock, which tracks with chronological age.

As I began writing this book, assessing bio age with the DNAmAge (or any other) epigenetic clock had been accessible only to researchers and was very expensive. Only a year later, this technology is becoming available and more affordable for both clinicians and individuals, empowering you to objectively assess the epigenetic effects of any diet or lifestyle interventions. (See the Resources, page 429, for more information on how to gain access to bio age testing.)

So that you can measure the changes you make to your bio age over the next eight weeks (and beyond), I am including three different ways to assess and keep tabs on your bio age. While none of them can match the accuracy of a bio age test that analyzes your individual DNA methylation patterns, they can give you a detailed look at your current state of health.

The first is the Bio Age Self-Assessment (BASA), which gauges how your daily habits and basic biometrics are collectively influencing your rate of aging. The second is the Medical Symptoms Questionnaire (MSQ), which is a standard tool in functional medicine that every patient at our clinic fills out regularly to give us a window into how our interventions are impacting overall health and quality of life. And the third is guidance on which basic blood tests to ask your doctor for (if you haven't had these done in the last three to six months), as well as how to interpret those results. While none of these tools replaces DNAmAge testing, taken together, they are a quick, low-cost way to objectively evaluate both the steps you're taking to improve your health (with the BASA) and the results of those steps (with the MSQ and the lab results).

I suggest taking both of these self-assessments—and, if you can, getting your bloodwork done—now, before you start implementing any Younger You program changes (be they from the Intensive or the Everyday version), so that you can capture your "before" and give yourself a baseline to help gauge your progress and incentivize you to stay on track.

Ideally, you'd do the BASA again in four weeks (halfway through the Younger You Intensive) and then again at the end of the eight weeks; and you'd do the MSQ every week during the Intensive so that you can evaluate the fruits of your efforts as you go, which should give you great motivation to keep going. I know that lab tests typically require a doctor's order to get, but if you are able, I suggest getting your blood tested again at the end of eight weeks.

You can also take the BASA and MSQ, and input the values of your blood work, in our Younger You app, the digital version of the Younger You program, which will keep track of your scores and, through our program nutritionists, give you personalized recommendations based on your results. And if you are interested in learning your bio age via a DNAmAge test, and learn more about the methylation patterns on some of the genes I mention throughout the book, including the nutrient-responsive tumor-suppressor genes, you can do that through our Younger You digital program as well. See Resources, page 426, for more information.

BIOLOGICAL AGE SELF-ASSESSMENT (BASA)

This subjective biological age self-assessment (BASA) questionnaire is a useful guide to show you what you're already doing right and where you can improve. To find your BASA score, simply answer the questions below and follow the directions at the end of the questionnaire to calculate your score.

How often to do this assessment:

- Before you get started
- Halfway through the Intensive (four weeks in)
- Once you've completed the Intensive (after eight weeks)
- Every two months thereafter

SECTION 1: Diet and Nutrition

1. How many servings (1 serving = 3 ounces) of vegetables do you consume on an average day (e.g., cruciferous, dark leafy, or colorful vegetables)?

    None (+3)
    1–3 (+2)
    4–6 (-2)
    7+ (-3)

2. How often do you consume at least one of the following nutrient-dense foods: nuts and seeds, fatty fish, eggs, liver?

    Once per month or less (+2)
    Once a week (0)
    2–3 times a week (-2)
    Almost every day (-3)

3. How often do you eat fermented foods or prebiotic-rich foods (e.g., lacto-fermented vegetables and legumes, kombucha, raw garlic, onion, leek, dandelion greens, etc.)?
>   Once per month or less (+2)
>   Once a week (+1)
>   2–3 times a week (0)
>   Almost every day (-2)

4. How often do you consume at least one of the following herbs, teas, and spices: rosemary, turmeric, garlic, green tea, oolong tea, curcumin supplement, EGCG supplement?
>   Once per month or less (+2)
>   2–3 times a week (0)
>   Daily (-1)

5. How many glasses of water do you consume on a daily basis?
>   0 (+2)
>   1–3 (+1)
>   4+ (-1)

6. On a typical day, what is the longest window of time you go without eating a meal?
>   9 hours or less (+1)
>   10–12 hours (0)
>   12+ hours (-1)

7. How often do you eat mindfully (e.g., away from distractions such as your phone or TV, chewing slowly, paying attention to flavors and textures of food, taking a break to breathe and check fullness)?
>   Never (+2)
>   Rarely (+1)
>   Sometimes (0)
>   Often (-1)

8. How many 4-ounce glasses of wine or alcoholic beverages do you consume in an average week?
>   More than 21 drinks per week (+2)
>   14–21 drinks per week (+1)
>   5–14 drinks per week (0)
>   Less than 5 drinks per week (-1)

9. How frequently do you eat deep-fried, broiled, or charred foods?
>   Almost every day (+2)
>   2–3 times a week (+1)
>   Once a week (0)
>   Once per month or less (-1)

10. How often do you consume refined flour or refined sugar (e.g., fast food, soda, packaged snacks, baked goods)?

> Almost every day (+2)
> 2–3 times a week (+1)
> Once a week (0)
> Once per month or less (-1)

SECTION 2: Lifestyle

1. How often do you engage in an activity you would consider to be "play" (e.g., playing tennis with a friend, playing a board game with your children or grandchildren, etc.)?

> Never (+2)
> Once per month (0)
> 1–2 times per week (-1)
> 3+ times per week (-2)

2. How often do you engage in moderate or high-intensity cardiovascular exercise (that gets your heart rate up, causes you to break a sweat, and have some difficulty in talking)?

> Never (+2)
> Once per month (0)
> 1–2 times per week (-2)
> 3+ times per week (-3)

3. How often do you do exercise that makes your muscles work as hard as they can (e.g., pushups, situps, lifting weights, using bands)?

> Once per month or less (+1)
> 1–2 times per week (-1)
> 3+ times per week (-2)

4. How many hours do you spend sitting every day?

> 8 hours or more (+2)
> 5–8 hours (+1)
> Less than 5 hours (-1)

5. How many hours do you sleep on an average night?

> 0–4 hours (+2)
> 5–6 hours (+1)
> 7–9 hours (-2)
> 10+ hours (+1)

6. How do you rate your quality of sleep (do you wake up feeling refreshed and well rested)?
> Poor (+2)
> Fair (+1)
> Good (-1)

7. How would you describe your overall level of toxin exposure (e.g., regular exposure to construction materials, gasoline, eating or heating food stored in plastic, cleaning chemicals, mercury dental fillings, lead paint)?
> Very high (+3)
> High (+2)
> Moderate (+1)
> Low (0)

8. Do you smoke cigarettes or live with somebody who does?
> 1 pack per day or more (+3)
> Half a pack per day (+2)
> 1–5 cigarettes per day (+1)
> None (0)

9. Were you ever a smoker? If yes, how long ago did you quit?
> Less than 1 year ago (+3)
> 1–5 years ago (+2)
> 6–10 years ago (+1)
> More than 10 years ago (0)

10. How much time do you spend in nature (hikes, hanging out in the yard, or visiting a city park all qualify)?
> Almost never (+2)
> 1–3 times per month (0)
> 1–3 times per week (-1)
> Daily (-2)

SECTION 3: Mental Wellness

1. How often do you experience high levels of stress?
> Daily (+2)
> Weekly (+1)
> Monthly (-1)
> Almost never (-2)

2. How do you most commonly cope with high stress levels?
> Meditation, breathing exercises, journaling, or talking it out (-2)
> Physical activity (-1)

Eating comfort food (+1)
Smoking or drinking (+2)
Tranquilizers or antidepressants (+3)

3. How would you rate your happiness?
Mostly unhappy (+2)
Sometimes unhappy (+1)
Generally happy (-1)
Mostly happy (-2)

4. How many strong and reliable relationships with others would you say you have?
None (+2)
Few (+1)
Fair amount (-1)
A lot (-2)

5. Is your job fulfilling?
Not at all (+2)
Somewhat enjoy it (+1)
Mostly enjoy it (-1)
Love it (-2)

6. How involved are you in the community at large?
Very actively involved (-2)
Moderately involved (-1)
Not so involved (+1)
Not at all (+2)

7. How often do you engage in creative activities?
Weekly (-1)
Daily (-2)

8. Are you currently learning new skills that stretch your brain? (e.g., learning a new language, taking up a new musical instrument, studying a new field)
Yes (-3)
No (0)

9. Do you feel like you have a sense of purpose in life?
Always (-2)
Sometimes (-1)
Rarely (+1)
Almost never (+2)

10. Do you engage in prayer, meditation, or breathing exercises?
> Daily (-2)
> Weekly (-1)
> Not so much (0)

SECTION 4: Anthropometrics

1. What is your waistline?
> MEN:
> Greater than 40 (+2)
> 37–39 (+1)
> 32–36 (0)
> Less than 32 (-1)
> WOMEN:
> Greater than 35 (+2)
> 33–34 (+1)
> 28–32 (0)
> Less than 28 (-1)

2. What is your BMI?

(Use the calculator at https://www.nhlbi.nih.gove/health/educational/lose_wt/BMI/bmicalc.htm; if your waistline doesn't add to your bio age, and you have a lot of muscle, your BMI will be falsely high, as muscle is heavy—if that's you, choose the next lowest answer.)
> 35+ (+3)
> 31–34 (+2)
> 20–30 (0)
> Less than 20 (+1)

3. Your blood pressure is two numbers. What is the **lower** number (diastolic)?
> 90+ (+2)
> 80–90 (+1)
> 60–79 (-1)

Calculating Your Results

To determine your subjective biological age

- Total up the numbers, positive and negative.
- Divide by ten (just add a decimal point; for example, if your total is -12, your score is -1.2).

- Subtract this number from (or add it to) your chronological age to find your bio age; compare it to your chronological age for a glimpse of how well you're doing now, and use it as a baseline to assess how your efforts are paying off in bio age reversal (or not).

MEDICAL SYMPTOMS QUESTIONNAIRE (MSQ)

Virtually every functional medicine practice the world over uses this questionnaire. We find it essential in tracking a patient's response to treatments. We used the MSQ in our study, and it will likewise be useful for you in gauging how you are responding to the Younger You program.

If you have a current diagnosis, this review of symptoms helps you and potentially your health-care provider see which of your systems are performing well, and which might be struggling. It will also help you see how changing your diet and lifestyle affects the number and intensity of symptoms.

Rate each of the following symptoms based on your experience in the past seven days, assigning them a point value based on the following scale. Focus less on your total score and more on how that number changes over the next eight weeks.

As you go, add up your total for each section in the space provided. When you're done, add up all the section scores for your total score.

How often to do this assessment:

- Before you embark on either Younger You program
- While you're on the Younger You program, once a week
- Once a month at a minimum thereafter

Point scale:

0 Never or almost never have the symptom
1 Occasionally have it, effect is not severe
2 Occasionally have it, effect is severe
3 Frequently have it, effect is not severe
4 Frequently have it, effect is severe

Digestive Tract

_____Nausea, vomiting

_____Diarrhea

_____Constipation

_____Bloated feeling

_____Belching, passing gas

_____Heartburn

_____Intestinal/stomach pain

Total _____

Ears

_____Itchy ears

_____Earaches, ear infections

_____Drainage from ear

_____Ringing in ears, hearing loss

Total _____

Emotions

_____Mood swings

_____Anxiety, fear, nervousness

_____Anger, irritability, aggressiveness

_____Depression

Total _____

Energy/Activity

_____Fatigue, sluggishness

_____Apathy, lethargy

_____Hyperactivity

_____Restlessness

Total _____

Eyes

_____Watery or itchy eyes

_____Swollen, reddened, or sticky eyelids

_____Bags or dark circles under eyes

_____Blurred or tunnel vision

(does not include near- or far-sightedness)

Total _____

Head

_____Headaches

_____Faintness

_____Dizziness
_____Insomnia

Total _____

Heart

_____Irregular or skipped heartbeat
_____Rapid or pounding heartbeat
_____Chest pain

Total _____

Joints/Muscle

_____Pain or aches in joints
_____Arthritis
_____Stiffness or limitation of movement
_____Pains or aches in muscles
_____Feeling of weakness or tiredness

Total _____

Lungs

_____Chest congestion
_____Asthma, bronchitis
_____Shortness of breath
_____Difficulty breathing

Total _____

Mind

_____Poor memory
_____Confusion, poor comprehension
_____Poor concentration
_____Poor physical coordination
_____Difficulty in making decisions
_____Stuttering or stammering
_____Slurred speech
_____Learning disabilities

Total _____

Mouth/throat

_____Chronic coughing
_____Gagging, frequent need to clear throat
_____Sore throat, hoarseness, loss of voice
_____Swollen or discolored tongue, gums, lips
_____Canker sores

Total _____

Nose

_____Stuffy nose
_____Sinus problems
_____Hay fever
_____Sneezing attacks
_____Excessive mucus formation

Total _____

Skin

_____Acne
_____Hives, rashes, dry skin
_____Hair loss
_____Flushing, hot flashes
_____Excessive sweating

Total _____

Weight

_____Binge eating/drinking
_____Craving certain foods
_____Excessive weight
_____Compulsive eating
_____Water retention
_____Underweight

Total _____

Other

_____Frequently ill
_____Frequent or urgent urination
_____Genital itch or discharge

Total _____

Grand total _____

Interpreting Your Results

Less than 10: Aging at an optimal rate: Although you're doing well, you still stand to benefit from the Younger You Intensive — our study participants were very healthy to begin with, and they still reversed their bio age by an average of over three years!

10–50: Aging at a typical rate: In my clinical opinion, any score over 10 is reason to pay attention (seriously, do you want to be aging at a "typical" rate in the United States, where so many of us are destined for the chronic diseases of aging?). Your scores should drop quickly on the Younger You Intensive.

50–100: Aging at a moderately accelerated rate: In our practice, typically, people respond positively, and quickly, to the Younger You Intensive—even those with a condition or disease—and we can tell because their MSQ scores come down. You can expect to see your numbers get better over the next eight weeks of the program, regardless of whether you have a diagnosed condition or not.

100+: Aging at a significantly accelerated rate: As with the previous category, you can expect to see your total come down quickly as you embark upon—and stay on—the Younger You Intensive.

FOR EVERYONE, NO matter your total score, notice if your points are clustered in one category or another. These may be explained by something short-term. If, for example, it's pollen season and your sniffles and sneezes are severe, that's why your Head and Nose scores might be high; it might also explain why your sleep is poor. Your scores should drop fairly quickly as the season changes. And if your condition is acute, like a head cold or a stomach bug, you will likely see your scores spike and then lower quickly. But if your symptom scores linger or even start to creep up, you want to monitor the situation.

If, during the eight weeks, you don't see a downward trend, the question is why: are there any foods you might be consuming that aren't on the diet—whether knowingly (continuing to drink beer, for example) or unknowingly (eating out at a restaurant and inadvertently ordering something with hidden dairy or gluten)? If you don't see a favorable downward trajectory and you're following the plan, or you're having trouble complying with any part of the plan, reach out to your care provider or to a practitioner whom you find through the avenues we list in the Resource section on page 426.

ASSESS YOUR BLOOD WORK RESULTS FOR CLUES
TO YOUR BIOLOGICAL AGE

Scientists and doctors are always looking for standard, affordable blood chemistries that will give us clues to your aging journey. And the fact is, there are quite a few tests that can provide important insights. While clinical lab tests such as these are not as rigorous as the DNAmAge test, they are still important and useful to assess both where your health is now and to gauge the effectiveness of any changes you make to your diet and lifestyle in the coming weeks.

These are some of the routine blood tests I order for my patients that are generally part of your annual physical and, therefore, you should have access to these results in your patient records. With the exception of DHEA-S, these labs are common and cheap, and their results offer a reasonable snapshot of how the body is performing at a physiological level in a given time period.

I included DHEA-S, which stands for dihydroepiandrosterone sulfate and is a precursor to testosterone, because in one interesting study it was a very strong predictor of bio aging in both men and women—the lower the DHEA-S, the higher the bio age.[2] I did not include homocysteine on this list because, although it's a key player in the methylation cycle and does tend to rise with chronological age, it's not predictive of bio age.

While I'm including standard and optimal ranges, you should also always check with your medical practitioner for interpretation, particularly if one or more of your values falls outside these ranges. (You can also enter your blood chemistry lab data into the Younger You digital program metabolic age calculator to receive a bio age score based on blood chemistry, chronological age, and sex. See the Resources section for more information.)

How often to get your blood tested:
- Before starting either Younger You plan
- Again after eight weeks of following the plan
- Twice a year after that

	STANDARD REFERENCE	OPTIMAL RANGE
Glucose**	70–100 mg/dL	70–84 mg/dL
Albumin**	3.4–5.4 g/dL	4–5.4 g/dL
Creatinine**	0.6–1.3 mg/dL	0.7–1.1 mg/dL
Potassium**	3.7–5.2 mEq/L	4.0–5.0 mEq/L
ALT**	4–36 U/L	10–30 U/L
AST**	8–33 U/L	10–25 U/L
Lymphocytes	20–40%	25–40%
WBC	4.3–15.3 umol/L	5–8 umol/L
HS-CRP**	0–3 mg/L	<= 1.0 mg/L
HbA1c	4.5–5.7%	<= 5.0%
Cholesterol*	100–199 mg/dL	180–200 mg/dL
LDL*	0–99 mg/dL	Under 100 mg/dL
HDL*	40–59 mg/dL	Over 55 mg/dL
Triglycerides**	0–149 mg/dL	Under 100 mg/dL
DHEA-S	Men: 25–510 ug/dL Women: 15–320 ug/dL	Men: 350 ug/dL–500 ug/dL Women: 275 ug/dL–400 ug/dL

** Fasting test

* Clinicians practicing functional medicine may say that your LDL, HDL, and/or cholesterol are fine at higher levels when other lipid lab values are in check.

Now that you have a clear picture of where you're starting from, it's time to implement the methyl donor + DNA methylation adaptogen + lifestyle practices = Y2 formula. This is where you can start making positive changes to your DNA methylation immediately—and start building long-term health.

5

THE YOUNGER YOU
INTENSIVE EATING PLAN

S USAN EXPERIENCED SOMETHING SO MANY MOMS FACE—SHE HAD
felt pretty healthy until she had her first child. Then the rigors of working motherhood had led her to skimp on sleep, skip exercise, use wine
to take the edge off her stress, and rely on carb-heavy foods like bagels,
sandwiches, and sweets to keep her energy up during the long days of balancing career and parenting. Now that her children were young adults and
out of the house, Susan had the bandwidth to focus on her own health,
which was clearly suffering. At fifty-seven and postmenopausal, Susan had
been experiencing pervasive fatigue, continual hunger, brain fog, blurred
vision, hair loss, constipation, and weight that had accumulated around
her middle. Investigating those symptoms had recently resulted in her
being diagnosed with LADA (latent autoimmune diabetes in adults), and
Hashimoto's thyroiditis.

When I first saw Susan, her fasting blood glucose was very high
(335 mg/dL, when ideally it should be below 90), with a hemoglobin
A1C of 12.1 (I like to see this number around 5 or lower). I took aim
at her blood sugar and prescribed her a low-carb, anti-inflammatory diet.
After two months, her blood sugar had dropped to 108, which was great.
However, her homocysteine was 14.0, which was not great—it suggested

she was having issues with all methylation, including DNA methylation. That's when I refined her prescription to be the full Younger You Intensive.

Our nutritionist helped Susan prioritize the many DNA methylation superstar foods; she also worked closely with Susan to help her develop a plan to stay on the program even on her frequent business trips to Asia. For travel, that guidance included tips for navigating restaurant food and a list of packable foods to take with her. We also worked a little bit on sleep hygiene to minimize jet lag—prescribing melatonin and a little extra magnesium glycinate. Guidance for minimizing toxin exposure and developing regular exercise habits and a relaxation practice rounded out Susan's diet and lifestyle plan.

After four months on the plan, her labs had improved remarkably: her fasting blood glucose was down to 82 and her homocysteine lowered to 7.1. Best of all, Susan had never felt better. Her sharp thinking returned. And, not for nothing, she looked great, too. Her eyes shone, the color in her cheeks returned, her hair started to grow in thicker, and her relief at knowing exactly what to do to address her health challenges was palpable. Susan's renewed energy also gave her the motivation to stick with the program over the long term. Seeing this transformation, from scared and overwhelmed to vital and empowered, never fails to give me goose bumps.

This is where your transformation begins, too.

Let's just pause for a moment, because this, right here, is the oldest your bio age—relative to your chronological age—is going to be. Following this eating and lifestyle plan is your ticket to a younger you. No matter what you're facing in your life or in your health, the Younger You Intensive will help you bring your most resilient self to the challenge.

In this chapter, I'm outlining the exact program that enabled our study participants to achieve the incredible result of shaving three-plus years off their biological clocks as compared to the study controls. Just a reminder that our study and the Younger You Intensive is an eight-week program. This is because, while epigenetic changes can occur after just one meal, in order for them to be lasting, you've got to stick with a DNA methylation–supportive plan for at least eight weeks. In fact, we measured our study participants' biological age at four weeks, and while things looked to be headed in the right direction, there weren't yet significant changes. You've got to stick with it.

It's also important to remember that the lifestyle components of the Younger You Intensive are also vital to its success; they all have powerful, documented anti-aging benefit, and we believe that our study participants achieved the age turnaround that they did because these practices were included in the program. But since diet is probably the single most important, make-or-break strategy for boosting and balancing DNA methylation, we're going to start with the eating plan first.

YOUNGER YOU INTENSIVE AT A GLANCE

- o This eating plan is rich in methyl donors and DNA methylation adaptogens.
- o The mainstay of the diet is vegetables—dark leafy greens, cruciferous vegetables, and antioxidant-rich colorful veggies (and some fruits); as a result the diet is high fiber and low glycemic.
- o The bulk of the calories come from healthy fats, in the form of nuts, seeds, and high-quality oils.
- o There are moderate amounts of high-quality, organic animal protein, which provide important methylation-supportive nutrients; vegetarians and vegans can readily adapt the plan to their needs.
- o The plan is somewhat lower carb, and contains no grains— *especially* no grains fortified with folic acid (basically any processed grain product—including wheat and rice flours)—no beans or legumes, no added sugars, and no dairy.

* * * * *

THE PILLARS OF OUR EPIGENETIC EATING PLAN

The Younger You Intensive diet is built on the foundations of what we know to be important elements of a healthy diet, including:

Low Sugar and Low Glycemic

High blood sugar is a fundamental imbalance that, like Mrs. O'Leary's cow, starts a fire that can burn down the entire town. Sugar and simple carbs in excess amounts are uniformly inflammatory and thus toxic to your body. In fact *all* of the chronic diseases of aging are associated with inflammation and caused or made worse by excess sugar. Sugar directly damages the tissue it comes in contact with and it induces the synthesis of fat and bad cholesterol. Visualize sugar glomming onto your organs, tissues, and cells, making them unable to work correctly. The results? Liver disease, high blood pressure, heart disease, diabetes, kidney disease, dementia, and of course, aging.

As far as methylation goes, research suggests that the impact of high blood sugar can influence DNA methylation patterns in a bad way, and do it quickly—even after one single high-glucose event. Worse yet, these negative changes last for a long time after blood sugar drops back to normal.[1] When scientists tested the effects of short-term glucose on human insulin-producing cells, they were blown away by the far-reaching changes to DNA methylation patterns on important genes associated with metabolism and inflammation.[2] Elevated blood sugar over the long term, which is measured via a hemoglobin A1C (HbA1c) blood test, is no better for your epigenome: high HbA1c levels correlate with epigenetic dysfunction, suggesting that high blood sugar directly damages DNA methylation.[3] Conversely, research also suggests that adopting a diet that reduces blood sugar in the short and long term is associated with improved epigenetics.

For all these reasons, the Younger You Intensive is low glycemic, which means that it includes foods that have a low impact on your blood sugar. Typically, low glycemic foods are high in fiber as well as low in sugar, as the fiber slows the digestion and absorption of any sugar, avoiding spikes in blood sugar.

Because high blood sugar leads to high levels of insulin—the hormone that cues the body to sweep sugar out of the bloodstream—eating a low glycemic diet also keeps insulin in a healthy low range, which is good because chronically elevated insulin drives many imbalances, from cardiometabolic diseases (including high triglycerides and cholesterol) to full-on type 2 diabetes. Not surprisingly, elevated insulin is also associated with imbalanced DNA methylation. (Our study participants lowered their triglycerides and cholesterol—clear evidence that they were following the program and reaping benefits.)

Keto Leaning

A ketogenic diet is lower carb, moderate protein, and higher fat, with the stated goal of getting your body into ketosis, or the state where it manufactures ketones for fuel from fat instead of burning glucose. (Again, we can see our participants succeeded in achieving ketosis because their triglycerides dropped significantly, showing us they were using fat as fuel.)

Ketones have a powerful anti-inflammatory benefit, and ketosis appears to have a beneficial influence on the epigenome. We also know ketones are highly beneficial in brain health—in refractory epilepsy, dementia, and Parkinson's disease,[4] for example. Further, the ketogenic diet is being used as an adjunct therapy in a wide variety of cancers, including breast and colon. I have no doubt that the underlying mechanisms for these conditions include epigenetic changes. In fact, one study discusses ketones not just as fuel for the body, but "signal molecules" with the ability to *reprogram* the epigenome, including DNA methylation.[5] I suspect as more research emerges, our appreciation of ketones will continue to rise.

While getting into ketosis is not a primary goal of the Younger You Intensive, we designed the diet to allow for some "background" ketones to be created by keeping simple carbs lower, fats higher, and protein moderate. This macronutrient ratio is also a great way to keep your blood sugar at a healthy level.

Beyond ketone production, healthy fats are helpful for DNA methylation because, oftentimes, consuming polyphenols (micronutrients found in plant-based foods, many of which are DNA methylation adaptogens) with fat yields better absorption, particularly for resveratrol and curcumin. Thus, eating plenty of fat with your vegetables (such as a salad with dressing, or a stir-fry with olive or medium-chain triglyceride [MCT] oil) helps your body absorb the nutrients that support DNA methylation.

Plant-Forward

Low-glycemic plants (meaning, nonstarchy vegetables and low-sugar fruits) are primary sources of methyl donors and DNA methylation adaptogens— the two categories of food that contain the ingredients we want in copious amounts. In addition, they are high in fiber, low in calories, and easier on the environment. As such, the vast majority of the foods included in the Younger You Intensive are vegetables, with a smattering of fruits. In fact, your target is to eat seven cups of various types of vegetables per day.

Eating a broad array of vegetables and fruit (in moderation) is also helpful because research suggests that eating polyphenols in combination is better than alone, particularly when it comes to exerting anticancer benefits.[6]

Moderate Amounts of Clean Animal Protein

That being said, the Younger You Intensive does include a moderate amount of clean animal protein, which is the highest quality that you can obtain. Ideally, it would be local, organic, and raised humanely, but this isn't always available or accessible. Just do the best you can. Pastured and/ or organic liver is a methylation superstar (so potent, in fact, that you only need to eat it a few times a week). And salmon, grass-fed beef, pastured chicken, organic pork, and organic lamb provide amino acids that are vital for DNA methylation. This plan does limit the amount of meat you should consume per day to 6 ounces total (unless you are over sixty or weigh over 175 pounds, in which case that amount can go as high as 10 ounces).

This small amount of quality animal protein we believe is safe and highly beneficial. Although there is research that links the consumption of animal protein to overall mortality, that is primarily talking about processed meats, such as hot dogs, salami, and sausages, which aren't included in this eating plan.

MACRONUTRIENT TARGET RATIOS

FOR THOSE OF YOU WHO THRIVE ON NUMERIC GUIDELINES, HERE IS THE BREAK-down of macronutrients for the Younger You Intensive; you'll see that we've also included macronutrient percentages in each of the recipes.

Fat: 45–50 percent of daily calories, from a blend of healthy monounsaturated, saturated, omega-3, and omega-6 fats.

Protein: 15–20 percent of daily calories, which come from organic and pastured meat, eggs and organic liver, nuts and seeds, and—to a much smaller extent—vegetables. (For vegetarians and vegans, we are including legumes as an additional protein source.)

Carbs: 30–35 percent of daily calories, nearly all of which come from green, cruciferous, and colorful vegetables and low-sugar fruits.

To calculate exactly how much protein per day you should be consuming, use the following formula:

If you are under sixty: You want to eat 0.66 grams of protein per kilogram of body weight.

If you are over sixty, or weigh more than 175 pounds (79.5 kg): You want to eat 1.0–1.2 grams of protein per kilogram of body weight.

For most people, this works out to 5 to 6 ounces (for under sixty) or 9 to 10 ounces (for over sixty or those who weigh more than 175 pounds) of animal protein daily (in addition to the protein contained in nuts, seeds, vegetables, and fruit). For vegan and vegetarians, this is about 40 to 50 grams of protein from beans, legumes, or protein powder per day (again, in addition to the protein found in other types of food). For vegetarians, this protein total can include eggs as well.

Caveat: If you are an athlete working on building muscle or are increasing your protein to detox from a sugar addiction, short-term protein increases are absolutely fine and helpful. But if you want to follow our study guidelines, stick with these lower protein recommendations during the eight-week Intensive.

· · · · ·

Organic Whenever Possible

Eating organic reduces toxin exposure and saves the body from having to use methyl donors to both protect the body (including the DNA) from chemical damage and to detox the pesticides, hormones, and antibiotics present in conventionally raised produce and meats. More on this on page 196.

Grain-, Legume-, and Dairy-Free

Grains, particularly gluten-containing grains, have a high inflammatory potential for some. They can also be high in carbohydrates, which pushes up blood sugar and insulin. In addition, many processed grains are fortified with folic acid, which as I covered in Chapter 3, can easily be over-consumed and can disrupt all biochemical methylation, including DNA methylation. Dairy—particularly cow dairy—can also be inflammatory and fairly high in sugar. And legumes, while generally a very healthy source of protein and fiber, are higher in carbs and, for a small subset of folks, might cause indigestion and even be pro-inflammatory.

In order to give your body some time off from as many potentially problematic foods as possible, I suggest avoiding grains, dairy, and legumes during the Younger You Intensive. That is, unless you're a vegetarian or vegan, in which case you can have some legumes—see page 114 for more information on modifying the plan to a completely animal product–free diet.

(Soaking, fermenting, and pressure cooking will render legumes more digestible, which is why beans and other legumes are part of the Younger You Everyday program. We just want to keep the diet as easy on your gut as possible during the Intensive.)

Moderate Intermittent Fasting

Intermittent fasting is a great way to keep blood sugar low, support the production of anti-inflammatory ketones, and kick in something called autophagy—a vital cellular detox and clean-up process. Eating early in the day and going to bed without a full stomach (and the task of digestion) is a potent preventative measure against diabetes, obesity, and other metabolic diseases. Research demonstrates benefits of intermittent fasting across most chronic diseases and on health span and life span. We know that at least some of this benefit is likely driven by epigenetic reprogramming, including DNA methylation.[7]

Both the Younger You Intensive and the Everyday incorporate a very doable intermittent fasting schedule of eating only between the hours of 7 a.m. and 7 p.m. If you don't naturally get hungry for breakfast until 9 or 10 a.m., that's great, too—just be sure you stop eating before 7 p.m. as you want your blood sugar to have a chance to fall and your metabolism to be done with digestion before you go to bed. And if you're a night owl and go to bed later than 11, you can adjust this schedule so that you still go twelve hours without eating overnight—just make sure to have your last bit of food at least three hours before you retire so that you don't go to bed with a full stomach, and ideally you're consuming most of your calories while it's light out, as research demonstrates that you burn more of your food, rather than storing it as fat, when you eat during the day and fast at night.[8] Obviously if you are a shift worker (I've been there, believe me!) you'll need to follow what's right for you. I certainly understand if your fasting time is daytime, when you're sleeping.

TURNING UP THE DNA METHYLATION POWER

To these foundational pieces, the Younger You eating plan adds in ortho-molecular nutrition guidelines designed to support your ability to optimize your DNA methylation by prioritizing the components of the formula I introduced in the previous chapter:

Methyl donors + DNA methylation adaptogens + lifestyle = Y2 (Younger You)

Consume Ample Vegetables

Methyl donors and DNA methylation adaptogens are found in abundance in many, many veggies, which is why you'll be eating a lot of them over the next eight weeks! As I mentioned earlier, the whole foods matrix is the most effective way to consume these all-important nutrients, especially in combination, as in a salad or stir-fry. All of the veggie examples listed below contain both methyl donor and DNA methylation adaptogen nutrients. For many, many more food options, refer to our Nutrient Reference, starting on page 407.

Your daily food intake should follow these guidelines:

2 cups dark leafy greens (measured raw, chopped, and packed)
   Choose from: beet greens, collard greens, dandelion greens, escarole, kale, lambsquarters, lettuce (endive, green, mesclun, raddicchio, red, romaine, spring—but sorry, iceberg doesn't cut it), mustard greens, purslane, spinach, Swiss chard

2 cups cruciferous vegetables (measured raw, chopped, and packed)
   Choose from: arugula, bok choy, broccoli, broccoli sprouts, Brussels sprouts, cabbage, cauliflower, collard greens, daikon radish, kale, kohlrabi, mustard greens, radishes, rutabaga, turnips, watercress

3 cups colorful vegetables
>   *Choose from:* artichokes, asparagus, bean sprouts, bell peppers
>   (red, orange, yellow, green), cucumbers, eggplant, green beans,
>   green peas, leeks, okra, onions, parsley, radicchio, radishes,
>   sea vegetables (kelp, spirulina, wakame), summer squash,
>   sweet potato, sweet red peppers, tomato (including sun-dried
>   tomatoes), watercress, yams, zucchini

1–2 medium beets

¼ cup sunflower seeds or seed butter (ideally raw)

¼ cup pumpkin seeds or seed butter (ideally raw)

6 ounces clean animal protein (10 if you are over sixty or weigh
more than 175 pounds)
>   *Choose from:* beef, bison, buffalo, chicken, Cornish hen, duck,
>   elk, goose, lamb, low-mercury fish (anchovy, bass, cod, fish roe,
>   flatfish, halibut, haddock, herring, mackerel, perch, salmon,
>   sardines, snapper, squid, tilefish, trout, whitefish), pork, rabbit,
>   quail, shellfish (clams, crab, lobster, mussels, octopus, oysters,
>   scallops, shrimp), turkey

**If you are vegetarian or vegan, you'll need additional protein from
beans and legumes** (see page 114 for more specific guidance).
>   *Choose from:* black beans, chickpeas, edamame, kidney beans,
>   lentils, protein powder, tempeh, and tofu (see page 137 for more
>   guidance on eating soy)

In addition, you have weekly targets for two methyl donor powerhouses:

Organic liver (3 3-ounce servings per week; these count toward your
daily animal protein total)
>   *Choose from:* organic beef, chicken, or lamb liver (see page 149
>   for insight on how to do this if you think you don't like liver)

Eggs (5–10 eggs per week; these are in addition to your daily animal
protein total)
>   *Choose from:* pastured and/or omega-3 enriched eggs from
>   chickens, ducks, or geese

You should also familiarize yourself with the twelve superfoods—the Dynamic Dozen (see page 142)—that do the heaviest lifting for supplying these methyl donors and DNA methylation adaptogens. Because they are such DNA methylation powerhouses, they should become your go-to foods for the next eight weeks, and beyond.

Layer in Extra DNA Methylation Adaptogens

These are the foods that have been the bedrock of traditional cultures around the world and that continually rebalance your DNA methylation portfolio by helping to add methyl groups where they are needed and remove them where they aren't.

In a DNA methylation twofer, the cruciferous family of vegetables provides both methyl donors and DNA methylation adaptogens. So just by eating your two cups of cruciferous veggies per day, you will be getting a nice amount of DNA methylation adaptogens. (Thanks to the wonderful complexity of nature, there are actually loads of foods that overlap these two categories . . . you can make a game out of perusing the lists of DNA methylation–supportive foods in the Nutrient Reference that starts on page 407 and finding the ones that deliver the most bang for your epigenetic buck if that's your idea of a good time!)

In addition to that, you want to eat at least two servings of other adaptogen foods a day (see the list of my favorites below on page 101)—and you can certainly have more, although you want to limit your fruit intake to two ½ cup servings per day while on the Intensive to keep the plan keto-leaning. Remember, it's the blend of multiple nutrients that provides the broadest base of benefit.

In addition to eating your adaptogens with a bit of fat, as I mentioned earlier, add a bit of freshly ground black pepper to your salads and stir-fries. Why? Because some DNA methylation adaptogens, particularly curcumin (turmeric), are better absorbed when combined with piperine, a compound found in black pepper that is released when the peppercorns are ground.[9]

SELECT DNA METHYLATION ADAPTOGENS

Note: Limit the servings of berries and tomatoes to no more than two per day, due to their sugar content. Again, for many more adaptogen possibilities, refer to the Nutrient Reference on page 407.

ADAPTOGEN	SERVING SIZE (AIM FOR 2 PER DAY, MINIMUM)
Blueberries (wild preferred)	½ cup
Capers	1 tablespoon
Cocoa powder	1 tablespoon
Coffee	1 8-ounce cup (before noon)
Dill	1 teaspoon, fresh, chopped, or ⅓ teaspoon, dried
Garlic	2 cloves
Green tea	1 8-ounce cup
Lemon	1 tablespoon juice or 1 teaspoon grated rind
Lime	1 tablespoon juice or 1 teaspoon grated rind
Mexican oregano	1 teaspoon, fresh, chopped
Oolong tea	1 8-ounce cup
Oregano	1 teaspoon, fresh, chopped, or ⅓ teaspoon, dried
Parsley	1 teaspoon, fresh, chopped, or ⅓ teaspoon, dried
Peppermint	1 teaspoon, fresh, chopped, or ⅓ teaspoon, dried
Rosemary	1 teaspoon, fresh, chopped, or ⅓ teaspoon, dried
Shiitake mushrooms	½ cup
Soy (organic edamame and fermented forms such as natto, miso, and tempeh—and only for vegans and vegetarians while on the Younger You Intensive, as soy is a legume)	1 tablespoon for natto and miso, ¼ cup tempeh, crumbled, ½ cup edamame
Strawberries	½ cup, chopped
Tomatoes	½ cup, chopped
Turmeric	1 teaspoon, dried, or 1 tablespoon, fresh, grated

Basically, for the next eight weeks, you are going to get all the green, cruciferous, and colorful veggies that you know you should have been eating all along. You're going to eat them with delicious dressings, sprinkle them with flavorful nuts and seeds, and accompany them with an egg or a deck-of-cards-size piece of pastured chicken or grass-fed steak. You're not going to worry about counting calories, because the healthy fats and the high fiber will naturally make and keep you full. You can still have your morning cup of coffee; all other times you're going to enjoy filtered tap or spring water or seltzer, or sip on green tea or a Golden Turmeric Milk, and enjoy how good it feels to be fully hydrated (without having your hydration negatively impacted by high-sodium processed foods).

Of course, it's a shift from the way most of us eat. I get that. It can take a few days to get into the rhythm of it, which is totally OK. To help you over the hump, my nutrition team and I have created recipes and a two-week meal plan for you to follow, which you can see on page 124. We calculated all the totals you could possibly calculate in that meal plan, from macronutrient breakdowns to amounts of methyl donor and DNA methylation adaptogens. If you like to cross your Ts and dot your Is, the meal plan is your road map.

But I know that some of you prefer to wing it. And that is totally possible—just follow the Cheat Sheet on page 122 to make sure you're hitting your daily targets for green vegetables, cruciferous vegetables, colorful vegetables, adaptogens, healthy fats, and clean protein. It really can be as easy as checking a box.

Think of it as a choose-your-own adventure. One is scripted, and one is more of an improvisation. You can also use our Younger You digital program for super easy tracking and support (see page 426 for more info).

Option 1: Scripted. Follow our menu plans—included on page 124—and get started; I've provided two weeks of meals, which you can repeat in order to get to eight weeks.
> *Pros:* This takes the thinking out of it, and our recipes are scrumptious!
> *Cons:* If you're working or raising a family or both, it is likely going to require some batch cooking, probably once on the weekend and once during the week.

Option 2: Improv. Use the Cheat Sheet on page 122 to make sure you're hitting your food targets each day.

Pros: This approach has a lot more freedom in it—you can look in the fridge and see which greens you feel like eating that day, for example. It's also a lot simpler. You can always use our recipes to inspire you and expand your healthy-cooking repertoire.

Cons: You have to make more decisions. At least until you get your sea legs. In our age of information overload and decision-fatigue, sometimes it's easier to just be told what to do.

There is no one right choice—just the one that works for you. Because our study participants met with nutritionists trained in the program on an ongoing basis, we learned that most of them were improvisers, using the recipe pack occasionally, but leaning heavily on our Cheat Sheet. Even though the official Younger You Intensive is eight weeks long, our patients, and many study participants, report that eating this way becomes fairly habitual. Ron, who was part of our study, reports that following the Intensive eating plan greatly broadened the range of vegetables he was eating, and that he has kept his vegetable intake up to approximately seven cups per day. Even when you aren't technically "on the program," once you've adapted to the daily targets, it's easy to adhere to without thinking about it too much.

A DAY IN THE LIFE: THE IMPROV VERSION OF A YOUNGER YOU

Morning: Drink a glass of water when you wake up and have a coffee at home. If you're hungry and it's after 7 a.m., have a Blueberry Beet Scone or an egg or two. If you're not hungry yet, it's fine to wait to eat until you are. Fill a seven-cup Pyrex container with at least five cups of your daily veggies, all chopped up—a mixture of greens and cruciferous and colorful veggies. (During the colder months, this salad can become a stir-fry that you cook in the morning—frozen veggies are OK to use, which minimizes prep time—and then put in the Pyrex container so that you can bring it to work.) To it, add a quarter cup of sunflower or pumpkin seeds, a handful of berries—frozen organic berries are great in the off-season—and 3 ounces of chicken, salmon, or hard-boiled egg on top (5 ounces if you're over sixty or weigh more than 175 pounds, or one of the vegan sources of protein discussed on page 114). Pour a serving of the Herbal Epigenetic Dressing (page 310) into a jar so that it is portable.

Midmorning: Have a cup of green tea at work. Eat a little bit of that huge salad/stir-fry around 9 or 10, or whenever you are hungry either for your first meal of the day or for a snack if you ate something earlier. Keep a big pitcher of water on your desk to ensure that you get half your body weight in ounces of water during the workday.

Lunch: Eat the rest of that massive salad/stir-fry.

Midafternoon: Sip on some Golden Turmeric Milk (page 386), eat a handful or two of nuts.

Dinner: Eat another two cups of veggies (the balance of the veggie and adaptogen requirement)—sautéed with garlic, olive oil, and MCT. Eat some pickled beets and have another 3 ounces of whatever protein is in the fridge (or 4 to 5 ounces if you are over sixty or weigh more than 175).

Dessert: A square or two of Lily's brand chocolate (sweetened with erythritol and stevia).

WHAT TO EAT (AND AVOID) ON THE YOUNGER YOU INTENSIVE PROGRAM: OR, OK, BUT WHAT THE HECK DO I EAT?

For an exhaustive list of donors and adaptogens, see the Nutrient Reference starting on page 407; here's a shorter, accessible list to get you started:

	LOTS OF . . .	NO. . .
Vegetables	Antioxidant-rich colorful vegetables, cruciferous vegetables, and dark leafy greens	Corn, fries, potato chips, processed vegetable snacks, white potatoes
Fats	Nuts and seeds: almonds, Brazil nuts, cashews, chestnuts, chia seeds, flax seeds, hazelnuts, hemp seeds, macadamia nuts, pecans, pine nuts, poppy seeds, sesame seeds (and tahini), walnuts Fruits: avocados, olives Oils: almond oil, avocado oil, coconut oil, flaxseed oil, MCT oil, olive oil, pumpkin seed oil, red palm oil, safflower oil, sesame oil, sunflower oil, walnut oil	Nuts and seeds: peanuts Oils: cottonseed oil, Crisco, hydrogenated fats, margarine, shortening, soybean oil, trans fats, vegetable oil

Animal Protein* * Unless you are vegetarian or vegan—see page 114 for guidelines on getting ample protein without eating meat.	Beef (grass-fed), bison, buffalo, chicken (organic), Cornish hen, duck, eggs (pastured and/or omega-3 enriched from chickens, ducks, or geese), elk, fish (wild-caught or responsibly farmed and low mercury), goose, lamb, liver (beef or chicken, organic), pork, quail, rabbit, shellfish, turkey	Any meat from animals raised with antibiotics or hormones, grilled meats and fish, fried meats and fish, high-mercury fish, processed meats including sausage, hot dogs, cold cuts, and canned meats
Dairy and meat alternatives	For everyone: unsweetened nondairy milks and yogurts, including almond, cashew, coconut, and hemp For vegetarians and vegans only: organic and/or fermented soy: edamame, miso, natto, tamari, tempeh, and tofu	All dairy, including milk, cheeses, yogurt, kefir, and butter All other soy, including soy sauce, soybean oil, soy milk, soy yogurt, textured vegetable protein; nondairy creamers
Fruit* * With the exception of avocado, lemon, and lime, limit your fruit intake to two ½-cup servings per day to minimize blood sugar spikes.	Apple, apricot, avocado, banana, blackberry, blueberry, blood orange, cantaloupe, cherry, clementine, date, grapefruit, grape, guava, honeydew, kiwi, lemon, lime, lychee, mango, nectarine, olive, orange, papaya, peaches, persimmon, pineapple, plums, pomegranate, raspberry, strawberry, tomato	Dried fruits, fruit juice, fruit snacks, fruit jellies and jams
Condiments	Avocado-oil mayonnaise, Baker's yeast, brewer's yeast, cocoa (70%+ dark, not Dutch processed), coconut aminos, mustard, nutritional yeast, salsa (no sugar added), tamari (low sodium), vinegars	Prepared sauces with sugar and additives, including BBQ sauce, honey mustard, ketchup, and teriyaki sauce; store-bought salad dressing
Sweeteners	Minimal amounts of natural no-calorie sweeteners that don't impact blood sugar, including erythritol, inulin, monk fruit, and stevia	Artificial sweeteners, coconut sugar, evaporated cane juice, high-fructose corn syrup, honey, maple syrup, molasses, and refined sugar
Drinks	Coconut water, coffee, green tea, herbal tea, oolong tea, seltzer, water (filtered, mineral, or spring)	Alcohol, fruit juice, soft drinks, including diet sodas

CUSTOMIZING YOUR CURRENT EATING PLAN
TO THE YOUNGER YOU PROGRAM

While the Younger You Intensive is designed to be its own stand-alone eating plan, it's also customizable to work with most other eating plans. In our practice, we prescribe highly individualized nutrition programs for our patients depending on their medical history, their presenting issues (auto-immune issues, gastrointestinal problems, hormone imbalances, allergies, heart disease, cancer, and so forth), and what their laboratory testing shows us they need or need to avoid. Regardless of the specifics, the Younger You principles are always included. I absolutely love and appreciate how the Younger You program is eminently layerable into any dietary pattern. There is no reason that I can think of not to incorporate the fundamentals of the Younger You program into any eating pattern you are adhering to. Below are the modifications we suggest for several of today's most popular diets.

Ketogenic Diet

The Younger You Intensive is "keto leaning," so if you follow the program to the letter it is possible that you will get into ketosis after a couple of days. But because it isn't super high fat, nor is the protein or carb or calorie count particularly low, if you want to be in full-tilt ketosis, you might need to tweak things in order to start producing ketones. If that is a priority for you, I suggest the following:

- Start by lowering or stopping the colorful fruits and replace those with more greens.

- You can also increase your fat intake, particularly MCT oil, for a few days.

- Once you are in ketosis, try slowly adding back colorful veggies and berries, as they are very important sources of DNA methylation adaptogens. Note that some colorful fruits and veggies may knock you out of ketosis—such as carrots—while others don't—like red and orange peppers. You'll need to gauge what you can consume based on your ketone production (I use a urine strip, and all I'm looking for is a small to moderate level of ketones).

- The more consistent you are with the mild intermittent fasting, exercise, sleep, and stress reduction, the easier it will typically be to stay in ketosis.

If you are on a strict low-calorie, low-protein, very-high-fat keto program (as an epilepsy intervention or as part of a cancer treatment program, say), you can absolutely incorporate Younger You–friendly foods, but your overall diet should be adjusted and managed by a practitioner versed in both protocols. It's essential that your dietary plan be nutritionally sufficient.

Paleo

The Younger You Intensive *is* a paleo program. No modifications are needed!

Elimination Diet

The Younger You Intensive is free of many common allergens, including peanuts, wheat, and dairy, but it does allow some forms of soy for vegans and vegetarians (listed on page 114), incorporates many tree nuts plus sesame seeds and shellfish, and relies on eggs—all foods that can be allergenic.

The easiest way to eliminate any allergens from the Younger You Intensive is to print the full list of included foods on page 104 and simply cross off any foods that you know you don't tolerate. You can do this with the recipes as well. If your elimination diet is very restrictive, get help from a knowledgeable nutritionist to help tailor the program so that you can ensure that your nutrient intake is sufficient and balanced.

A good way to monitor if the Intensive is triggering your allergies or sensitivities is to repeat the medical symptoms questionnaire (MSQ) on page 83 every seven days. If your score isn't trending downward, it could be that there's an allergen in the diet that you're reacting to, or that you have an underlying gut dysbiosis that needs to be remedied. In either case, it's helpful to work with a functional medicine practitioner and/or nutritionist to find the eating plan that is right for you.

Anti-inflammatory Diet

With no processed foods, added sugars, grains, legumes (unless you're vegan), or dairy, plenty of antioxidant-rich vegetables and select fruit, and good fats and proteins, the Younger You Intensive is potently anti-inflammatory.

Note that the Younger You Everyday plan does incorporate gluten-free grains, clean dairy, and legumes, but for most people, these foods don't promote inflammation. If that's not the case for you, continue to avoid your problematic food group when you follow that version of the program.

Low-FODMAP Diet

A full low-FODMAP diet layers easily with the Younger You Intensive program. In my experience, it's rare that all of the carbohydrate categories (fermentable oligo-saccharides, di-saccharides, mono-saccharides, and polyols) are problematic. In our practice, after a short-term full FODMAP elimination, we will have our patients try one group at a time to identify the type(s) that causes a reaction. Generally, only one or two categories of carbs require a longer period of elimination.

One note of caution: A long-term low-FODMAP diet can become nutrient insufficient and/or negatively influence the microbiome. If you've been on a low-FODMAP diet for more than a month, seek out a practitioner (ideally trained in functional medicine—see the Resources section on page 426 for guidance on where to find one) who can help resolve underlying issues.

Mediterranean Diet

Both Younger You plans are Mediterranean-friendly. The Everyday version, with its legumes, whole grains, and dairy, is most closely aligned, although the greens and cruciferous and colorful veggies that the Intensive relies on are also part of the Mediterranean diet. You'll just need to make sure you eat more fish for your animal protein than red meat while on the Intensive or Everyday to stay within the confines of the Mediterranean guidelines, and of course include lots of fabulous olive oil, too.

Vegetarian or Vegan

You can incorporate legumes into the Younger You Intensive—see page 114 for a more detailed discussion and look for recipes marked with a "VGT" for vegetarian or "V" for vegan in the recipe section.

Autoimmune Protocol Diet, Autoimmune Paleo Diet, and Wahls Protocol

These diets, in their most restrictive phases, require the removal of several foods included in the Younger You Intensive, including nightshade vegetables, eggs, nuts, and seeds. Simply omit these from the list on page 104 and the recipes. Long-term adherence to these more restrictive protocols should be tracked by a practitioner to ensure nutrient sufficiency.

Time-Restricted Eating, Intermittent Fasting, or Caloric Restriction

The Younger You plans recommend mild time-restricted eating (aka intermittent fasting), eating only between the hours of 7 a.m. and 7 p.m. (or what's known as a 12:12 structure). If you are currently following a different intermittent fasting schedule, such as 16:8 (eating only during an eight-hour window during the day) or 5-2 (eat five days, fast two), you can still follow the Younger You Intensive during your eating windows. The big caveat here is, can you sustain such restriction over the long haul? Be mindful and realistic: you don't want to be so restricted that you lapse into disordered eating, which I see in my practice every day. For most people, a 12:12 pattern is something they can stick to a majority of the time over a sustained period, but I encourage you to see what works for you.

QUICK TIPS ON UPPING YOUR VEGGIE INTAKE

HERE ARE A FEW WAYS TO SNEAK IN AN EXTRA SERVING OF FRUITS AND veggies during the day:

- ○ **Drink them.** Spinach, chard, and beets—not to mention beet greens, don't throw them out!—are *great* in smoothies.
- ○ **Have veggies for breakfast.** It's a thing! Add a side of greens to your egg(s), or toss in steamed or lightly sautéed spinach,

broccoli, tomatoes, peppers, mushrooms, zucchini, olives, onions, and/or garlic to an omelet, or treat yourself to a warm cauliflower rice bowl with more veggies on top.

o **Make them grab-able.** Take a container of precut cucumbers, broccoli, cauliflower, bell peppers, zucchini, jicama, carrots, or celery with you whenever you leave the house, or just keep them at the ready in the fridge for when hunger strikes. I find if I put cut veggies out on the counter before dinner, my daughter and I both happily eat them—kind of a pre-dinner that doesn't spoil our appetites.

o **Blend 'em.** Stick some veggies in the Nutribullet to add to your tomato sauce or tahini dip—it's an easy hack that amps the nutrition while not altering the taste.

o **Add at the end.** Toss as many extra veggies as you can into soups. Most extra veggies added toward the end of the cooking process won't change the taste of a dish.

o **Turn them into confetti.** Here's a great way to add a pile of veggies without a lot of prep. Chop an assortment of veggies in a food processor, then save them in the fridge (in a glass container) to sprinkle on salads raw, or wilt and serve as a side.

o **Roast them.** Prep a pile of roasted veggies at the beginning of the week so you can easily toss them into salads and soups, use them as a side dish, add them to your scrambled egg, or eat them as a snack.

• • • • •

SUPPORTING PLAYERS IN THE YOUNGER YOU EATING PLAN

While the foods that contain methyl donors and methylation adaptogens are the stars of the show, there are several character actors that round out the cast of DNA methylation superstars.

Hydration

What you drink is a key piece of optimizing your DNA methylation. It's vital that you stay adequately hydrated, which means we recommend drinking enough ounces of water, seltzer, or herbal tea per day to equal about half your body weight in pounds—the standard guideline used in functional medicine. That means, if you weigh 150 pounds, you need to aim for 75 fluid ounces of noncaffeinated, nonalcoholic, unsweetened beverages every day.

Hydration is a crucial piece of detoxification—without consuming ample amounts of water, your toxic load will be higher, and toxins are an impediment to healthy DNA methylation—something I cover more in depth in Chapter 6. Beyond that, hydration is also crucial for reducing oxidative stress.[10]

It's important that the water you drink either be filtered or spring (from a glass, not plastic, bottle). I recommend carbon-block filters, such as those made by Aquasauna or Multipure, because they will keep out most toxins and retain most trace minerals, although you will need to change the filter regularly so that it functions well and doesn't get contaminated with bacteria.

In addition to water, other DNA methylation–supportive beverages include:

Chamomile tea (another adaptogen rock star along with all the other teas listed here)

Coconut water (so loaded with potassium)

Green tea

Oolong tea

Other herbal teas, such as ginger, hibiscus, and rooibos

Seltzer (limit to two 12-ounce servings per day)

Turmeric tea, often known as golden milk, so long as it is sweetened only with stevia (see our recipe on page 386)

COFFEE IS A DNA METHYLATION ADAPTOGEN!

FOR THOSE OF US (ME INCLUDED) WHO ARE LOATH TO GIVE UP COFFEE, know that it's a DNA methylation adaptogen, thanks to two amazing polyphenols it contains: caffeic acid and chlorogenic acid. Likely due to this fact, coffee, like green tea, has been solidly associated with longevity. Looking at the research, it seems like you could consume quite a bit of coffee without negative effects and probably some good benefit. The tricky part is that for most of us (including me), the caffeine content in both green tea and coffee comes at the cost of lost sleep, or poor-quality sleep, which is definitely damaging to our DNA methylation and gene expression in the brain.

HERE'S WHAT I RECOMMEND FOR COFFEE LOVERS:

o Go organic

o Limit to one or at most two cups

o Finish your last cup before noon

o Drink it black and unsweetened, or with MCT oil for an extra serving of healthy fat

. . . . .

Fermented and Prebiotic Foods

While functional medicine views the body as a synergistic whole, if our field were forced to choose one organ system to prioritize, it would be the gut. It interacts with all the other organ systems—the endocrine system, the cardiovascular system, the nervous system, the brain, and especially the immune system, about 70 percent of which is housed around your GI tract. The population of microbes in your gut, aka your microbiome, are fundamental drivers of health. If they are friendly and comprised of the right players, they contribute to digestion, blunt inflammation, make loads of nutrients—including the short-chain fatty acid butyrate, vitamins B_1 and B_2, and the methyl donors folate and B_{12}—in addition to making other helpful, bioavailable molecules from the foods you eat.[11] To this last point, our gut critters are required to activate many key methylation adaptogen polyphenols. In short, the gut microbiome plays a direct role in your DNA methylation. The healthier and more robust your gut microbiome, the better your DNA methylation will be.[12]

Yet in the majority of patients I see, and in the general population, our microbiomes and our overall gut health are suffering. Why? The reasons are far reaching and include excessive hygiene (a lack of exposure to dirt, nature, and plants); overuse of medications (such as antibiotics, nonsteroidal pain relievers, and acid blockers); nutrient-poor, calorie-high diets; limited breast feeding and high rates of Cesarean section deliveries; toxin exposures (pesticides on foods, chemicals in plastics); and of course loads and loads of stress that directly shuts down our ability to digest. I strongly suspect that these changes have created negative influences in our younger generation's epigenomes, contributing to the meteoric rise in inflammatory illnesses such as autoimmunity and allergic disease.

For all these reasons, it's vital to support your gut health, and both the Younger You Intensive and Everyday programs help you do that, by removing many common allergens and toxins that can irritate your gut (see more about allergens on page 252) and adding in prebiotic food options like garlic, blueberries, cruciferous veggies, greens, onion, flax seeds, leeks, asparagus, cocoa, and others (can you already see that a number of prebiotics are methyl donors and DNA methylation adaptogens, too? How cool!). We further support your friendly microbiome population with a probiotic supplement (see page 209 for more info) and with a daily recommended intake of fermented foods—ideally, a little bit with most of your meals. That means sauerkraut, kimchi, coconut kefir, kombucha, and traditionally made pickled vegetables, including pickled beets (my favorite, and yet another way to kill two DNA methylation requirements with one stone!). While you can buy these foods at the store, you have to make sure they contain live cultures. A good indicator of this is if they are refrigerated (not on the room-temperature shelves) and cost more than you think they ought to, because traditional fermentation takes a lot longer than simply adding vinegar (the method most commercial packaged pickles use).

Here's a guide to serving sizes for different types of fermented foods:
- Pickled beets (¼ cup)
- Sauerkraut (½ cup)
- Kimchi (½ cup)
- Miso (1 tablespoon)
- Coconut kefir (1 cup)
- Kombucha (1 cup)
- Olives (yes, olives are always fermented) (5 olives)

CONSIDERATIONS FOR VEGETARIANS AND VEGANS

Although technically the Younger You Intensive is bean- and legume-free, if you are vegetarian or vegan, you can and should absolutely include them so that you get adequate protein while following the plan. Aim for 40–50 grams of additional protein—from legumes, beans, and plant-based protein powders—to compensate for the animal protein you're not eating. Use this table to assess how much of these foods to eat each day to meet that protein target.

Black beans	1 cup	15.2 grams
Chickpeas	1 cup	14.5 grams
Kidney beans	1 cup	15.3 grams
Lentils, cooked	1 cup	17.9 grams
Protein powder*	2 tbsp	15 grams
Tempeh, organic	1 cup	15 grams
Tofu, organic	½ cup	10 grams

Also know that you are getting protein from your daily allotment of pumpkin seeds, sunflower seeds, and vegetables, as well as the nuts that are allowed on the Intensive.

In addition, there are certain methylation-supportive nutrients that vegetarians and vegans will need to give a little extra attention to in order to ensure sufficient intake while on the Younger You Intensive. This is because they are found primarily in animal-based foods, or they are present in lesser-quantity in plant foods. These include B_{12}; choline; the sulfur-containing amino acids methionine, cysteine, and taurine; the omega-3 fatty acids EPA and DHA; and minerals zinc, iron, and selenium. Preformed fat-soluble vitamin A (retinol) is derived from animal products, but may be converted in the body from certain carotenoids. A vegan not converting carotenoids well (as can happen in hypothyroidism) may require supplemental vitamin A.

---

* See page 436 in Supplements for a list of vegan protein powders we recommend to our patients and page 126 for a sample one-day vegetarian/vegan menu

Some nutrient deficits may be addressed in the vegan diet with the increased seed and nut intake, sea vegetables (nori especially), shiitake and enoki mushrooms, and the green, colorful, and cruciferous vegetables that are the mainstays of the Younger You Intensive eating plan. Still, in my experience, even vegans and vegetarians on the Younger You Intensive benefit greatly from a few specific supplements—refer to page 210 for a list of those.

In addition, there are two nutrients that vegans can be deficient in that are easy to get from foods:

- Selenium, which you can easily get from Brazil nuts. One Brazil nut contains 96 ug, or 175 percent of the RDI. Think of the Brazil nut as an edible supplement.
- Zinc is also easy to get from foods if you're intentional—refer to page 420 for a list of zinc-rich foods.

FOODS TO AVOID

Just as important as what to add to your diet are the things to be avoided. While eating foods high in methyl donors and DNA methylation adaptogens will definitely help, it's a little like adjusting your sails when you have holes in your boat. You may move a little faster in the direction you want to go, but you're sinking as you go. While yes, even if you only eat one healthy meal a week it is still beneficial, if you make that same choice the majority of the time, it will potently bias you (and your epigenetics) toward long-term longevity and all the things that accompany it, such as maintenance of a healthy weight, lower risk of disease, and a longer health span.

Inflammatory Foods

Aging and inflammation—the body's immune response to anything it deems an invader—are as conjoined as the double helix of DNA. In fact, in the scientific literature, they call it "inflammaging." In a nutshell: aging creates inflammation. And inflammation, in turn, drives all of the diseases of aging. It needn't be huge amounts of inflammation in order to be damaging, either. Pesky—but chronic—low-grade inflammation is a problem, too. And nothing turns on inflammation (high or low) more efficiently than a lousy diet. Even transient poor nutrition can have long-lasting impact on the expression of pro-inflammatory genes. Then, if these bad patterns continue, new daughter cells are created that house the same pro-inflammatory epigenetic instructions.

What's worse, we can inherit this tendency toward epigenetic inflammation from previous generations. Many of us need to double down on a healthy diet because of the choices of our recent ancestors (I fall into this camp) or the disease risks we have in our family (cardiometabolic diseases are in mine), especially if we want our health span and life span to be optimal (I am also a member of this group).[13]

You probably already have an inkling that there are certain foods and food combinations that are highly unhealthy because they promote inflammation. These foods include sugar, refined carbs (such as flour, bread, pasta, pastries, and muffins), ultra-processed vegetable seed oils (such as canola), and processed or poor-quality meats (like deli meats, sausages, and hot dogs). When we combine high sugar, refined carbs, and high fat, it's a triple whammy of inflammation.

When you eat a highly processed food, there is a complex cascade of damaging events that occur body-wide. But specifically, let's focus on the immune system: your white blood cells assess the food and register it as foreign. In response, your body will trigger the release of immune system molecules that kick off an inflammatory response. We know this thanks to a famous 2004 study where researchers gave healthy adults either a fast-food-style breakfast of an egg or sausage muffin with two hash browns (refined carbs and poor-quality fats) or a glass of water. No surprise that the greasy, salty, and probably, let's admit, delicious breakfast took more of a toll on the body, but what was surprising was just how bad it was. The people who ate the greasy breakfast experienced a significant increase in reactive oxygen species (i.e., free radicals) and C-reactive protein, which is used as a gauge to measure the extent of the body's inflammatory response, and an upregulation in nuclear factor kappa-B, or NF-kB, which goes into the nucleus of the cell, lands on the DNA, and tells the gene to blast out inflammatory compounds. In other words, the body responded to the fast-food meal as foreign and dangerous, like it would to a toxin such as mercury, a flu virus, or a strep bacteria. And these changes lasted for longer than three hours; just long enough for the next meal to come along and do the same thing all over again.[14] This study showed the exact mechanisms by which the standard American diet of fast, processed, nutrient-poor, fried foods put us on a moving sidewalk to disease. Again, this 2004 study was before scientists were routinely looking at epigenetic changes. If they repeated this study today, I suspect we would see changes to the genes regulating inflammation, resulting in turning on these inflammatory genes for far longer than the meal lasted; maybe even for days longer, as we've seen in animal and cell epigenetic research.[15]

On the other hand, when you are choosing foods that are low in sugar, unprocessed, and high in methylation adaptogens and methyl donors, you provide your body with a whole different set of information that's nourishing and balancing to your DNA. As a result, inflammation is lowered, epigenetic processes are enhanced, and your cells no longer need to defend and repair after every meal. They become programmed for optimization instead, and your physiological function gets better as your biological age gets lower.

Sugar

I know, I know. By now you're probably sick of hearing the advice to stop eating sugar. Here's the thing: it's wildly damaging, and highly inflammatory. And what sugar your body can't immediately use for energy, which is *most* of it, unless you're running a marathon or you are a member of a highly physical profession, it stores as fat. This fat gets tucked inside your cells, your organs, and most visibly, your abdomen. That fat around your middle is especially inflammatory. As such, it's linked to all the top causes of disease and death, including diabetes, Alzheimer's disease, heart disease, and cancer. And aging. But we already knew that.

Now we have a new lens on why sugar is so destructive in the body: it disrupts epigenetic methylation, and not in a good way. A 2008 study showed that a single high-glucose event had lasting negative effects on methylation of a gene found in cells from the endothelial lining of the aorta that regulates NF-kB.[16] The researchers administered large amounts of glucose to both endothelial cells from mice in vitro and to live non-diabetic mice. In both cases, the NF-kB gene experienced increased expression, which opens the faucet on inflammation, aging, and all of their associated diseases. Worse yet, these effects lasted at least six days past the time it took to metabolize the glucose. Although the study only looked for changes for six days, so who knows how long those effects really lasted? Granted, it was a study performed on rodents so we can't say for sure that the same thing happens in humans in the same way, but we know for sure lasting epigenetic changes do happen in humans and can happen quite rapidly sometimes. And in healthy (not diabetic) human cell studies, we see glucose exposure leading to far-reaching, negative changes to insulin- and glucose-regulating genes via DNA methylation.[17]

In some ways, knowing this makes it easier to stay away from sugar nearly all the time, which is ultimately helpful, because sugar is one of those foods where it's very, very hard to have just a little. It's almost easier to avoid it altogether; that way your taste buds, your brain, and your gut microbiome will reacclimate and that longing for a sweet taste will abate.

While on the Intensive, you want to limit your sweets consumption to two ½-cup daily servings of fruit, particularly low-sugar, epi-nutrient dense fruits such as wild berries, and natural sweeteners that don't impact your blood sugar—you can find these listed in the chart on page 105. Once you're on the Everyday program, you can expand this to small amounts of natural forms of sugar such as dates, honey, blackstrap molasses, and maple syrup, but just for now, use the Intensive as an opportunity to reset yourself away from sweet and more toward nutrient rich.

That said, there are ways to keep your sweet tooth satisfied during the eight weeks of the Younger You Intensive. Berries are great DNA methylation adaptogens, as is cocoa. The recipes for No-Bake Sunbutter Chocolate Squares (page 377) are totally tasty, as is our Rosemary Lemon Tart (page 382), which is my family's go-to celebratory treat—it's always a hit!

It's like that old punitive saying, "A moment on the lips, forever on the hips," except when it comes to sugar, it's about health span, not your jeans size: "A moment on the lips, a really long time on the epigenome."

Artificial Sweeteners

While there isn't specific research that sheds light on artificial sweeteners' effect on DNA methylation—yet—there are still compelling reasons to avoid them as part of your Younger You plan. Artificial sweeteners still cue insulin (even though they don't contain glucose, which is the typical trigger for the release of insulin) and light up pathways in the brain that seek reward. As a result, eating artificial sugars can cue cravings for sweets and make it harder to make healthy food choices. They can also be disruptive to gut health.[18] We counsel everyone in our practice to avoid them.

Nonorganic Foods

There's no debating it: living and eating as cleanly as possible is important for healthy epigenome and DNA methylation. This means that eating organic and clean sources of foods as often as possible will help protect epigenetic expression (including DNA methylation and the DNA genetic material itself). While some environmental toxins occur elsewhere, a number of them are found in our food supply and food packaging materials (I talk more about environmental toxins in Chapter 7).

Organic foods, on the other hand, aren't exposed to most toxins in the first place. In addition, organic foods have been shown to have higher nutrient levels than their conventional counterparts, meaning they also have more methyl donor nutrients and especially DNA methylation adaptogens than chemically grown foods. These increased epi-nutrients include the polyphenols that help protect the plant from pests—and our genes from disordered DNA methylation (more on this starting on page 195).

The unfortunate reality is that the presence of toxins is so pervasive in our modern environment that doing whatever you can to lessen the amount you are exposed to in the first place—by eating organic, for example, filtering your water, and avoiding plastics and nonstick cookware (again, more on these strategies in Chapter 7)—is not only a wise strategy for promoting health, it's urgently necessary.

Before you despair that toxins are unavoidable, know that research, particularly by Bernhard Hennig, a professor of nutrition and toxicology at the University of Kentucky, has shown that many nutrients that are supportive of healthy DNA methylation and are mainstays of the Younger You Intensive as well as the Younger You Everyday, such as omega-3 fats, curcumin, and EGCG, can lessen the inflammatory damage caused by environmental toxins such as polychlorinated biphenyl compounds (PCBs). So, avoid what toxins you can, and know that the dietary changes you're making will help protect you from those you can't.[19]

Charred Foods

Cooking foods at a high enough heat to sear them, crisp them, or leave grill marks may have a tasty result. But those bits of food that turn dark brown during the cooking process are packed with compounds—known as *advanced glycation end products (AGEs)*—that are pro-oxidant, pro-inflammatory, and damaging to cells and DNA. And since the entire aim of the Younger You Intensive and Younger You Everyday is to equip the body to fight inflammation, oxidation, and other damage by turning on the genes that help in these efforts, eating a seared burger—even one made with beets and grass-fed beef—works against you. Instead of cooking your clean animal protein in a dry pan at high heat (or on a grill), you want to cook at a lower temperature with some moisture involved, as this minimizes the formation of AGEs. In addition to what you eat, the Younger You Intensive guides you to change how you cook what you eat and to embrace slow-cooked methods, like braising or using a slow cooker or the ever-popular Instant Pot.

Alcohol

I know many of you reading this will be holding out hope that red wine is supportive of healthy DNA methylation because of the high levels of the antioxidant resveratrol you've heard about. Sigh . . . that is not the case. (As a former red wine lover myself, I feel your pain.)

Alcohol is not sanctioned for the Younger You Intensive, because despite how much of the well-known DNA methylation adaptogen resveratrol may or may not be in your nightly glass (or two), alcohol impairs DNA methylation. It does so by inhibiting the enzymes used in the methylation and folate cycles, which results in a potentially significant reduction of SAMe (the body's main methyl donor), lowers folate absorption, and directly inhibits the enzymes that methylate our DNA.[20]

I know that giving up alcohol for the rest of your life is a big ask—although many people do it and find it helpful and discover other ways to relax and celebrate—so certain alcohol is OK in very moderate amounts on the Everyday version.

Considerations Before You Jump In

In general, both the Younger You Intensive and the Younger You Everyday are exceedingly healthy eating patterns. But any time you start a new diet and exercise regimen you want to consult with your primary care provider.

There are two particular instances where you may need to take more care in adopting the Younger You Intensive:

- If you have trouble digesting fat, have a predisposition to gallstones, or have had your gallbladder removed, you might need to adjust your macronutrient ratios to eat less fat.

- If you have a family or personal history of kidney stones, this eating plan may contribute to the formation of kidney stones because the diet is high in oxalates. Oxalates are organic acids that occur naturally in many plant foods; they are especially high in several foods that form the mainstay of the Younger You Intensive and Everyday, namely spinach, beets, raspberries, and soy (which is part of the Intensive only if you are a vegetarian or a vegan). Once in your body, oxalates bind with calcium and can contribute to the formation of kidney stones. Consuming plenty of citrate, from citrus fruits, and good hydration lower the amount of oxalates in your blood, and this diet prioritizes both of those—squeezing lemon and lime into your water covers both bases. However, if kidney stones are part of your history or you have kidney disease, you should consult with your doctor to see if this plan is appropriate for you.

GETTING STARTED

Ideally, you would start the Younger You Intensive at a time when you aren't super busy. You want extra time at the grocery store to see which veggies look the most tantalizing and fresh and to cook up a few recipes. Also, if you have been eating a standard American diet, you may experience some detox symptoms, such as fatigue, brain fog, gassiness, or bloating. There is a lot of fiber and prebiotic foods on this eating plan; it's appropriate to expect that as your microbial population adjusts you might feel a little bit worse before you feel better. Really prioritize your hydration and your intake of healthy fats, which will help ward off any sugar cravings that might flare up now as well.

These symptoms should pass after a few days; if they don't, consult with your health-care provider, a functional medicine practitioner, or a nutritionist to assess and address what's going on for you.

⬤ CHEAT SHEET OF YOUNGER YOU INTENSIVE FOOD TARGETS

IF YOU PREFER TO DO THE IMPROV VERSION OF THE YOUNGER YOU INTENSIVE, these are your daily guidelines.

For a more scripted version, see our sample two-week menus on pages 124–127. (There is also a one-day version for vegetarians and vegans on page 126.)

EACH DAY:

__ 2 cups dark leafy greens, measured raw, chopped, and packed (see list on page 98)

__ 2 cups cruciferous vegetables, measured raw, chopped, and packed (see list on page 98)

__ 3 cups additional colorful vegetables (see list on page 99)

__ 1–2 medium beets, cooked or raw

__ ¼ cup pumpkin seeds or pumpkin seed butter

__ ¼ cup sunflower seeds or sunflower seed butter

___ Two-plus servings of DNA methylation adaptogens (see list on page 101)

___ Two 3-ounce servings of clean animal protein (see list on page 99) (unless you're over sixty or weigh more than 175 pounds, then two 5-ounce servings; or vegan or vegetarian, then you want to get 40–50 grams protein from beans, legumes, or protein powder—refer to page 99)

___ 5 tablespoons of healthy fats (see list on page 104)

___ One-plus servings fermented foods (see list on page 113)

___ Half your body weight in fluid ounces of water, herbal tea, or seltzer (limit seltzer to 24 ounces per day)

EACH WEEK:

___ Three servings of liver (3 ounces per serving), preferably organic*

___ 5–10 eggs, preferably free-range, organic, and omega-3 enriched*

  * On days when you eat liver and/or eggs, those count toward your daily clean animal protein target; one egg is roughly approximate to 1 ounce of meat.

GENERAL GUIDELINES:

o Eat organic as much as possible

o Stay hydrated (.5 ounce of water, sparkling water, or herbal tea per pound of body weight per day)

o Give yourself a twelve-hour fast each day, typically between 7 p.m. and 7 a.m.

o Include healthy oils (coconut, olive, flaxseed, and pumpkin seed)

o Avoid sugar, dairy, grains, folic acid–fortified foods, legumes/beans, charred foods, and alcohol

o Minimize plastic food and beverage containers and nonstick cookware

· · · · ·

TWO-WEEK MEAL PLAN

For those of you who prefer a scripted version, here are two weeks of meals that have been chosen by my team of nutritionists to meet all the daily targets included on the Cheat Sheet (recipes start on page 285).

	DAY 1	DAY 2	DAY 3
Breakfast	Berry Muesli	Salmon and Spinach Omelet	Matcha Coconut Crunch
Snack	Baked Spinach and Artichoke Dip + celery sticks Beet Bubbly	Sunflower and/or pumpkin seeds Beet Bubbly	Celery sticks Beet Bubbly
Lunch	Warm Salmon and Roasted Cauliflower Salad + side of steamed broccoli	Mix-and-Match Rainbow Salad + broccoli + chicken	Mix-and-Match Stir-Fry + protein of choice
Snack		Golden Turmeric Milk	Luscious Liver Pâté wrapped in cabbage
Dinner	Rosemary Chicken with Tomato, Avocado, and Bacon + side of arugula	Mediterranean Stuffed Pork Tenderloin with Green Beans + steamed snap peas	Not Your Mama's Burger with Kohlrabi Mash + Turmeric-Pickled Daikon
Dessert		Raspberry Cacao Truffles	

	DAY 8	DAY 9	DAY 10
Breakfast	Savory Onion and Chard Muffins + steamed mustard greens	Energy Boost Green Smoothie + No-Bake Golden Energy Balls	Berry Muesli
Snack	Broccoli + cauliflower florets + seeds Beet Bubbly	1 boiled egg with raw broccoli florets	Oolong tea

DAY 4	DAY 5	DAY 6	DAY 7
Blueberry Beet Scones	Matcha Coconut Crunch	Green Eggs and Shiitake Ham	Blueberry Beet Scones
Calming Herbal Tonic Soft boiled eggs + side of steamed kale	Luscious Liver Pâté with seed crackers + orange peppers Beet Bubbly	Sunflower seed butter + broccoli and radishes	Luscious Liver Pâté + carrot sticks
Mix-and-Match Rainbow Salad + chicken	Not Your Mama's Burger with Kohlrabi Mash + side of steamed spinach	Mix-and-Match Stir-Fry + protein of choice	Rosemary Chicken with Tomato, Avocado, and Bacon + side of spinach
Green or oolong tea	Beet Bubbly	Green or oolong tea	Green or oolong tea
Warm Salmon and Roasted Cauliflower Salad	Mix-and-Match Stir-Fry + leeks + chicken	Mediterranean Stuffed Pork Tenderloin with Green Beans + Oven-Baked Beet Chips	Mix-and-Match Stir-Fry + cauliflower + chicken
			Rosemary Lemon Tart + berries

DAY 11	DAY 12	DAY 13	DAY 14
Veggie-Wrap Breakfast Burrito	Energy Boost Green Smoothie + No-Bake Golden Energy Balls	Savory Onion and Chard Muffins + kale	Veggie-Wrap Breakfast Burrito
Luscious Liver Pâté + red peppers	2 hard-boiled eggs + celery	Sunflower and/or pumpkin seeds and Red Cabbage, Beet, and Pomegranate Slaw Beet Bubbly	Iced oolong tea

continues

continued

	DAY 8	DAY 9	DAY 10	
Lunch	Wild Mushroom Ragout	Mix-and-Match Rainbow Salad + protein of choice	Wild Mushroom Ragout + Swiss chard	
Snack	Berries and seeds	Oven-Baked Beet Chips and Luscious Liver Pâté	Red Cabbage, Beet, and Pomegranate Slaw	
Dinner	DNA Methylation Minestrone	Simple Pan-Fried Steak with "Creamed" Greens + zucchini	Mix-and-Match Stir-Fry + chicken + Beet Bubbly	
Dessert			No-Bake Sunbutter Chocolate Squares	

SAMPLE ONE-DAY VEGETARIAN/VEGAN MENU

To give you an idea of a vegan-friendly version of the Intensive, here is a meal plan that excludes animal protein and includes legumes.

Breakfast: Berry Muesli

Snack: No-Bake Golden Energy Balls + Oven-Baked Beet Chips

Lunch: Lemon Garlic Broccoli Rabe and White Bean Stew

Snack: Beet Bubbly; celery sticks with Baked Spinach and Artichoke Dip

Dinner: Crispy Garlicky Tempeh with Cauliflower Rice + side of steamed kale

TAKING THE YOUNGER YOU INTENSIVE ON THE ROAD

I'll tell you what: gone are the days when an indulgent meal with drinks at the airport appeal to me. I eat a modified Younger You Intensive most of the time and since I feel so good on it, it's pretty rare that I want to deviate, especially with the stress of travel. Further, I don't want my kiddo eating

DAY 11	DAY 12	DAY 13	DAY 14
Spiced Salmon Cakes with Vegetable Fries + side of spinach and cauliflower	Mix-and-Match Rainbow Salad + chicken	Cauliflower-Crust Pizza + side of arugula	Mix-and-Match Stir-Fry + beet + chicken
Sunflower and/or pumpkin seeds	Beet Bubbly		Sunflower and/or pumpkin seeds
Simple Pan-Fried Steak with "Creamed" Greens + Brussels sprouts	Spiced Salmon Cakes with Vegetable Fries + spinach and cauliflower	DNA Methylation Minestrone	Cauliflower-Crust Pizza + side of spinach
			Rosemary Lemon Tart

the airport food, either, so I love packing foods. That said, airports are more and more meeting consumer demand for healthier choices. Recently, Iz and I were at LaGuardia, and since she was being such a travel rock star, I said she could pick out some chocolate for the flight. Needless to say, I was pretty thrilled that she went straight for the stevia-sweetened Lily's.

While preparing your own meals at home is the easiest way to make sure you hit all your Younger You eating plan targets, it's not always possible. Also, I get that eight weeks is a long time. For some of us, it's rare that we're home for fifty-six days in a row, except perhaps while in the midst of a pandemic.

Before I dive into my best tips for staying on the program while traveling, I just want to say that taking a short trip and sticking to your eating plan is a great reward in itself—it helps you see how possible it is to eat differently even when conditions aren't wholly under your control. And if you typically come home from vacation feeling like you've put on a few pounds and need a vacation to recover from your vacation, you'll love feeling like you can seamlessly move back into your regular, healthy-eating ways without feeling like you need to make up lost ground! Here are some ways to keep yourself on track no matter where you are:

- Stock up on snacks before you go. (See the list that starts on page 157.)

- Check out a restaurant's menu online *before* you go. Generally, sticking to a protein entrée (chicken, fish, beef) with a nonstarchy vegetable side is a good bet, as is ordering a large salad, or even two salads. Also, roasted cruciferous veggies are a big thing right now and show up on most menus—order two servings and hit your numbers easily. Just remember that super-crispy stuff probably has advanced glycation end products, so eat them only occasionally. You can also call ahead to see what modifications are available.

- Bring a full glass water bottle with you wherever you go. If you are in a hotel with a gym, you can usually get unlimited filtered water there.

- Consider staying in accommodations that have a kitchen, whether that's an Airbnb or a residence-style hotel. While you *can* stick to the plan at restaurants, if you're eating multiple meals out a day, it gets harder to stay on course and easier to order the pasta.

- Bring an assortment of teas (green, hibiscus, oolong, chamomile) with you.

- Consider bringing some spices with you—especially rosemary and oregano—to add to the meals you prepare in your home away from home. I bring a jar of rosemary with a grinder top that my mom found for me at T.J. Maxx wherever I go—rosemary is tasty and super easy to add to pretty much anything.

- Find a grocery store near your lodgings to stock up on fresh, precut veggies, prepared beets, almond milk, etc. If you don't have a fridge, you can stock up on pumpkin and sunflower seeds and/or get cut veggies to snack on.

- Make muffins for your travel day (the Savory Onion and Chard Muffins on page 301 are great for this). Pack sunflower and/or pumpkin seeds; green apples and blood oranges also make great travel snacks as they aren't likely to get squashed in your bag, as do hard-boiled eggs or celery sticks and almond butter.

ONCE YOUR EIGHT WEEKS ARE UP

Truthfully, you can't expect the biological age reversal that we know the Younger You Intensive is capable of creating to last if you go back to old eating habits once these eight weeks are through.

In order to maintain the benefits these eight weeks create, you have two options:

1. **Keep going with the Younger You Intensive.** The Intensive eating plan is a wonderfully healthy way to eat all of the time—it doesn't carry any risks of developing nutritional deficiencies over the long term, as do some eating plans, such as keto.
2. **Stay true to the basic formula but loosen the reins a bit with the Younger You Everyday.** Once you're done with these first eight weeks, you can shift gears into the more lenient Younger You Everyday—a long-term maintenance plan that the patients we see in our clinic who don't require the Intensive for some reason are given.

The choice is yours.

If you stay with the Intensive version, you won't continue to tick younger and younger indefinitely (do you *want* to go back to your teen years??). You *will* position yourself to be the best, youngest you that you can be—staving off that sixteen-year drop. Quite honestly, we don't know what happens to bio age after more than eight weeks on the Intensive, because we haven't studied it . . . yet. We *will* be gathering data that we can analyze via the Younger You digital program (from those participants who explicitly choose to share their data with us). See page 426 for more information.

And if you decide to shift into the Everyday, while your bio age likely may not continue to trend downward, you will slow your rate of aging and avoid the accelerated aging that the typical American diet all but guarantees. If you choose the Everyday, know that you can, and should, return to the Intensive again and again. **I recommend recommitting to the Younger You Intensive at least once, and ideally twice, a year;** once at the start of winter and again at the start of summer.

Remember, the Younger You Intensive isn't just an eating plan—it also has lifestyle components that are key for DNA methylation optimization. Because I know the eating plan is a bit complex and, depending on what your diet was like before you started it, perhaps a big adjustment, I've kept the lifestyle recommendations as simple as possible, and the same as what we included in our study. There are also a few supplements that will help ensure you get the baseline of necessary nutrients. We'll cover all of those soon. First, let's look at the Younger You Everyday, so that you can decide which version of the program is the right one for you at this time.

6

THE YOUNGER YOU
EVERYDAY EATING PLAN

THE EVERYDAY VERSION OF THE YOUNGER YOU PROGRAM FOLLOWS the same formula as the Intensive—methyl donors + DNA methylation adaptogens + lifestyle practices—just at more doable levels and with a more inclusive list of allowed foods.

The Everyday is what we prescribe to many of the patients in our clinic who either don't need an Intensive intervention at this time or who *did* need an Intensive intervention and are now ready for an eating plan that will help them maintain the benefits they have achieved.

Where the Intensive is very specific and prescribed, the Everyday is more fluid. I think of it as a continuum, and your starting point and your goals will dictate exactly what it looks like for you. There are three primary paths to the Everyday that I see in our practice:

- **As a starting point.** It could be that you have been eating the standard American diet and want to take some baby steps toward improving your nutritional status and your health. In that case, you can start by following the list of swaps I include on page 154 and prioritizing the Dynamic Dozen foods I list starting on page 142. Even though it's just a few changes here and there, this introductory version of the

Everyday will provide your body with more of the nutrients it needs for balanced DNA methylation.

- **As a finishing point.** On the other end of the spectrum, maybe you've just finished up the Intensive, and you've adjusted to the diet and you'd like to retain all the benefits you've just created, but you'd also like to expand your diet to include legumes, a few grains, a little alcohol, and maybe a little organic dairy. If that's the case, start at Younger You Everyday: What's Different, on page 135. This is where most of our study participants ended up: they had adjusted to the high vegetable intake, and had learned to cook liver and eat beets, so they kept that going, but they also added a few more food options (and the occasional drink).

- **As a foundational eating plan.** Or maybe you're right in the middle. You want to make your diet healthier for you and your genes and slow your rate of aging without having to follow an eight-week protocol (or perhaps you're already on an eating plan for a particular condition or disease and are looking to cover your DNA methylation bases, too, by layering in principles of this program). If this is you, I've outlined a Cheat Sheet for the Everyday version for you that is essentially a "lite" version of the Intensive—eating four to five cups of green, cruciferous, or colorful veggies a day instead of the seven required on the Intensive, for example. You can see it on page 160.

No matter which approach you choose, when you couple it with the lifestyle strategies I share in Chapter 7 that are integral to both the Intensive and the Everyday, and the supplements I cover in Chapter 8, it can add up to a big impact on your DNA methylation—and, thus, your risk for disease and accelerated aging—over time.

There's only one note to consider here: We haven't yet studied the Younger You Everyday's affect on bio age. Thus it may not provide the quickest or most dramatic results on your biological age and overall health—the Younger You Intensive program does that. But the Everyday does make improved methylation easy to attain for everyone, no matter how busy you are or what your diet and lifestyle have been up until this point.

WHICH VERSION IS RIGHT FOR YOU?

THE YOUNGER YOU INTENSIVE DIET IS A BETTER FIRST STEP FOR YOU IF

○ You want to rapidly, powerfully turn back the biological hands of time through balancing your DNA methylation; because the Intensive is the jumpstart that gives quick results (maintain your results with the Everyday plan over the long term, which is what many of our study participants did—they kept their veggie intake high and kept eating beets and liver, but also added in some beans, grains, and/or alcohol).

○ You are dealing with a chronic condition or disease and want a fast-acting diet and lifestyle strategy to address the root cause of your issue.

○ You want to lower cholesterol and triglycerides, move into ketosis, lower blood sugar, and/or lose weight (if needed).

○ You want to turn off pro-aging inflammation ("inflammaging") while boosting immune resilience.

○ You want to improve folate status without folate supplements.

○ You want to lower homocysteine and improve inflammatory markers without relying on methyl donor supplements, as our patients have done.

○ You've got gut dysbiosis, leaky gut, or food allergies/intolerances or sensitivities; because the Intensive removes most common allergens (except for nuts and eggs) and provides plenty of fiber to improve digestion and nourish your friendly microbes, it will give your gut a chance to heal while simultaneously bolstering DNA methylation.

THE YOUNGER YOU EVERYDAY VERSION IS BETTER FOR YOU IF

○ You want simple ways to upgrade your health without having to completely overhaul your diet.

○ You've already done the Younger You Intensive and want to keep your benefits going while also giving yourself more dietary choices.

○ You want a gentle transition into the Intensive, as the Everyday makes it easy to start by making basic swaps to get more DNA methylation–supportive nutrients into your diet and take some of the DNA methylation-harming nutrients out. Once you've made some changes in your typical eating pattern, following the Intensive guidelines won't feel as intense.

○ You want to upgrade your already pretty healthy diet so that it is geared toward optimizing DNA methylation but are not overly concerned about making significant reductions in your bio age; rather, you're looking for a foundational diet that you follow the majority of the time.

Remember that both the Everyday and Intensive dietary patterns readily layer into any program you're already doing.

· · · · ·

YOUNGER YOU INTENSIVE VS. YOUNGER YOU EVERYDAY AT A GLANCE

	YOUNGER YOU INTENSIVE	**YOUNGER YOU EVERYDAY**
Primary goal	Reversed biological age	May slow the rate of aging down, but not necessarily reversing it
Macronutrient ratios	Fat 45–50% / Carbs 30–35% / Protein 15–20%	Fat 40–45% / Carbs 35–40% / Protein 15–20%
Green, cruciferous, and colorful veggies	7 cups a day	4–5 cups a day
Clean animal protein (unless vegetarian or vegan)	Two 3–4-ounce servings per day (unless you're over sixty or weigh more than 175 pounds, then two 5–6-ounce servings per day)	Two 3–4-ounce servings per day (unless you're over sixty or weigh more than 175 pounds, then two 5–6-ounce servings per day)
Eggs (unless vegan)	5–10 a week (aim for 10 if you're not eating liver)	5–10 a week (aim for 10 if you're not eating liver)
Liver (unless vegetarian or vegan)	Three 3-ounce servings per week	One 3-ounce serving per week

Beans and legumes	None (unless vegetarian or vegan, then enough to meet your 40–50 grams of protein daily requirement—protein powder can also help you meet this target)	One to two ½-cup servings per day, preferably soaked or soaked and sprouted (unless vegetarian or vegan, then enough to meet your 40–50 grams of protein daily requirement—protein powder can also help you meet this target)
Organic dairy	None	If tolerated, up to two servings per day (serving sizes vary)
Healthy fats	At least 5 tablespoons per day	At least 3 tablespoons per day
Grains	None	Up to ½ cup per day
Nuts and seeds	Up to ½ cup of nuts per day ¼ cup each of sunflower and pumpkin seeds per day	Up to ½ cup of nuts per day 2 tablespoons each of sunflower and pumpkin seeds per day
Beets	1–2 medium beets per day	3 medium beets per week
DNA methylation adaptogens	Two-plus servings per day	One-plus servings per day
Hydration	Half your body weight in ounces of water, herbal tea, or seltzer (limit to 2 glasses per day)	Half your body weight in ounces of water, herbal tea, or seltzer (limit to 2 glasses per day)
Coffee	No more than 2 cups, before noon, no dairy or sweeteners	No more than 2 cups, before noon; adding a little organic cream, half-and-half, or natural sweeteners is OK
Alcohol	None	Max one drink per day (5 ounces wine, 12 ounces beer, or 1½ ounces spirits)
Intermittent fasting	Go twelve hours between your final meal of the day and the first meal of the next day—typically this means 7 p.m. to 7 a.m., but you can adjust to your sleep and wake cycle	Go twelve hours between your final meal of the day and the first meal of the next day—typically this means 7 p.m. to 7 a.m., but you can adjust to your sleep and wake cycle

YOUNGER YOU EVERYDAY: WHAT'S DIFFERENT

In general, the Younger You Everyday is a pretty even mix of low-glycemic carbs; protein from nuts, seeds, beans, legumes, and clean animal sources; and healthy fats. It has a higher level of carbs in total than the Intensive version, with more of those carbs coming from certain grains (nongluten and non-folic-acid-fortified), and beans and legumes lend some extra carbs to the eating plan in addition to protein.

Like the Younger You Intensive, the Everyday version still relies on green, cruciferous, and/or colorful vegetables, clean animal protein, healthy fats, nuts and seeds, lots of fresh herbs and spices, and plenty of hydration. (See the "What to Eat [and Avoid]" list in the previous chapter, page 104, for choices in all these categories.) But there are categories of foods that are part of the Everyday eating plan that aren't included in the Intensive version—beans and legumes, grains, and dairy, as well as *very* moderate amounts of natural sugars and alcohol. Here's more about each of those.

Beans

Beans are wildly nutritious, and people who live a long time generally eat beans. They're rich in many methylation-related nutrients including magnesium, potassium, folate, choline, and sulfur compounds, as well as a great source of fiber, which supports a happy and healthy microbiome.

The only reason beans and legumes aren't on the Intensive (for everyone except vegans and vegetarians) is that they are higher in nonfiber carbs and may, in some, promote insulin resistance. In addition, many folks have a hard time digesting them—although soaking helps with digestibility, which is why I strongly suggest that you soak or even sprout beans before eating them. (See page 402 for instructions.) And for a very small subset of folks, beans might prompt inflammation because they have high levels of lectin—a phytochemical that impedes the bioavailability of nutrients and can irritate the digestive tract. The beans on the Everyday plan include:

Adzuki beans	Fava beans	Red beans
Black beans	Great northern	Red lentils
Black lentils	beans	Soy (see the
Black-eyed peas	Green lentils	next page for
Brown lentils	Kidney beans	guidelines on
Cannellini beans	Mung beans	eating soy)
Chickpeas/	Navy beans	Split peas
Garbanzo beans	Pinto beans	Turtle beans

Note: Eden brand soaks their beans, then pressure cooks them in their cans and even adds a bit of the sea vegetable kombu to improve digestibility. If you don't have time for soaking, seek out this brand, which is available at most grocery stores.

THINGS TO KEEP IN MIND WHEN EATING SOY

I KNOW SOY HAS GOTTEN A BAD RAP FOR ITS LECTIN CONTENT, POTENTIAL negative estrogenic effects, and for the genetically modified soy that abounds in processed foods. However, we also know that

o Soy isoflavones genistein, diadzien, and equol are potently and beneficially epigenetically active.
o Equol is protective against dementia.
o Soy consumption is associated with a protective effect against breast cancer (perhaps in part because of the isoflavones' beneficial effect on demethylating tumor-suppressor genes).
o Dr. Randall Jirtle demonstrated that genistein eliminated the toxic effect of in utero BPA exposure on agouti mice offspring (by acting like a methyl donor).
o The modest estrogenic effect is helpful for women in perimenopause.
o Soy is helpful for bone health.
o It's also a good source of protein.

My read on the literature is that, correctly chosen, soy is a smart food.

When opting to eat soy, make sure that it is organic, as most conventional soy is genetically modified and highly contaminated with pesticides, and preferably fermented—which includes varieties such as tempeh, miso, tamari, natto, and pickled tofu—as fermentation makes the nutrients in soy more bioavailable.

· · · · ·

Grains

When chosen carefully, whole grains can be a valuable source of magnesium and B vitamins, which are important for DNA methylation, and chromium, which improves blood sugar management. Some grains, such as oats, provide sulfur, which is important in the methylation cycle and our antioxidant and detoxification systems. Whole grains are also an excellent source of fiber, which, again, is great for your microbiome.

That being said, there are two types of grains I recommend greatly minimizing (or even avoiding altogether if you can)—those that contain gluten, and those that are fortified with folic acid. So many people don't tolerate gluten well, and the incidence of celiac disease—an autoimmune condition that can be triggered by gluten—has been increasing 7.5 percent a year for the last several decades according to a 2020 review of eighty-six studies (rates are higher for women and children than men).[1] And I covered the danger in over-consuming folic acid (the synthetic form of folate) on page 54.

Another very important reason to minimize grain consumption—or at least approach it carefully—is that for many of us (myself included) grains can aggressively spike blood sugar, especially processed grains such as wheat flour. Finally, grains do contain lectins, and if you've determined yourself to be sensitive to these antinutrients, you'll want to take care in consuming them.

GRAINS TO PRIORITIZE

Amaranth	Rice (basmati, bran, brown, wild)
Buckwheat (technically a seed)	Rye (particularly dark rye)
Millet	Sorghum
Oats (look for gluten-free oats)	Tapioca
Quinoa (technically a seed)	Teff

GRAINS TO MINIMIZE/AVOID

Barley	Spelt
Bulgur	Wheat
Kamut	

You can also soak your grains before cooking to improve their digestibility and nutrient bioavailability (I share soaking instructions on page 402).

GREAT ALTERNATIVES TO TYPICAL GRAIN PRODUCTS

Pasta made from red lentils, chickpeas, or mung beans (a huge favorite for kids, including mine)

Shirataki noodles (made from the konjac plant)

Almond flour

Coconut flour

Cassava flour

Arrowroot flour

Tapioca flour

Paleo baking flour (generally a mix of almond, coconut, and cassava flours and tapioca starch)

• • • • •

Dairy

Dairy from cows, sheep, and goats can be a great source of methylation nutrients, especially methionine and B_{12}. Other nutrients in fairly good amounts include protein, calcium, phosphorus, selenium, and zinc. Butyrate is a very important short-chain fatty acid found in dairy. Also, most dairy sold in the United States is fortified with D_3 and vitamin A (as palmitate). However, you do want to keep your dairy consumption fairly low, organic, and rbGH-free, and consider leaning on goat or sheep sources, which are easier to digest and are generally less inflammatory. The casein family of proteins found in all dairy sources is problematic for many individuals. In our practice, we see a lot of instances of dairy allergy or sensitivity, which contributes to everything from eczema to migraine and inflammatory arthritis. And the milk sugar lactose is frequently a cause of gas and bloating in individuals with genetic lactase (the enzyme that digests lactose) deficiency or acquired lactase deficiency, as commonly seen in adult-onset irritable bowel syndrome (IBS) or small intestinal bacterial overgrowth (SIBO). Anecdotally, some patients in our clinic report dairy consumption on a low-carbohydrate diet contributes to weight-loss resistance and/or difficulty getting into ketosis.

The form of dairy I feel the least conflicted about recommending is ghee, a form of butter that has been clarified to remove the dairy proteins (including the problematic casein). This renders it very hypoallergenic and most often well tolerated even by people who are sensitive to dairy. It is also a good source of butyrate, which nourishes cells in your digestive tract and directly modulates genetic methylation to favorably alter gene expression. (Clinically, we have not seen ghee inhibit ketosis or contribute to weight-loss resistance.)

If you tolerate dairy, stick to moderate amounts (no more than two 1-tablespoon servings per day, unless otherwise noted below) of the following dairy products:

Butter

Cottage cheese (¼ cup)

Cream

Ghee

Goat cheese

Gruyère cheese

Kefir

Milk (½ cup)

Parmigiano-Reggiano cheese

Romano cheese

Yogurt (unsweetened, ¼ cup)

Sweeteners

In general, sweeteners of any kind aren't great for health because they raise inflammation and drive oxidative stress that can cause injury at the molecular and cellular level and contribute to the development of long-term diseases. That's why there are no added sweeteners included on the Younger You Intensive.

Since the Everyday is designed to be more doable, even something you can stick to over the long term, you can have small amounts of natural sweeteners, listed below. Just keep it to no more than 1 teaspoon at a time, and no more than twice per day. For some people, the sugar alcohols erythritol and xylitol cause gas and bloating; if this is your experience, avoid these noncaloric sweeteners.

Blackstrap molasses

Cane sugar, unrefined

Cocoa (70%+ dark, not Dutch processed)

Erythritol (a few drops)

Honey

Maple syrup

Monk fruit

Stevia (a few drops)

Xylitol (a few drops, and keep it away from pets as it's toxic to dogs)

(A Little) Alcohol

When you're on the Younger You Intensive, alcohol really is a no-no, as it's known to deplete methylation reserves and interfere with healthy epigenetic methylation patterns. However, this is the Everyday version. And everyday is real life. I don't expect you to never have a drink again unless that's the choice that makes the most sense for you.

If you do consume alcohol, keep it to a minimum. This means no more than one alcoholic drink per day for women and men. If you can drink less, or none at all, that's even better, because drinking alcohol does directly inhibit the methylation cycle, but I understand that we live in the real world.

For clarity's sake, one alcoholic drink is equivalent to five ounces of wine, twelve ounces of beer, or one and a half ounces of spirits. When you imbibe, I suggest drinking organic or biodynamic wine so that you minimize pesticide exposure (just as you would when selecting a food to eat). Red wine contains a small amount of resveratrol, an antioxidant *and* a DNA methylation adaptogen, but don't let this fact convince you that your red wine is a health food—many other foods contain significantly more resveratrol; see page 411 in the Nutrient Reference for a list. Or enjoy a grain-free spirit such as vodka or tequila, because they are low carb and, thus, take less of a toll on your body to metabolize because they don't spike your blood sugar the same way, say, a beer does. Obviously, most beer contains gluten. In the best of all worlds, if you are a devoted beer drinker, you'll find a beer you like that doesn't contain it.

And when you have those drinks, I suggest counterbalancing that DNA methylation inhibition with a super methylation-supportive snack or meal either before (a snack of sunflower and pumpkin seeds), during (a big helping of greens with dinner), and/or the next morning (a blueberry smoothie).

Intermittent Fasting

Because the intermittent fasting portion of the Younger You Intensive is so moderate and doable, I recommend you continue it on the Everyday version, as well. To refresh your memory, that means finishing up your last meal at 7 p.m. and then not eating again until 7 a.m. the next morning. If you are more of a night owl, you can push both of these times back to one that suits you better, making sure to finish eating at least three hours before bed. If you are already regularly going longer than twelve hours overnight without eating, that is fine. Keep it up.

Foods to Continue to Avoid

Charred/fried/grilled foods
Artificial sweeteners
Added sugars (except for those few exceptions I just listed)

And although these aren't foods, per se, they influence the chemical content of your food and beverages, so avoid these too: plastic food storage containers, plastic water bottles, and nonstick pans (more on this in Chapter 7).

You also want to continue to eat organic as much as you possibly can.

MEET THE DNA METHYLATION SUPERFOODS, AKA THE DYNAMIC DOZEN

I find it's more helpful to focus on what you *can* eat instead of what you *can't*. So allow me to introduce you to what I affectionately call the Dynamic Dozen. These are the top twelve foods that get your DNA methylation machinery humming. Some of them will be familiar to you, some you may love, and some, honestly, you may question. (I mean, I get that liver isn't exactly a popular food.) But when you learn why these foods are so powerful — and try our recipes that incorporate them — I think you, too, will be a fan, and you'll be inspired to weave these foods into your regular rotation.

Just know that, in addition to being DNA methylation superstars, the foods in the Dynamic Dozen are what's known as *pleiotropic*, which is a fancy way of saying they do lots of good things. (In Greek, *pleio* means many and *tropic* means effects. Pleiotropic is most often used to describe single genes that influence multiple biological characteristics; I use it here to refer to one compound or food having a broad array of benefits.) They're anti-inflammatory, anticancer, and in many cases, antiviral. And remember, some of them are both methyl donor and DNA methylation adaptogens (especially cruciferous vegetables), meaning they offer double the benefits to bio age.

There are of course *many* other DNA methylation–rock star foods, so don't stop with just these twelve! See page 407 for the full list.

#1: Green Tea
DNA methylation adaptogen
In addition to being a beneficial anti-aging player via a variety of ways, green tea is anti-inflammatory, antioxidant, anticancer, and neuropro-tective (to name a few). I am sure some of these important mechanisms of green tea are enacted via epigenome regulation. Many of the world's longest-lived humans are avid, daily green tea drinkers.

You probably have heard that green tea is healthier than black tea. While they are both made from leaves of the same plant, *Camellia sinensis*, black tea leaves are exposed to the air and allowed to oxidize and turn darker in order to intensify their flavor. Green tea leaves are protected from exposure to the air; that's why they are much lighter in color. This difference in process leads to different nutrient profiles. While both black and green tea are high in the antioxidants known as flavonoids (which are a subgroup of the category of antioxidants known as polyphenols), green tea is significantly higher in a handful of important flavonoids epigallocatechin-3-gallate (EGCG), which is a powerful DNA methylation adaptogen. Green tea is also lower in caffeine than black tea and less dehydrating.

How to consume it: Of course, you can brew tea out of green tea. To get the maximum amount of EGCG, let it steep for ten minutes in hot water that has just kissed the boiling point (this provides about 100 mg EGCG per cup, although, be warned, it will intensify the taste; if steeping this long makes green tea unpalatable to you, steep it as long as you can and still find it drinkable). Matcha is a powdered form of green tea, and you can also make tea out of it, or a delicious Matcha Latte (page 387), or use it in your cooking. Check out our recipe for Matcha Coconut Crunch on page 293—it is truly a delicious way to get not just your EGCG but also other superfoods such as seeds, all in one bowl (or handful—it's good enough to eat straight!). And the Matcha Gummies on page 374 make EGCG's goodness extremely portable and palatable if you don't want to drink an entire cup.

Alternatives: White tea, oolong tea, and black tea, which have varying amounts of EGCG (although less than green tea does); other EGCG sources are listed on page 409 in the Nutrient Reference.

#2: Turmeric

DNA methylation adaptogen

Known as the "king of spices," turmeric has many potent effects on your biochemistry and your health, including preventing cancer as well as neurological and inflammatory diseases.[2] Of course, I am most excited about its impressive ability to modulate genetic expression by changing levels of DNA methylation, which is a primary way that turmeric exerts its powerful effects.

A constituent of turmeric is curcumin, which is a powerful DNA methylation adaptogen. In cell studies, curcumin looks to be able to both add *and* reverse excess or erroneous methylation marks on your DNA, like the clean-up crew for life's inevitable biochemical messes. While turmeric's bright yellow color may stain your fingers and your cookware, it's worth the potential cleaning mishaps.

How to eat it: You can buy turmeric fresh—it looks a lot like fresh ginger, only smaller, and is often found in the produce section of the grocery store. You can also buy it powdered, but if you choose this option, spring for organic. Some conventional brands add things like lead (seriously) to keep it looking bright yellow, and it's not the color that's beneficial, it's the curcumin. You don't want your DNA methylation superfood to expose you to toxic metals, right? You can add turmeric to eggs, salad dressings, stir fries, soups, and stews (my favorite is our Creamy Coconut Curry recipe on page 342), or even make a tasty beverage out of it—see page 386 for our Golden Turmeric Milk recipe (I drink it almost every day!). Just be sure to have it with a little healthy fat and freshly ground black pepper, which makes the curcumin more readily used by your body.

Alternative: Curry powder

#3: Blueberries

DNA methylation adaptogen

Blueberries are rich sources of DNA methylation adaptogens, including anthocyanins, chlorogenic acid, ellagic acid, and quercetin. Plus, they're sweet while still being low-sugar and low-glycemic, making them a natural fit on the Younger You program.

How to eat them: Luckily most berries aren't a hard sell—they are delicious on their own, especially when they are in season, and you can eat up to one cup of them per day (and more if your blood sugar isn't impacted by them; less if it is). When they're not in season, frozen wild or organic versions are great additions to smoothies and Younger You–approved grain-free baked goods, like the Blueberry Beet Scones on page 305. I also throw fresh or frozen blueberries in glasses of water or on my salad. Whenever possible, choose wild berries, as they typically have higher levels of DNA methylation adaptogens than their cultivated counterparts.

Alternatives: Blackberries, black currants, raspberries, and strawberries are all rich in DNA methylation adaptogens, too.

#4: Rosemary

DNA methylation adaptogen

Rosemary is a stealth contender in the health-food world—it doesn't get near the attention that turmeric, garlic, or ginger do, but it's definitely worthy of your adoration and a place in your daily diet. Rosemary is a potent antioxidant and anti-inflammatory, it's anticancer and provides neuroprotection (boosting memory and cognitive performance) and pain relief.[3] It's even been shown to be as effective as minoxidil (aka Rogaine) in regrowing hair.[4] But most importantly for our purposes, it's a powerhouse DNA methylation adaptogen, thanks to abundant amounts of rosmarinic acid and ursolic acid, among others. It's also super easy to grow on a patio (although more challenging to keep alive on a windowsill, at least in my experience). Choose fresh rosemary or dried whole-leaf rosemary that you chop or grind just before using, as they have significantly higher levels of rosemarinic acid than powdered dried rosemary.

How to eat it: Rosemary goes with so many things—roasted vegetables, soups, meat dishes, soups, stews. If you don't like its woody texture you can put it in one of those spice containers that has a built-in grinder. You can also buy one with black peppercorns or sea salt in it and add a little rosemary, as the piperine present in freshly ground pepper may help the rosmarinic acid be better absorbed. You can also brew a tea with it by steeping two teaspoons of the whole leaves (whether dried or fresh) in hot water, then garnishing with a squeeze of fresh lemon or orange. Or try my favorite Rosemary Lemon Tart for a "legal" sweet way to enjoy it (page 382)!

Alternatives: Peppermint, spearmint, sage, thyme, lemon thyme, and oregano are also good sources of rosmarinic acid.

#5: Cruciferous Vegetables

Methyl donors and DNA methylation adaptogens

Cruciferous vegetables are rich sources of sulfur-containing compounds known as glucosinolates (maca is another source). Once ingested, glucosinolates are metabolized by your digestion and your gut microbes into other compounds, including indoles, thiocyanates, and isothiocyanates. These biologically active derivatives are known to prevent cancer, reduce inflammation, turn on our body's antioxidant system, balance our microbiome (they're antimicrobial), improve estrogen metabolism (important for men as well as women), and support detoxification. One isothiocyanate getting a lot of attention in the epigenetic world is sulforaphane. In addition to the benefits of isothiocyanates, sulforaphane is a powerful DNA methylation adaptogen that has been shown to support epigenetic changes that are potently anticancer, anti-inflammatory, and neuroprotective.[5,6]

Thanks to glucosinolates' tremendous beneficial influence on the epigenome overall, not just DNA methylation, the Younger You program prescribes eating a lot of them. For comparison, the USDA suggests eating four cups of cruciferous vegetables *per week*.[7] On the Younger You Everyday, you'll be eating two cups *per day*. (If that sounds like a lot, consider that's measured raw, not cooked, and lightly packed.)

How to eat them: Highly versatile, cruciferous vegetables are equally great eaten raw, roasted, or sautéed.

Examples: arugula, bok choy, broccoli, broccoli rabe, Brussels sprouts, cabbage, cauliflower, collard greens, daikon radish, horseradish, kale, kohl-rabi, radish, rutabaga, turnip greens, turnips, wasabi, and watercress

#6: Beets
Methyl donor

Beets get a bad rap, but they are so loveable. Not only for their sweet earthy taste, but also, and especially, for one specific phytonutrient they contain: betaine. This important methyl donor plays a big role in keeping the methylation cycle humming (fundamental for DNA methylation fitness). Beets are also high in vitamin C (a DNA methylation adaptogen), fiber, potassium (needed in the methylation cycle, too), protein, folate (another methyl donor), and manganese. They help lower blood pressure, fight cancer, and support detoxification. They are smart for so many reasons!

On the Younger You Everyday, I advise eating a minimum of three medium beets per week. While red beets are the most widely available, all beet varieties (such as golden beets) have unique polyphenol profiles that contribute to their lovely colors. It's my recommendation that you eat a variety of different types of beets, as you're able to source them. And if you can't stomach eating any variety of beet regularly, opt for a beet supplement (see page 434). (True story: red beets will also turn your poop bright red, which can be startling, I admit, but a good way to gauge how long it takes for your body to digest and eliminate a meal.)

And while I'm selling you on beets, I can't neglect raving about beet greens! Don't throw these out: they are chock-full of antioxidants and nu-trients, with more iron than spinach and loads of protein, phosphorus, zinc, fiber, vitamin A, vitamin C, and calcium.

How to consume them: Beets are great roasted or boiled and eaten ei-ther on their own or in salads. They're also good grated, raw, and used in slaws or even folded into burgers (see our Not Your Mama's Burger on page 349). You can also get betaine by drinking beet juice, which is a great addition to seltzer or sparkling water (see the Beet Bubbly on page 388), or even to our Blueberry Beet Scones (recipe on page 305). Isabella and I both love them boiled, peeled, and drizzled with a little olive oil (or half extra-virgin olive oil, half MCT oil) and balsamic. As for those beet greens, you can use them instead of spinach in many recipes or stir-fry them with olive oil, garlic, and salt; you can also add them to smoothies.

Alternatives: Quinoa, spinach, and lambsquarters are also excellent sources of betaine.

#7: Eggs

Methyl donor

Once considered the "bad egg" of the nutrition world, the humble egg—especially a pastured, organic, and omega-3-enriched egg—is a DNA methylation darling because it is arguably the best food source of choline. And choline is a vital methyl donor (in addition to brain food, mood food, liver food, pregnancy food, and so on), albeit one that works in a bit of a backdoor way. Choline is tough for your body to make and sucks up S-adenosylmethionine (SAMe), the universal methyl donor that donates the methyl groups that get laid down on the genome, along the way. Indeed, choline is considered "conditionally essential" because it is so hard to make and pretty much no one eats enough in their diet. So if you supply the body with choline through food, you preserve SAMe, and in so doing, you plug up a hole in the methylation process, leaving yourself more SAMe available for DNA methylation.

On both the Younger You Intensive and Everyday, we suggest eating a range of between five and ten eggs per week. You can go on the lower end of that spectrum if you're willing to eat liver (the other primary source of choline) once or twice a week. If liver is just a no-go for you—although I truly do believe our Luscious Liver Pâté recipe (page 326) can convert most nay-sayers—then you can double up on your weekly eggs. That being said, eggs *are* a common allergen. And of course, vegans don't eat them. I list some alternative sources of choline below.

How to eat them: Poaching is the healthiest way to prepare an egg. Aside from the standard directives to hard boil, scramble, or fry eggs, my best advice is to eat them with other members of the DNA methylation Dynamic Dozen—add a teaspoon of turmeric to scrambled eggs, sauté greens in the same pan, or try our Green Eggs and Shiitake Ham (recipe on page 297). You can also pop a hard-boiled egg on a salad, or eat it on its own as a snack.

Alternatives: Grass-fed beef, wild salmon. Plant-based sources of choline include: soybeans (must be organic), lentils, cauliflower, Brussels sprouts, broccoli, shiitake, and flax seeds. If you are a woman who's considering pregnancy, you need choline (the recommended daily intake for pregnant women is 450 mg and 550 mg for lactating women—likely more than you're eating, especially if you are vegan); while the foods listed above do indeed provide some choline, supplementation might be appropriate for you (see pages 213 and 220 for more information).

#8: Organic Liver

Methyl donor

Liver is such an astonishing powerhouse source of methylation-friendly nutrients, I really should have put it in the number-one spot on this list. If everything else here is one of the Supremes, liver is Diana Ross. But I know I would probably scare you off if I did that. I get that liver is not exactly popular, and that perhaps right about now you're envisioning the liver and onions your mom or grandma used to try to force on you as a kid. But please, hear me out. *No other food matches liver's broad-spectrum methylation support.* It provides a surprisingly high amount of natural folate and B_{12} (more than a day's supply), other B vitamins, betaine, choline (almost a full day's supply), methionine and cysteine (which is converted back to methionine or into our body's chief antioxidant, glutathione), as well as zinc. Every single one of these nutrients supports the methylation cycle. Additionally, liver has a lot of preformed vitamin A (which is important for DNA demethylation). There are, however, two caveats with liver: 1. If you have been diagnosed with too much iron, don't eat it, as it is rich in iron; 2. It is a detox organ, so you always want to choose organic and/or grass-fed (for beef liver). And if you can't find clean liver, I recommend using liver capsules instead (see page 433).

How to eat it: I really think our Luscious Liver Pâté (page 326) will make a liver believer out of you! Otherwise, you can add it to soup (see our DNA Methylation Minestrone, page 355) or mix a little bit of it into hamburgers, meatballs, or meatloaf. You can also stick to chicken, lamb, or calf liver, which typically have a milder flavor than beef liver. I grew up eating liverwurst and still like it with mayo (I hold off on the bread). Ron, the study participant I mentioned earlier who is still eating his daily seven cups of vegetables, swears by breading chicken livers in a little paleo flour that's been seasoned with paprika and garlic powder and pan-frying them—he calls them "the new chicken fingers." I understand that liver can be a struggle. Just know that any amount of it that you eat is a win.

Alternatives: The nutrient density of liver requires that you double down on all of the other Younger You super nutrients if you are going to avoid it. Plan B: consider taking liver in supplement form (see Resources for our suggestions).

#9: Seeds

Methyl donors

Pumpkin seeds and sunflower seeds are powerhouses of DNA methylation, since they are rich in zinc, methionine, cysteine, magnesium, potassium, B_3, B_6, folate, and betaine. They're also great sources of polyunsaturated fatty acids. On the Younger You Everyday, you'll be eating one tablespoon each of pumpkin seeds and sunflower seeds every day, which is surprisingly easy to do.

How to eat them: Seeds are a great addition to salads. You can also eat them by the handful, or try them in a blend (see our Cinnamon Nut Crunch, page 371). For a different texture, you can also use sunflower seed or pumpkin seed butter, which are just like peanut butter. There are quite a few different brands on the market, and some contain sugars or added oils, so make sure to look for one that only contains seeds and salt. You can also easily make them at home with a little time and a food processor. Go for raw rather than roasted whenever possible.

Alternatives: Sesame seeds and tahini also pack a DNA methylation wallop.

#10: Salmon

Methyl donor

Oh salmon, how do I love thee? Let me count the ways. You are a great source of the omega-3 essential fatty acids DHA and EPA, and DHA helps indirectly to regulate the methylation cycle. You also deliver healthy amounts of vitamins D and A, which modulate the function of enzymes involved in both methylation and demethylation. You are also an excellent source of the methyl donor B_{12} (with a massive 236 percent of recommended daily intake!), as well as other important methylation nutrients choline, zinc, magnesium, and potassium. *Plus* you offer selenium, biotin, niacin, iodine, and phosphorous. This potent cocktail of nutrients makes the omega-3s more bioavailable, meaning that eating salmon is more effective at elevating levels of DHA and EPA than taking fish-oil supplements (as fish oil typically only contains omega-3s, other fats, and some vitamin A and D).

While wild caught salmon is great, I'm also a fan of very cleanly sourced, humanely raised farmed salmon, of which some varieties have more omega-3s than wild caught. (Note that organic fish farming is not yet regulated by the FDA, so if you're buying "organic" I suggest carefully reviewing just what the producer is doing to make sure it is indeed organic and regulated by a reputable certification body.) Correctly raised farmed salmon has an abundance of good nutrients and is very low in toxins. I regularly eat super-clean farmed salmon that I buy at Whole Foods (Izzy loves it as much as I do). It tastes great, and most importantly the standards used in raising the salmon are humane and the diet is very clean. In addition, the nutrient levels are verified by a third party.

How to eat it: Salmon is so darn easy to cook—just sprinkle with a little salt and pepper and sauté in a small amount of avocado oil until opaque throughout. It goes great with greens (I think you'll find most things go great with greens!). If you want a little more flavor variety, try the Spiced Salmon Cakes with Vegetable Fries on page 337.

Alternatives: Whitefish, roe, and oysters are other DNA methylation superfoods from the sea. If you are vegetarian or vegan, get omega-3s from flax and chia seeds and walnuts; you may also want to consider supplementing with DHA- and EPA-containing algae. I assure you, these fatty acids are *that* important.

#11: Shiitake Mushrooms

Methyl donor and DNA methylation adaptogen

Shiitakes offer a winning combo for supporting DNA methylation. They modulate the activity of enzymes involved in methylation and have been shown to reduce excess levels of homocysteine.[8] They are also a good source of the methyl donors folate and choline; plus vitamins D, B_2, B_3 and B_6. And they act as a DNA methylation adaptogen. Good sources of zinc and potassium, shiitakes are also packed full of polysaccharides called beta glucans. These are anti-inflammatory, antioxidant, and immune rejuvenating.

I realize mushrooms can be a hard sell for some folks—I think shiitakes are the least "mushroomy" mushrooms, especially when you sauté them until they are just barely golden brown, with a little salt and a splash of coconut aminos (see page 404 in the Nutrient Reference for more about this savory ingredient). Cooked this way, they almost taste like bacon, with a great savory flavor that perfectly embodies the so-called fifth taste known as umami.

How to eat them: Sauté them and add them to salads, soups, scrambled eggs and frittatas, stir-fries, and curries.

Alternatives: Other forms of mushrooms show up in multiple places on the Nutrient Reference that starts on page 407—enoki and reishi, for example—so experiment with those if you are so inclined. Supplementing with shiitake is a reasonable alternative; it can be taken as powder or in capsules. Dried mushrooms have been used for centuries in traditional Chinese medicine. Just make sure you're buying a pure, organic product that has been standardized for beta glucans concentration and clearly states that on the label. I generally avoid products with the term "mycelium" in the ingredient list—it should say "fruiting body" on the label.

#12: Spinach

Methyl donor

Really, all dark leafy greens are methylation superstars, but I'm calling out spinach on this list because it has a mild taste that blends well with other flavors, making it a great starter green. All greens are rich sources of folate and betaine, which are methyl donors, and they're terrific sources of minerals, including iron, calcium, and magnesium. For the Younger You Everyday, you'll be eating one cup of dark leafy greens per day. But consider that two cups of raw greens cooks down to about one-third of a cup—you can totally do this. (Also, I include a list of ways to make sure you get your daily veggie allotment on page 109.)

How to eat it: Sautéed with a bunch of garlic; steamed and sprinkled with lemon juice; torn up and thrown into smoothies, soups, stews, stir-fries, and curries; or raw with a dressing made of healthy fats.

Alternatives: kale, Swiss chard, collard greens, dandelion greens, mustard greens, beet greens—or my favorite, broccoli rabe

FOOD SWAPS FOR HEALTHIER DNA METHYLATION

I've seen the power of even baby steps in improving diet make a huge difference in symptoms and overall well-being. One patient, Terri, a woman in midlife, had arthritis, hives, and complained of having gained weight that she couldn't lose. Although I suggested she meet with a nutritionist to develop a personalized eating plan, she didn't keep the appointment and didn't follow the Everyday dietary guidelines very well. But she did stop eating between 7 p.m. and 7 a.m., and she switched as many of her foods to organic as she could. Her pain and her hives both improved considerably, and she even lost a little bit of weight, without making any other changes. Best of all, she raved about how much better she felt. While I love to see patients make huge strides and adopt a top-notch diet, the truth is, not everyone is motivated to do so. Yet even small steps can truly add up.

Many of my patients find the easiest way to start making changes to their diet is to swap out things they're already consuming with something that packs more of a DNA methylation punch. The following fifteen swaps will go a long way toward bathing your genes in the ingredients they need for optimal expression and making sure that they are methylated in just the right amounts (not too much or too little). Copy this chart and stick it on your fridge for an easy reminder!

SWAP OUT	FOR
Coffee or black tea	Green tea or oolong tea
Bananas	Berries—especially blueberries, raspberries, and strawberries
Potatoes	Beets, kohlrabi, carrots, or sweet potatoes
Typical hamburgers	Grass-fed burgers, wild salmon burgers
Vegetable oil, soybean oil, cottonseed oil, canola oil, grapeseed oil, safflower oil (for cooking)	Avocado oil, coconut oil, MCT oil
Regular olive oil	Organic extra-virgin olive oil—bonus points for rosemary infused—only for drizzling on salads or cooked foods, not for cooking
Potato chips and other bagged snacks	Roasted beet chips, roasted chickpeas, seaweed snacks, kale chips, plantain chips, sunflower seeds, or pumpkin seeds
Hot chocolate	Turmeric-rich golden milk
Pasta	Quinoa or legume pastas
Sausage	Sautéed shiitake mushrooms (or if you want real sausage, get a clean-sourced product; fresh organic chicken sausage is good and fairly easy to find
Iceberg or regular lettuces	Spinach, arugula, kale, chard, and collard greens as a base for salads
White or brown sugar	Stevia, monk fruit, inulin, erythritol, honey, or maple syrup
Peanut butter	Almond butter, sunflower butter, or pumpkin seed butter
Cereal	A grain-free, nut- and seed-heavy granola (such as our Matcha Coconut Crunch), a porridge made from quinoa, or an egg dish (such as Green Eggs and Shiitake Ham)
Conventional produce and meat	Organic produce, meat (pastured and/or grass-fed whenever possible), and fish (wild caught or third-party-verified, clean farm-raised)

WONDERING WHAT TO EAT? KEEP THESE PRINCIPLES IN MIND

I've got a Cheat Sheet and a sample weekly menu for you at the end of this chapter that helps show what the Everyday eating plan looks like. But it's also helpful to keep these few principles in mind as you decide what to eat on your plan (especially if you are following the Everyday as a foundational eating plan and aren't transitioning out of the Intensive or are merely looking to swap in more DNA methylation-foods).

- **Focus on incorporating a variety of nonstarchy veggies that support methylation:** Prioritize the consumption of three types of vegetables: cruciferous, leafy green, and colorful, as they are rich in methyl donors and, particularly in the case of cruciferous vegetables, DNA methylation adaptogens. (To reiterate, many foods contain nutrients that are both methyl donor *and* adaptogen—cruciferous vegetables are just one example of this wondrous fact.) That includes things like leeks, daikon radish, asparagus, bok choy, Brussels sprouts, broccoli, broccoli rabe, kale, collard greens, spinach, Swiss chard, and peppers of all colors. A simple way to incorporate these veggies is with a big chopped salad or in a stir-fry. Season/flavor with olive oil, salt and pepper, and perhaps a squeeze of lemon for zing (or use our Herbal Epigenetic Dressing for even more DNA methylation support and flavor).

  One thing to keep in mind is that these vegetables are all low-glycemic, meaning they don't have a big impact on your blood sugar. Most potatoes, squashes, and corn rank higher on the glycemic scale, so keep those to a minimum.

- **Increase your healthy fat intake** by including a combination of avocados, nuts, and seeds—particularly sunflower seeds, pumpkin seeds, and sesame seeds, which are all rich in methyl donors. Add cold-pressed oils of these foods to your meals to keep the healthy fat content high. All nut and seed oils should not be heated; instead, use as finishing oils. Avocado oil (naturally refined), however, can be used for high-heat cooking.

- **Make your animal protein organic.** Animals can pass on all the contaminants found in their feed, so make sure that any animal protein you eat is at least organic, and ideally grass-fed and pasture-raised. It will help you keep more toxins out of your diet, and will protect your body's ability to methylate your DNA in a balanced way.

- **Get plenty of the Dynamic Dozen.** These are the twelve foods and beverages that offer the biggest boost to balanced DNA methylation that I listed starting on page 142. Think of them as your new best-friend foods! These are the foods to prioritize, even on days (or during weeks) when you're not otherwise focused on supporting your epigenome. Just put them on your regular shopping list so that you have them on hand at all times. Some require a little prep (like the liver), while others are grab and go (like the nuts and seeds).

- **Eat fermented foods daily, ideally a little with most meals:** Healthy gut microbes are crucial for optimal health and balanced DNA methylation. They reduce inflammation, promote healthy digestion, make the polyphenols (the plant compounds that fuel DNA methylation) in your food bioavailable, and can even make methyl donors, such as folate. Making a habit of eating some fermented foods most days helps keep your microbiome and your genetic expression healthy.

  Options for fermented foods include sauerkraut, kimchi, kefir, kombucha, pickles, olives, and fermented beets (make sure that these have no added sugar and are fermented traditionally so that they are high in probiotics—generally, you can tell by looking at the ingredient list; traditionally fermented veggies often only have salt and other herbs in them and develop their telltale tang over time as they ferment, while "quick pickles" rely on vinegar for that puckery taste). Two good choices are fermented products from Farmhouse Culture and Bubbies. Just make sure that what you buy is from the refrigerated section rather than the room-temperature shelves. You can also make your own—see the recipes for Turmeric-Pickled Daikon on page 312 and Lactofermented Vitamin D Mushrooms on page 313.

- **Add in prebiotic foods:** Prebiotics nourish your microbiome by providing the fiber that your good gut bugs rely on for food and are also a great daily addition to your diet. Good sources of prebiotic fiber include apples, asparagus, cocoa, dandelion greens, flax seeds, garlic, inulin, Jerusalem artichoke, jicama, leeks, onions (raw or cooked), and seaweed. Jerusalem artichoke works well sautéed with olive oil and some rosemary. The dandelion greens sauté easily with some olive oil and lemon. Jicama is ideally suited to grating raw and adding to salads.

- **Up your intake of DNA methylation adaptogens.** Honestly there are *so many* polyphenol-rich DNA methylation adaptogens it should be easy to eat these—even multiple types—at every meal. I included a list of the top ones on page 101—go back and review that to find the few that you can commit to having on a regular basis. But don't stop there. My nutritionist team and I have scoured nutrients databases and the scientific literature to generate a compilation of these wonderfully nutritive foods—it's so exhaustive that it quickly grew to many pages, and so we included it in the Nutrient Reference on page 407. Read it over, circle some of your faves, and star the ones perhaps you haven't tried before but are game to try. I cannot tell you how much I love this resource. I am certain it's the most comprehensive listing of DNA methylation and epigenetically bioactive nutrients anywhere to date. (In fact, much to the chagrin of our publisher, I kept adding to our Nutrient Reference list as new science was released, right up until we went to press!)

EPIGENETICALLY FRIENDLY PREPARED FOODS

As much as I adore and espouse whole foods, I get that sometimes you just want to grab something off the shelf and rip open a bag, or shake a bottled dressing on your burger or salad. The following products are DNA methylation friendly—eat them in moderation (because, of course, I prefer that you primarily get your nutrients from whole foods, not things that come in a wrapper, box, or bag).

Protein Bars

EPIC bars (there are a variety of flavors; find your favorite)
Go Raw Pumpkin Seed Sprouted Bar
Bulletproof Collagen Protein Bars (especially the Vanilla Shortbread and Fudge Brownie flavors—my personal favorites)
Health Warrior Pumpkin Seed Bars
RXBARs
BHU FIT Vegan or Paleo Protein Bars

Condiments

Sir Kensington's Avocado Oil Mayo, Vegan Mayo, or Avocado Oil Vegan Mayo

Primal Kitchen Avocado Oil Mayo

Primal Kitchen salad dressings (made with avocado oil)

Bragg salad dressings (I especially love the organic olive oil)

Primal Kitchen Organic Unsweetened Ketchup

Hellmann's Real Ketchup sweetened only with honey

Seafood

Wild Planet sustainably caught sockeye salmon, mackerel, and
sardines

Safe Catch tuna—their Elite line is lowest in mercury

Vital Choice canned seafood

Here are some labels to look for on farmed and wild-caught seafood:
MSC certified sustainable seafood
ASC certified farmed responsibly
Naturland
Whole Foods Market Responsibly Farmed

Wraps/Tortillas

Blue Mountain Organics Wraps, available in raw basil, raw tomato,
and raw curry flavors

NUCO Organic Coconut wraps

Siete Almond Flour Tortillas

Siete Cassava Flour Tortillas

Chips and Chip Alternatives

SeaSnax organic seaweed

EPIC Pork Rinds

LesserEvil Paleo Puffs

Barnana Organic Plantain Chips (my daughter would live on these if
I let her)

Nut- and Seed-Based Snacks

Nut butter pouches, from Justin's or Yumbutter

Go Raw snacks: Flax Snax, Sprouted Bites, Sprouted Cookie Crisps

Flackers Flax Seed Crackers
Simple Mills Crunchy Toasted Pecan Cookies

Dark Chocolate

Just make sure to choose chocolate that is 70 percent cacao or higher, preferably dairy-free and low sugar or sugar-free (sweetened with stevia or erythritol). Some of the brands that make bars that meet this criteria are listed below, but there are others—read the label carefully.

Rawmio
Alter Eco Dark Blackout
Lily's
Evolved

Crackers

Mary's Gone Crackers—the whole line is gluten-free
Simple Mills Almond Flour Crackers—they have many flavors and
varieties, all delicious

Bone Broths

Bonafide Provisions
Kettle & Fire
Cauldron Broths
Epic Bone Broth

Ice Cream

Van Leeuwen Vegan Ice Cream
NadaMoo!

WEEKLY MENU FOR THE YOUNGER YOU EVERYDAY

(Recipes begin on page 285)

	DAY 1	DAY 2	DAY 3
Breakfast	Zucchini Banana Muffins + coffee + coconut cream	Salmon and Spinach Omelet	Matcha Coconut Crunch
Snack	Herbed Beet Yogurt Dip + celery sticks	Seeds + berries Beet Bubbly	Luscious Liver Pâté on Nut and Seed "Everything" Bread
Lunch	Spiced Butternut Squash and Red Lentil Soup	Mix-and-Match Rainbow Salad + chickpeas + quinoa	Turkey Meatballs + sautéed kale + rainbow carrots + wild rice
Snack	Iced oolong tea	Golden Turmeric Milk	Beet Bubbly
Dinner	Broccoli Pesto with Pasta (using chickpea noodles) + steamed kale + pumpkin seeds	Spiced Butternut Squash and Red Lentil Soup Glass of red wine	Broccoli Pesto with Pasta (using chickpea noodles) + pumpkin seeds
Dessert			

CHEAT SHEET OF YOUNGER YOU EVERYDAY PROGRAM FOOD TARGETS

EACH DAY:

___ 2 cups dark leafy greens, measured raw, chopped, and packed

___ 1 cup cruciferous vegetables, measured raw, chopped, and packed

___ 1–2 cups additional colorful fruits and vegetables (limit fruit consumption to two servings a day, as they can be high in sugar)

___ 2 tablespoons pumpkin seeds or pumpkin seed butter

___ 2 tablespoons sunflower seeds or sunflower seed butter

___ One-plus serving of DNA methylation adaptogens (see list on page 101)

DAY 4	DAY 5	DAY 6	DAY 7
Zucchini Banana Muffins	Cranberry-Apple-Cinnamon Oatmeal + coffee	Green Eggs and Shiitake Ham + green tea	Cranberry-Apple-Cinnamon Oatmeal + oolong tea
Soft boiled eggs topped with Herbed Beet Yogurt Dip	Nut and Seed "Everything" Bread with berries	Sunflower seed butter + broccoli	Luscious Liver Pâté + snap peas
Mix-and-Match Rainbow Salad + salmon	Epigenetic Chili	Colorful Quinoa-Lentil Salad + pumpkin seeds	Turkey Meatballs + steamed veggies + black beans
Iced oolong tea	Beet Bubbly	Golden Turmeric Milk	Iced oolong tea
Colorful Quinoa-Lentil Salad	Mix-and-Match Rainbow Salad + chicken	Epigenetic Chili Glass of red wine	Mix-and-Match Stir-Fry + chicken
	No-Bake Chocolate Almond Cups		No-Bake Chocolate Almond Cups

___ Two 3- to 4-ounce servings of clean animal protein (unless you're over 60 or weigh more than 175 pounds, then two 5- to 6-ounce servings; see list on page 99)*

___ 3–5 tablespoons of healthy fats (see list on page 104)

___ One-plus servings fermented foods (see list on page 156)

___ Half your body weight in fluid ounces of filtered or spring water, herbal tea, or seltzer

EACH WEEK:

___ One serving of liver (3-ounce serving), preferably organic**

___ 5–10 eggs, preferably free-range and organic**

___ Three medium beets

* If you are vegetarian or vegan, aim for 40–50 grams of additional protein from beans, legumes, or plant-based protein powder

to compensate for the animal protein; see page 114 for a chart to help you hit this target.

    ** On days when you eat liver it counts toward your daily clean animal protein target.

· · · · ·

GENERAL GUIDELINES

- Eat organic as much as possible
- Eat between 7 a.m. and 7 p.m. (or finish eating three hours before bed if you go to bed after 11:30 p.m., and don't have your first meal until twelve hours after your final meal)
- Include healthy oils (coconut, olive, flaxseed, and pumpkin seed)
- Avoid folic acid–fortified foods (including nearly all commercial products made out of wheat, such as bread, pasta, and baked goods), vegetable oils, fried foods, and charred foods
- Keep alcohol consumption to two drinks per week or less
- Minimize plastic food and beverage containers, nonstick cookware

Just as with the Intensive, the Younger You Everyday isn't complete without the addition of a few powerful lifestyle practices, which I'll cover in the next chapter.

7

THE YOUNGER YOU
LIFESTYLE PRESCRIPTION

SINCE THERE'S MORE TO YOUR LIFE THAN MEALTIMES, THERE'S ALSO more to the Younger You plans than food. The truth is, the way that you take care of yourself beyond what you eat has incredible power to positively influence your DNA methylation and your epigenome.

In this chapter, you'll learn how to optimize your exercise, stress reduction, sleep, and connection to others so that your DNA methylation engine is firing on all cylinders. Every one of these pieces I share is moderate and doable and has been road tested by our patients, our study participants, and even our staff and family members. Best of all, these are the types of practices that take all the good inputs you've been giving yourself with your DNA methylation-supporting food choices and lend them even more power. When you combine high-quality nutrition with sleep, movement, and relaxation—the lifestyle practices from the formula I introduced on page 98—you function at your best. And you feel *amazing*.

EXERCISE

Exercise is an anti-aging elixir that spins the biological clock in reverse: when you look at the lifestyle habits of healthy centenarians, a commonality among all of them is that movement is a foundational part of their life.

And in general, it needn't be intense—gardening, walking, dancing, or bike riding are truly all it takes to tick the box on your requirements for exercise.

Exercise is the ultimate form of hormesis (beneficial stressor). It turns on physiologic processes for cellular repair, detoxifies you through your sweat, burns pro-inflammatory fat for fuel, and builds heart muscle. In fact, *not* exercising takes as big a toll on life span as smoking.

A big reason that movement is such a vital component of health and longevity is that it nourishes the epigenome.[1] It acts like yet another epi-nutrient by turning bad genes off and turning on genes we want activated, and giving you the DNA methylation patterns of a younger person.[2]

Specifically, positive, exercise-induced DNA methylation changes have been found on genes that are related to the following:

- Obesity, diabetes, and fat storage (this particular study showed profound, beneficial changes in type 2 diabetics who started exercising in just six months!)[3]
- The inflammatory response and inflammation-associated diseases[4]
- Learning, memory, and neuroplasticity (the ability of brain cells to form new connections)[5]
- Suppressing cancer—and this effect is more pronounced the older you are[6]

Some of the epigenetic changes that exercise produces happen really quickly. A 2012 study found that nonexercising healthy adults experienced *immediate* (albeit transient) DNA methylation changes—genes associated with metabolism were turned on—*after a single exercise session.*[7]

Exercise has a significant effect on DNA methylation, and at least some of the methylation patterns on specific genes known to be favorably influenced by exercise are handed down generation to generation (called "imprinted genes"). Specific imprinted genes that are favorably influenced by exercise include those in cancer prevention, insulin sensitivity, and muscle. Could your resilience to developing diabetes come from your grandmother's lifelong tai chi practice? Or the very low incidence of cancer in your family be the result of your family history in the hard work of farming? Or the ease with which you build muscle be a benefit of your parents' and grandparents' love of the outdoors? Research suggests yes.[8]

That being said, there is such a thing as too much exercise. Again, there's a U curve of benefit. For one example, the process of generating the energy it takes to fuel all that exertion naturally creates free radicals that your body needs time (and nutrients) to be able to quench. Pushing up to and beyond your limit, too often, especially when you are not well-conditioned, can turn this beneficial stressor into a harmful one; intense, frequent exercise could have a pro-aging influence if not conducted correctly. Just as with food, you want to be in the sweet spot.

A reasonable starting goal—what we asked of our study participants, and the requirement for the Intensive program—is to aim for a minimum five sessions per week of at least thirty minutes at a moderate exertion level. We think that this exercise prescription is enough to keep your DNA methylation in a good place.

As far as what kind of exercise to do, we told our study participants to do something they loved, and suggested brisk walking, light jogging, hiking, dancing, yard work, bicycling, and swimming as activities to consider.

Whether you are doing the Younger You Intensive or the Everyday, that's your assignment now, too: at least thirty minutes of doing some form of exercise you love, at least five days a week. This not-too-structured, not-too-intense kind of exercise program is great for getting you into the groove of moving regularly—and that consistency is the most important piece (*not* the intensity).

Even if you're not a typical exercise aficionado, there is a way to incorporate movement into your life. My patient Jenny is a prime example. A fifty-five-year-old female with IBS and a self-admitted "allergy" to exercise, when Jenny was prescribed the Intensive program, the diet, sleep, and meditation pieces were all doable and she starting reaping rewards immediately—she had better GI function, lower C-reactive protein levels, lower cholesterol, lower blood sugar and fasting insulin, and better mood. It was all going quite well, except for exercise. For Jenny, the solution was using the app Couch to 5K, which connects you to others who also share a goal of being able to run five kilometers, no matter how sedentary you are when you start. She also found that chatting with someone on the phone during her training time, whether they were exercising or not, really helped. The exercise—and the community—aspect also boosted Jenny's mental health, and she began tapering her antidepressant medication. And interestingly, it wasn't the goal of the 5K that motivated her, it was the daily gentle jog and walk and community that provided her the most reward.

If you have mobility challenges, such as chronic illness or pain, a well-designed exercise protocol can provide respite from your pain and fatigue. Our patient Paul, even with his intense neuropathy, found that using the weight machines at the gym helped his body feel significantly better. Exercise can reduce pain through multiple avenues—it strengthens muscles, which then leads to better-supported joints, whether they are your knees or your vertebrae; it improves circulation and oxygenation, which means inflammatory waste products are swept away; it releases endorphins and endocannabinoids, endogenous chemicals that are extraordinarily potent natural pain relievers; and it lifts mood.

There are brilliant physical therapists, exercise physiologists, biomechanists, yoga instructors, and fitness trainers who can guide you through any physical limitations you may have. I have one patient with severe kyphosis who worked with a yoga instructor on appropriate stretching and strengthening moves, and her spinal curvature improved so significantly that she's gained back two inches in height (a feat verified by her orthopedist)!

If five sessions a week sounds like a lot to you, or you're not currently exercising at all, your simple goal is to do *something* to get moving at least three times per week, and gradually increase that number of weekly sessions to five. Just know that our study findings suggest you don't need to go for the burn. There's no need to hit the weight machines at the gym to the extent that you can barely move the next day, or go for a run when you've hardly been walking, so that your heart starts pounding. In fact, doing so can be counterproductive as it will increase inflammation *and* potentially dissuade you from making movement a regular part of your life.

Your goal is to reach an intensity of 60 to 80 percent of maximum perceived exertion (PE)—that means you're still able to carry on a conversation, although you might be sucking a little bit of wind in order to do so. You don't need to wear a heart rate monitor or fancy biometric tracking device, as research suggests that using PE alone is about as reliable as using fancy tracking equipment.

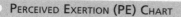
Perceived Exertion (PE) Chart

Target Zone	Intensity (% maximum exertion)	Feels Like...
Maximum	90-100%	Very exhausting for breathing and muscles. Sustainable for less than 5 minutes.
Hard	80-90%	Muscular fatigue and heavy breathing. Sustainable up to 10 minutes.
Moderate	70-80%	Light muscular fatigue, easy breathing, moderate sweating.
Light	60-70%	Comfortable, easy breathing, low muscle load, light sweating.
Very Light	50-60%	Very easy for breathing and muscles.

• • • • •

There's really not one right way to hit these moderate goals. My patients, staff, our study participants, even my mom all have a slightly different take on what they do and when to ensure that they move their bodies for at least thirty minutes, at least five times a week.

One study participant began walking to work, which was thirty minutes each way and perfectly fit the guidelines of thirty to sixty minutes, five days a week. Another, who was not very active, began going for a twenty- to thirty-minute walk with his son two or three nights a week. While he didn't completely hit his exercise goal, making that initial commitment made him realize how good it felt to get regular movement, and he said it was something he would continue after the study was through.

For a couple of our study participants, this level of activity was much less than they were used to. In fact, one participant had to delay the start of his eight weeks because he had a rock climbing trip planned where he would be climbing several hours a day. I don't want to talk anyone out of a beloved hobby, such as rock climbing, but I share his story because I know some of you are reading this book because you are fitness enthusiasts. There is a popular belief that more exercise is better, but there comes a point (that is still being defined) where it might work against your overall health. I definitely don't want to stop you from going after your highest fitness goals. I just hope that knowing that sleep, relaxation, and connection also play such a vital role in the health of your epigenome, you'll consider these other levers to be as important as working out, and perhaps—if it's correct for you—redistribute some of the time you spend exercising on these other endeavors. The good news is that by measuring your bio age using the various tools in the book plus a periodic look at your DNA methylation biological age, you will be able to find your exercise sweet spot.

Believe me, I understand the lure to intense exercise: I was a competitive cyclist during medical school, and it was one of the happiest, and most arduous, times in my life. I was also sick with sinusitis during that time quite often because I was always pushing myself scholastically and on the bike—I didn't understand the importance of recovery then. I've not had sinusitis once since graduation, which also coincided with the end of my competitive cycling career.

Riding is still my sport of choice, and I still like to get my heart rate up and work up a good sweat, but I have dialed the intensity and duration down somewhat. Now riding outdoors in as many weather conditions as possible is my sanity; it gets me outside where I can see (and smell) the change of seasons—the freshly mowed lawns and flowers of summer, the musky sweet grapes and colorful leaves of fall, and the bracing cold of winter. If I'm alone, I can listen to podcasts, engage in an active meditation practice, call in to a work meeting, check in with family, or just enjoy the silence. And if Isabella is sitting in her seat on the back of the bike, I can savor the sounds of her humming "Baby Shark."

Because sitting is the new smoking, I also invested in a treadmill desk at work that I walk on, very slowly, for one or two hours a day, or that I just use as a standing desk. And I've built a few core exercises and some gentle yoga poses into my getting ready for bed wind-down routine. They keep my lower back supple, strong, and pain free and help me relax a bit before sleep.

My mom is all about finding the right time of day to slot in her exercise based on her energy level. She goes for a walk in the early mornings, after coffee and meditation but before breakfast.

Mom says she goes even when she doesn't feel like it by telling herself she'll just go around the block, and she ends up nearly always walking around several blocks before she heads back. She said that listening to an audiobook—especially a good mystery—helps get her out the door. She also listens to a book in the afternoons when she does her leg-strengthening exercises, and when she watches the news at night she'll do some arm weights. Mom is also a passionate gardener, an activity she engages in most days during the warmer months. It's a good blend of doing the forms of exercise she loves, and for those types that aren't as fun (lifting arm weights, for example), she does them while doing something she does enjoy (although I don't know if "enjoy" is the right term to use for watching the news).

Karen, the COO of our practice, loves a loose schedule. While she's committed to exercising five or six days per week, she varies what she does, alternating between walks, weights, YouTube exercise videos, dancing, and yoga. She says that committing to a number of weekly sessions while maintaining flexibility around when and what she does works best.

It also helps to work movement into your workday wherever you can, whether that's walking to work or having a moving meeting. Karen and I have a regular weekly meeting during which I am on my bike and she's getting her fitness in—in the fall, I can often hear her raking leaves, and other times, she's on her treadmill desk, too.

There really is no one right way to get your moderate amounts of exercise, just as long as it's consistent. There's only the way that works for you. If you can exercise outdoors, you'll also get fresh air, but if a virtual experience (such as riding a Peloton bike) gets you active, use it. If exercising with others makes it more fun for you, by all means, set up a regular walking date or commit to a group class. I see this all of the time in my practice:

patients transitioning into an exercise routine do it best with a community, even a virtual one, some even using a free conference call line or an online video meeting to share workout time with others. But if you prefer solitude so you can hear yourself think, that's great, too. Whatever gets you moving.

When you're ready, you can add in bursts of more intense exercise, such as the aptly named high-intensity interval training (HIIT), where you alternate periods of pushing hard for a short amount of time (somewhere between thirty seconds and one minute, typically) with periods of rest (generally for about half the time you go all out). HIIT has a body of research that suggests that it provides extra benefits. Research has shown HIIT to be effective at:

- Boosting brain power[9]
- Burning fat[10]
- Lowering insulin resistance[11]
- Improving markers of cardiovascular health[12]

"High intensity" means you are going "all out" and reaching 90 percent or higher perceived exertion—your breathing is strained, it's impossible to keep up a conversation, and your muscles are fatiguing quickly. The good news is that you only maintain this level of intensity for two minutes or less. You can either incorporate your HIIT into your regular workout—walking up a few hills as quickly as you can, if you're walking, or sprinting if you're jogging—or you can perform a workout that is specifically designed to intersperse short intervals of exertion and rest—like the famous seven-minute workout. If you choose to do HIIT workouts, they should be in addition to, not in replacement of, your five thirty-plus-minute exercise sessions per week.

The take-home message here is that when it comes to exercise, what's most important is that you do something you can stick with, like my mom's faithful daily gardening or my patient Jenny's daily walk/jog. The thing you do day in and day out outweighs what you do every once in a while, even if that once in a while thing is the trendy exercise du jour. We have to start—and perhaps stick with—"good enough" and trust that even moderate efforts will improve health span. Our study suggests that it will. Some is always better than none.

Guidelines for DNA Methylation–Friendly Exercise

To recap, here's your exercise prescription:

- A duration of thirty to sixty minutes
- A minimum of five times a week
- At an exertion level of 60 to 80 percent of your max capacity—you can still have a conversation, but you're breaking a light sweat and your breathing may be noticeable
- As you're ready, add in one or two HIIT sessions a week; either incorporating them into your existing workout or adding an additional workout or two (because they can be as short as seven minutes, you can do HIIT workouts on the same days that you do your thirty-plus minutes of moderate exercise). Also: if you need additional support or motivation to do HIIT, look no further than YouTube; there are all sorts of HIIT videos, targeted specifically to beginners, older people, five-minute programs, and more.

Setting the Stage for Exercise Success

Any consistent new habit involves more than just a decision to start. It also requires some forethought. Here are the issues you need to think through to set yourself up for success:

- **What motivates you?** Give some thought to what you know helps you do the things you say you want to do. Do you need company (even virtually)? Accountability? Flexibility? Brainstorm ways to give yourself the conditions you need to be successful. Also think about the good feelings movement brings; the sense of accomplishment, the visual changes that getting in shape produces, and the turning on of the DNA methylation patterns of a younger you.
- **Finding the time.** Knowing that you're looking for blocks of time that are a minimum of thirty minutes long (you also need to factor in time to change clothes before and after, and perhaps shower, although at this moderate level of exertion you likely won't sweat much, if at all), get out your calendar and ask yourself when you have the most flexibility for fitting in exercise. Put it in your calendar

just as you would any other meeting or appointment—that way you can protect that time and even get a reminder to go do it.

- **Figuring out what you like to do.** Make a list of the physical activities you enjoy.
- **Securing supplies.** Is there anything you need to buy or repair in order to be able to do your favorite activities regularly? If you choose walking, an activity tracker, a comfortable pair of walking shoes, and some gear appropriate to your typical weather conditions can really help you get out the door. If you want to get back into playing tennis, do you need some new balls?

STRESS AND THE EPIGENOME

I know you've heard this message before, but it is vital that you're tending to how you respond to stress. Stress is inevitable, but managed poorly, stress will drive aging forward like gasoline poured on a fire. As I mentioned in Chapter 3, a full 25 percent of the methylation sites that are evaluated in the DNAmAge clock we used in our study are on gene regions that get turned on in response to stress (specifically, the glucocorticoids, like cortisol, which is released under stress, can turn the genes on). These stress-stimulated genes are associated with diseases driven by inflammation including cancer, heart disease and, of course, aging itself.[13] I know it's a bit of a complex phenomenon, but the take-home is that stress plays a very large, direct, but underappreciated role in driving aging, and aging-related diseases, forward.

Stress-altered epigenetics increases inflammation, dysregulates blood sugar, and imbalances our immunity. Stress can also lead to methyl donor drain, as we use up our precious SAMe—the universal methyl donor manufactured and then used in the methylation cycle (see page 422 for more about this vital process) in the process of metabolizing adrenaline.

The brutal truth is that some of us come into the world with epigenetic stress programming from previous generations' experiences that makes us more sensitive to its ravages. If you feel that you are quick to anger, overreact, or dive headfirst into overwhelm or fear, perhaps your epigenetics have been modified in such a way that your glucocorticoid response has been heightened or your oxytocin is blunted. You might have a baseline lower stress threshold that came from experiences in your lifetime, or perhaps your stress response was inherited (or a combination of both).

One animal study showed these stress and trauma-induced changes can be passed down through a full four generations;[14] and still another animal study showed fear responses (associated with significant anatomical changes to brain neuron size) were passed down for at least two generations![15] Wow.

In humans, the Överkalix, Dutch Hunger Winter, and Project Ice Storm studies all showed negative effects of maternal stress, both physical and emotional, on the DNA methylation of their offspring that, in some cases, was shown to last at least three generations. (I can't help but wonder what DNA methylation effects the COVID-19 pandemic will have on some mothers, kids, and the babies that were born in 2020 and 2021.)

Why is there such a huge relationship between early stress and lasting DNA methylation changes and the outcomes they produce? When we are little, DNA methylation patterning is wide open; it's a sensitive time for programming our response to the world. We are being shaped by environment in a powerful, direct way. There are two important genes at play in particular: oxytocin (or the oxytocin receptor)—the love hormone I cover on page 200—gene and glucocorticoid associated genes, which modulate the stress response. If mom's oxytocin activity is robust, she'll want to tend to baby, allowing for baby to develop a stress resilience that can last a lifetime. But if her oxytocin activity is low because her oxytocin receptor gene is hypermethylated, such as can be seen in postpartum depression or times of heightened stress, or due to mom's own history of mistreatment, her loving contact with baby may also be low, which can then result in hypomethylation of baby's glucocorticoid genes, which allows them to be turned on readily, increasing baby's stress sensitivities.

It all begs the question: in those of us with this inheritance, are we also predisposed to the chronic diseases of aging and accelerated aging? Unfortunately, I strongly suspect that the answer is yes, although that research has yet to be done. While we're waiting for the science, we already know that adopting these lifestyle habits will support healthy stress responses and a beneficial restructuring of DNA methylation patterns.

In the Project Ice Storm study, lead researcher Suzanne King and associate investigator Moshe Szyf found that both emotional and physical stress can lead to heritable epigenetic changes that result in immune dysregulation (i.e., inflammation, that fundamental driver of aging) in the offspring. The mothers who were pregnant during that ice storm were more likely to have children with autism, asthma, or negative changes to white blood cells, and these changes were triggered by changed DNA methylation patterns on the genes that code for immune system proteins responsive to glucocorticoids—a category of stress hormones that includes cortisol.

The Project Ice Storm study wasn't the first time Szyf demonstrated that stress negatively impacts offspring. In fact, he's been studying this phenomenon for decades: In his seminal research using rodents, he and co-investigator Michael Meaney found that maternal grooming, or lack thereof, changed DNA methylation patterns regulating glucocorticoids in the hippocampal region of the brain in offspring that persist into adulthood. Those without sufficient grooming experienced a heightened stress response that other rodent offspring with sufficient early life nurturing didn't experience (conversely, those that were groomed acquired a more balanced DNA methylation pattern on those same genes and thus a more balanced response to stressors).[16] Thus, another key way that stress influences DNA methylation is by lowering the brain's stress response threshold. Meaning, it takes a smaller stressor to elicit a bigger release of cortisol and adrenaline.

One other gene that can be differentially methylated in infants whose mothers experienced trauma in their childhoods is brain-derived neurotrophic factor (BDNF), whose healthy expression is essential for brain development in childhood and healthy function throughout the life span.[17] Fortunately, BDNF expression can be nurtured by following the Younger You program, as many DNA methylation adaptogens—green tea, blueberries, grapes, extra-virgin olive oil, chocolate, turmeric, and fatty fish—and lifestyle practices—sleep, exercise, and meditation—increase it.

One small piece of good news is that some research shows that the DNA methylation changes that are due to childhood stress don't always appear to be heritable. A 2019 study found that mothers who had stressful childhoods had a consistent pattern of imbalanced DNA methylation at key genes, including increased glucocorticoid receptor methylation (the stress response that's associated with aging and the chronic diseases of aging) even in adulthood, but their newborns didn't share that pattern.[18]

Healing from Trauma

We can't talk about reducing stress as part of reversing bio age without also addressing trauma. Being from Sandy Hook, where the pain and trauma of the mass shooting that happened at our elementary school is still palpable, and thinking about all of the pain, suffering, and loss that occurred during the COVID-19 pandemic, as well as the generations of trauma that BIPOC Americans have endured, I am constantly wondering how we can transform the biological embedding of traumatic experiences.

Just as stress gets biologically embedded in our epigenome, so does trauma. (Recall that biological embedding is the process by which emotional events are incorporated into our epigenome—either through our own experience or the experience of previous generations.)

If you've experienced traumatic stress—in utero, in infancy, or childhood, or throughout your life—and/or you have PTSD, it can alter the DNA methylation patterns in your brain, in some cases leading you to experience less stressful events as more stressful. Meaning, a small- to medium-size stressor occurs, and you have a large, extra-large, or Everest-size reaction to it. Or, conversely, loads of stress over the course of a lifetime can create a blunted response to stressful events, causing a shutdown.[19] In either case, whether you're hypersensitive to stress or your receptors are dulled to it, the chronic surge of cortisol still drives aging and age-related diseases via changes to DNA methylation.

When we look at the research on DNA methylation in those with symptoms associated with PTSD, across the studies, there are always abnormal methylation patterns on genes associated with cortisol and the hypothalamic-pituitary-adrenal (HPA) axis (the feedback loop between the brain and the adrenal glands that regulates the stress response) plus inflammatory genes; and often in this population, we see negative changes to feel-good brain hormones like oxytocin, BDNF, and serotonin.[20]

Kids mistreated in early childhood, in what's known in the literature as adverse childhood events (ACEs) or childhood maltreatment (CM), were found to have hypermethylated—and thus turned off—oxytocin receptor genes, which was associated with less gray matter volume in the left orbitofrontal cortex region of their brains as compared to kids who didn't experience CM. These changes were associated with a distorted attachment formation. There are plenty of other instances showing hypermethylated oxytocin genes resulting from early life adversities, including lack of maternal care, low socioeconomic status, and abuse. These changes appear to carry forward into adulthood, prompting difficulty with connection, emotional processing ability, and other challenges.[21]

An interesting 2020 review paper looking at DNA methylation patterns in PTSD confirmed that the genes that are involved in trauma responses are consistently associated with glucocorticoid activation, inflammation, and genes that code for the enzymes that make DNA methylation possible. Meaning, the effects of trauma on DNA methylation will push you toward inflammation, a heightened stress response, and disordered DNA methylation, all of which can accelerate aging and open the door to the diseases of aging.[22]

There is good news here, though, and it is this: because DNA methylation is a player in the effects of trauma, the Younger You program should help remedy them. While the results of animal studies aren't guaranteed to apply to humans, they do illuminate how DNA methylation works. One hopeful piece of trauma-related news came when Dr. Moshe Szyf published a paper in *Molecular Psychiatry* looking at DNA methylation patterns in mice. Those who displayed behaviors indicative of PTSD had noticeably—and consistently—different DNA methylation patterns in the nucleus accumbens region of the brain than those who didn't. Using SAMe and vitamin A, two nutrients that we know influence DNA methylation, Dr. Szyf and his team were able to return the DNA methylation patterns in the affected mice's brains back to normal.

Of course, when you are in a full trauma response it can be hard to shop for and prepare the healthy foods in the Younger You plans and to find the time and motivation for things like exercise, meditation, and sleep. Your financial reality may make paying more for organic produce not an option, but know that any piece of the Younger You Intensive you can adopt—drinking a cup of green tea, cuddling with a pet or loved one, taking a prebedtime melatonin to help you get seven hours of sleep, getting out for a ten-minute walk, for example—will help you avoid falling into a post-trauma DNA methylation slump.

While we—collectively and individually—absolutely must do what we can to reduce unnecessary trauma, it's scientifically impossible to completely insulate ourselves from it altogether. There *is* a powerful opportunity around trauma, however, and that is to study the epigenetic patterning around post-traumatic growth and resilience—what it is, how to nurture it, and how to supercharge it in times of hardship so that trauma doesn't have such a long tail.

And here is where the research simply hasn't caught up yet. As the authors of the review I just mentioned point out: "There are not studies examining post traumatic growth. This lack of literature is consistent with observations of a pathogenic research bias in trauma literature."

What we do know thus far is that there are epigenetic patterns associated with surviving and thriving after stress. What if we could encourage the development of those patterns in order to support ourselves and our family in recovering from and coming back stronger after stressful, even traumatic times? It's a lovely idea, to be sure, but also a very good possibility: in my 2017 podcast with Dr. Moshe Szyf, he said he is hopeful that we will be able to develop epigenetic diagnostics and therapeutics that will help us correct the biological embedding of trauma onto our epigenome. A possible scenario might be that, rather than having to relive trauma through talk or behavioral therapy, we could identify and gently nudge the epigenetic patterns of trauma back into balance with a noninvasive DNA methylation–supportive program, avoiding emotional debilitation and mood-altering psychotropic medications—and we might even be able to correct this in utero, long before any chance of expression. We will have to see how it shakes out, but the thought of improving overall health *and* releasing generations-old trauma is certainly tantalizing. In the meantime, incorporate as many of the Younger You guidelines as you can to rewire your genetic expression away from being trauma impaired.

Countering Current Stress

Beyond the epigenetic patterns you inherited and what you experienced in your earliest life, the stress that you're experiencing currently, whether it's PTSD, job strain, death of a loved one, illness, or the effects of a global pandemic, can all negatively influence DNA methylation patterns contributing to aging and stress-associated illnesses.[23]

This sounds like a bummer, I know. Whose parents and grandparents didn't experience stressful times, perhaps even trauma? And who among us isn't stressed in our current realities? But really, the enormous impact that stress has on the epigenome is a call to action. Your stress levels *require* your attention in order to bring them down.

I know that stress feels like a ubiquitous and completely unavoidable aspect of life; something you might be able to futz with around the edges, but not something you can make a significant change to, without winning the lottery, or retiring, or moving to a secluded island (or maybe all three). For many of us, it's often not until we have a realization or experience of its brutal toll on our health that we find the motivation to do anything about it.

The key takeaway here is that it is possible to nudge yourself out of this epigenetic pattern caused by, and which can contribute to, stress. The Younger You principles are an excellent preventative and restorative measure for anyone who has experienced trauma and fears that these experiences may have become biologically embedded. The eating plan will help keep DNA methylation in a more balanced place, and the lifestyle components of the program—meditating, cuddling, getting regular exercise— will help retrain your stress response so that stress has less of a negative impact on your DNA methylation in the first place. In particular, a consistent relaxation practice may have the potential to have a profound effect not only on your biological age, but also on the associated, chronic diseases of aging by favorably influencing those same HPA axis, immune, and feel-good hormone genes that I mentioned earlier. Recall in Chapter 3, I said tai chi practice significantly slowed age-related DNA methylation losses in a study of five hundred women; a sixty-day relaxation response practice likewise lowered DNA methylation age in a healthy population. Those who meditate—both experienced and inexperienced—can favorably alter DNA methylation patterns (the more experience, the more profound the change, however).[24] Yoga, qigong, and mindfulness are all capable of favorably influencing the epigenome.[25] It's really quite extraordinary what it looks like we can do by applying some intention and attention to stepping out of the powerful river of stress.

The icing on the cake is that as you turn down your stress, you'll not only be biologically younger, but also your day-to-day experience of stress will drop, in sometimes profound ways, as my patient Sean experienced.

Sean, a man in his thirties, had a very stressful job at a hedge fund (where he was also very successful). He came to see me because he was experiencing regular migraine headaches. Sean's first morning salivary cortisol levels (the stress hormone that, when released in excess over the long haul, wreaks havoc on health) were high and imbalanced enough that, along with a few other findings he had on labs, I was concerned about a heart attack—early heart attacks were in his family history, and similar morning cortisol patterns have an association with cardiovascular events. It wasn't until I showed Sean the hard laboratory data of his cortisol patterns that he got motivated to meditate every morning.

Sean's consistent practice helped his cortisol come down dramatically, but it also got him to deeply rethink how he was choosing to live his life. In what he viewed as a life-or-death decision, he ultimately changed careers to one that was more fulfilling—fostering small business development. De-stressing also remedied his cortisol levels and his migraines.

To be clear, the only de-stressing requirement of the Younger You Intensive is that you practice meditation for a minimum of ten minutes, twice a day (and as long as twenty minutes at a time if it's feeling good and you want to keep going) for the next eight weeks. But don't be surprised if regularly stepping off the hamster wheel and empowering your body to experience how good relaxation feels leads you to rearrange your life so that there's more room for relaxation and less room for stress.

ARE YOU STRESSED OUT? A FEW COMMON AND LESS COMMON SIGNS

LOOK AT YOUR NAILS. ARE THEY RAGGEDY AND CHEWED? ARE THE cuticles picked? (The medical term for this practice is creepily apt: autocannibalism). When I think I'm doing well at life, all I need to do is take a peek at my cuticles to confirm—they sometimes tell me a whole other story.

Are you yawning, sighing, or feeling like you need to catch your breath? Stress triggers shallow breathing, which can result in air hunger.

Having trouble thinking of words? Or conversely, can you not stop talking, crying, thinking, or ruminating? Stress impairs cognitive function, and can cause problems with memory, mood, and anxiety. This is at least in part because chronic stress and trauma can lead to imbalanced methylation of one of our key genes involved in memory and learning: BDNF. As previously mentioned, meditation and exercise both can improve BDNF availability.

Are you more tuned in to odors, or are certain smells bothering you? Humans are animals, and we use our sense of smell to sniff for danger. If you're stressed, your physiology is going to turn up the sensitivity of your olfactory system.

Are you getting a lot of tension headaches? Holding your breath or breathing shallowly results in low oxygenation of your muscles. Which leads to tightness. Which leads to tension headaches.

Are your muscles sore? In addition to low oxygenation, stress causes your muscles to tense in preparation for fleeing or fighting.

Have you been having heart palpitations? The fight-or-flight response raises your heart rate.

Are your eyelashes or eyebrows looking scant? Some folks deal with stress by pulling them out, in a practice known as trichotillomania.

· · · · ·

What I'm going to tell you to do about your stress is the same thing that Sean and our study participants did, and that is meditate.

You probably already know that meditation helps with emotional regulation and can even change the size of certain areas of the brain. Meditation also gives your brain a break from all the emails, texts, and to-dos that keep your nervous system in a heightened state. But you may not realize that meditation also supports healthy DNA methylation. This likely has to do with meditation's ability to reduce psychological and physiological stress. When you're in a stressed-out state, your adrenals pump out the hormones epinephrine and norepinephrine, which require methylation to be made, metabolized, and excreted. That means there are fewer methyl donors on hand for DNA methylation. In fact, a 2017 study found that long-term meditators had a younger epigenetic age than people who had never or rarely meditated.[26]

Clearly, it's time we all get our meditation on: twice a day, for a total of twenty to forty minutes, as part of the Younger You Intensive.

It's common to resist the very idea of meditating, or breathing, almost like a two-year-old throwing a tantrum (something I know a lot about at this point in my life). But once you metabolize just how pervasive an effect stress has on your health and your biological age—and how much meditation truly can benefit you—you'll be motivated to actually meditate and not just read about it.

If you already have a meditation practice, booyah for you! I hope that knowing that your practice helps promote healthy DNA methylation and reduces biological age will inspire you to keep going. If you *don't* already have a meditation practice, now is the time to start. You don't even have to know *how* to meditate. I'm including the exact directions that we supplied to our study participants on page 183. I suggest following them during the eight weeks of the Younger You Intensive if at all possible. But if you need a little more in-the-moment guidance, or are following the Younger You Everyday, there are many meditation apps that can talk you through it. An added bonus of using a guided meditation app is that it will track your sessions, which helps keep you accountable. Some good ones include:

- Oak
- Buddhify
- Insight Timer
- Headspace
- Calm
- University of Wisconsin's Healthy Minds app (completely free and research-based! I use their guided active mediations when I am biking)

It's really as simple as taking a seat. You—your sanity and your health—are worth that time. And every time you do, you'll be reclaiming a portion of those sixteen-plus years at the end of life that too many of us spend sick.

YOUR RELAXATION PRESCRIPTION

In our research study, we prescribed a twice-daily meditation session of ten to twenty minutes inspired by Dr. Herbert Benson's classic book *The Relaxation Response*. This recommendation was evidence based: a 2019 study demonstrated that sixty days of relaxation practice, twenty minutes twice per day, could significantly reduce biological age as measured by the Zbieć-Piekarska clock (which is a different DNA methylation clock than the DNAmAge clock that we used) in otherwise healthy people.[27] Because we recognized that twenty minutes twice a day was a big ask, we gave our participants a range of ten to twenty minutes for each session. Aiming for ten minutes makes the practice more doable, and once you are actually sitting, you may get into a groove and decide to stay longer than ten minutes.

When you are following the Younger You Intensive, this is your prescription, too—two daily meditation sessions of ten to twenty minutes each. If you are on the Younger You Everyday, aim for a minimum of ten minutes of meditation, done once per day, every day, or as many days as you can manage. Meaning, if you miss a day, don't throw in the towel—just get started again the next day.

There are, of course, many other practices that induce relaxation, such as tai chi, yoga, qigong, and breath work. You can sign up for these or for a meditation class that meets in person or virtually. The community aspect of these group settings can make the discipline of meditation easier, and it can also feel like less of an effort to get into a quiet, focused state—you can just ride the vibes in the (virtual) room. And practicing relaxation with others helps you feel that connection to others that's also so vital to emotional, mental, and DNA methylation health (I'll talk more about the benefits of connection on page 199).

If you prefer breath work to straight-up meditation, these apps are helpful:

- Stop, Breathe & Think
- MindShift CBT
- Just Breathe
- Breethe
- Box Breathing

Another option is HeartMath, which is an evidence-based program that can improve symptoms of stress, depression, and anxiety by helping you synchronize the rhythms of your brain and heart by optimizing your heart rate variability (HRV). The Inner Balance trainer, in particular, offers guided meditation that gives you feedback in real time about the effect your efforts are making on your heart rate and emotional state. It requires you to purchase a small sensor that clips to your ear. We frequently recommend HeartMath to our patients and they have found it very impactful in helping them shift out of long-held states of stress.

While not a meditation app per se, I have also come to rely on my Ōura Ring, which is a biometric tracker that measures all of the lifestyle components tracked in our study, including meditation, exercise, sleep, and sleep quality (in addition to heart rate and heart rate variability, which is a measure of how quickly your heart recuperates after exposure to stress). Seeing my body respond to meditation in the form of improved heart rate variability and overall heart rate is validating and motivating for me, a self-professed data hound. Many of us have some tool that can track our efforts, whether it's a Fitbit, smartphone, or Apple Watch. While they're not precise measurements, the trends these devices capture can offer beneficial insight and keep us heading in the right direction.

Just as with exercise, the most important criterion of your relaxation practice is that it be something you enjoy, so that it will be easy to make it a long-running part of your life. For the duration of the Younger You Intensive, I advise you to do the same exercise that our study participants did, outlined in the box below. If you are starting with the Younger You Everyday, this meditation practice is a great place to start if you don't already have something you love. Get some consistency under your belt with this, and then you can branch out if you like.

YOUR DAILY RELAXATION PRACTICE

ADAPTED FROM THE RELAXATION RESPONSE, *BY HERBERT BENSON, MD*
Let go of the idea of doing it correctly, or even of relaxing fully. This is a practice; you are *practicing*. Absolve yourself of any expectations of nailing it.

Try to resist the urge to set an alarm, as hearing it may undo some of the relaxation that you've cultivated. It's OK to open your eyes to check the time.

Sit comfortably in a quiet place (although if your best time to meditate is while riding the train to work—use it).

Close your eyes.

Breathe normally, through your nose.

Starting at your feet, check in with each body part and invite it to relax. Continue until you reach the top of your head.

Now rest your attention on your breath. Every time you breathe out, say the word "one" silently to yourself. Breathe in, breathe out, "one." Breathe in, breathe out, "one."

When stressful or distracting thoughts barge in, redirect your attention to your breath and to saying the word "one" as you exhale.

Keep going for 10 to 20 minutes.

Repeat the practice twice a day.

· · · · ·

TIPS FOR MAKING RELAXATION A CONSISTENT PART OF YOUR DAY

It's OK to Work Your Way Up

If twenty minutes feels too long, you can start with as little as three minutes. Once you sit down and get started, you're likely to keep going. Also, your body will start to crave more and more relaxation once it gets the experience of it. Again, an app like Calm or HeartMath or an Ōura Ring can track your time for you, so you don't have to expend any mental energy peeking at the clock.

Find the Time You Can Commit To

Many study participants found it helpful to do their relaxation practice right after waking up and just before going to bed. But for those with kids, the morning was typically too hectic. In that case, we advised them to do it just before or after breakfast, exercise, or dinner—whichever worked best for their schedule. Tying it to something else you're already doing—even brushing your teeth!—makes you much more likely to do it. For me, alone time is sometimes drive time or bike time. There are a couple of public parking lots in my town that are not busy that I can tuck into for a meditation session if needed.

Don't Stress About Getting It Wrong

The number-one rule of stress relief is that you can't let it stress you out. Anytime your mind tries to convince you you're doing it wrong (which it will, over and over), because your attention wanders or you get impatient, just notice that it's happened and go back to repeating the word "one" on your exhales. Learning how to notice that you've gotten off track and then starting again is essential to becoming versed in meditation and is a valuable life skill that will serve you elsewhere.

SLEEP

Sleep is a fundamental component of health overall and healthy DNA methylation in particular. Yet it's well documented that as we age, our sleep changes, and that these changes start as early as our thirties. Most significantly, the all-important, restorative deep sleep (the form of sleep we need to prevent age-related diseases and decline) decreases significantly over time. Also, the total duration of sleep drops off and it becomes more fragmented as we have more frequent wake-ups. In fact, as Matthew Walker, of the Sleep and Neuroimaging Laboratory at UC Berkeley says, "Sleep changes with aging, but it doesn't just change with aging; it can also start to explain aging itself."[28] Let that sink in! Additionally, all of the chronic diseases of aging have strong causal links to poor sleep. These facts, along with the epigenetic research into sleep and DNA methylation, make it clear why paying attention to sleep is so important to biological age and why it was something that we included in our study. Fortunately, there are ways to improve sleep—regardless of your age.

Whether you are doing the Younger You Intensive or the Everyday, your assignment is the same we gave to our study participants—to get at least seven hours of sleep per night. If that's lower than you typically get, you can feel good about knowing that you've already got this box checked (and certainly don't start sleeping less than you normally do just because I name seven hours a night as a goal!).

As I covered in Chapter 2, sleep is an important part of the Younger You program, because it is a powerful—and fast—influencer of DNA methylation and the epigenome. As I also mentioned in Chapter 2, sleep is the component of a healthy lifestyle that I struggle with the most. The upside for you is that my questionable track record of getting good sleep has motivated me to train for better sleep skills as if I were training for a marathon. Let's just say, I've learned some things. Namely, rather than looking for the one thing that will revolutionize your sleep, prepare to try several smaller adjustments to your daily routine. In my own experience and the experience of my patients, a lot of little changes add up to a lot of restful slumber.

The Stages of Sleep, and Why They Matter

While yes, the total duration of your sleep is important, the quality of those hours also matters. A lot.

There are four distinct phases of sleep that repeat throughout the night in a series of cycles. Each cycle lasts between 70 and 120 minutes—the first cycle of the night is the shortest; cycles then extend from there.

On average, you'll go through four to six sleep cycles in a night; although this number is affected by your age, how well you've been sleeping in general, and whether or not you've had alcohol, which tends to decrease REM sleep and contribute to middle-of-the-night waking. (This is yet another reason that alcohol isn't great for you, and why it is altogether excluded from the Younger You Intensive and allowed only in minimal amounts on the Younger You Everyday.)

Each of the phases of the sleep cycle are essential. They are as follows:

- **Dozing off:** This phase only lasts for a few minutes, and while your brain and muscle activity is slowed (except for some random twitches), you can still wake up easily.
- **Light sleep:** In this transitional stage, your core body temperature drops, your muscles relax, and your heart and respiration rates slow down. In transition sleep, you're preparing for deep sleep; you can still wake up fairly easily. In the first cycle of the night, you're in this stage for about twenty minutes. This phase gets longer in subsequent cycles, to the point that about half your total sleeping hours are spent in light sleep.

- **Deep sleep:** This is the most restorative stage of sleep, when your body cleans, rejuvenates, and repairs itself. In the brain, the glial cells dump their toxic load and the glymphatic system clears out the waste. There's also cleanup and rebuilding happening throughout the body, including in the muscles. This is more rationale for not eating after 7 p.m. — because the body has plenty of other tasks to tend to, and if it's busy digesting, the less focus and energy it will have for renewal. In deep sleep, blood pressure drops, heart rate variability stabilizes, your muscles are very deeply relaxed, and your pulse and breathing slow even further. We tend to spend more time in deep sleep earlier in the night; these phases get shorter in subsequent sleep cycles. All told, deep sleep should comprise up to 20 percent of total sleep time. Deep sleep decreases as we age.

- **REM sleep:** Perhaps the best-known sleep cycle, REM is when your most vivid dreams occur. REM sleep is associated with memory, learning, and creativity. In fact, your brain activity in REM sleep is nearly as high as it is when you are awake. All the muscles in the body, except the muscles of respiration and vision, are immobilized. Your first REM stage of the night is short—just a few minutes. But the duration of REM sleep grows throughout the night. Typically REM sleep comprises about 25 percent of total sleep time. REM sleep also decreases with age.

Tips for Getting More, Higher-Quality Sleep

There are some things you want to do on a daily basis to invite restorative sleep, and some things that you do once that will then support your ability to sleep from there on out. The one-time things include:

- **Make your room dark.** Light exerts a profound suppressive effect on the pineal gland's release of melatonin, thereby shortening the body's internal recognition of night duration.[29] Even something seemingly innocent, like a digital clock, can interfere with your sleep. It's well worth the investment to hang room-darkening shades, switch out your digital clock that's always on to one that only displays the time when you push a button, or buy a quality sleep mask if the first two things aren't an option. I invested in beautiful room-darkening, top-down, bottom-up blinds for me and my daughter. They allow lots of light by day (and exposure to morning light also helps regulate your internal clock, so you want to open those curtains and get outside as early as you can) and create lots of dark by night.

- **Keep things cool.** Your body temperature naturally drops during light sleep, so if your room is too hot, it can keep you awake. You may need to adjust your bedding—swapping out a heavy down comforter for a sheet, blanket, and quilt arrangement that will allow you to find just the right amount of cover to keep you cool. Or you may need a fan or an air conditioner, or to turn down your radiator or crack a window, to keep your bedroom in a temperate zone. I love a cool mist humidifier at night all year long for its cooling and moisturizing benefits. In fact, I've become so attached to sleeping with humidity that I use a tiny bedside USB-port travel humidifier when I'm staying in a hotel.

- **Eat—and don't eat—for sleep.** Turns out good sleep has an optimal diet: higher fat and lower carbs, which is in alignment with the Younger You Intensive. Sleep metabolism prefers the slow burn of fats rather than high-energy carbs. That being said, sleep is impaired when you go to bed on a full stomach. Why? A full stomach will inhibit sleep, and especially deep sleep. Your heart rate will not drop to where it needs to be for detoxification and repair and rebuilding; rather, you'll be directing energy toward digesting food, something we're designed to do during the day. It's yet another reason to stop eating by 7 p.m. each night, or if you are more of a night owl, at least three hours before you go to bed.

- **Secure some form of blue-light blocker.** Blue light is a primary component of sunlight, and we evolved to not have any blue-light exposure once night fell. Because blue light is stimulating, and because it is emitted by all the various screens in your life, you want to minimize your exposure to it after the sun has gone down. Your best first choice for minimizing your after-dusk blue-light intake is to turn off the screen after the sun sets. I know this is hard, and sometimes impossible, to do, so your second-best choice is to minimize or block the blue light that your screen emits. You can download an app such as f.lux, adjust your display settings on your device to shift into night mode at sunset, or buy blue-light blocking glasses to wear during any nighttime device usage. These glasses are ubiquitous now—I've seen them at office supply stores and the drugstore, although you can always find more stylish options online.

- **Consider wearing a sleep tracker.** Having struggled with poor sleep on and off for decades, I did not have confidence that I'd ever become a "good" sleeper. Knowing that, one of the first tools I found useful was a wearable sleep tracker. Seeing the amount and types of sleep you got last night as data points, and not relying on your perception of how well you slept—or didn't sleep—helps make the quest for a better night's sleep less fraught. Seeing that I achieved a good amount of deep sleep every night was eye opening—and comforting. And I can see that I do much better when I've exercised earlier in the day versus later in the day or not at all (as research suggests, this helps specifically deep sleep).[30] I can also see that when I eat late at night (and especially carbs late at night), forget it. My sleep stinks. The sleep tracker also reminds me when bedtime is approaching, which is a great cue to do my evening relaxation practice and make sure I'm getting to bed early enough—which, turns out, is the most important thing we can do to get enough total sleep, and specifically deep sleep. Which means that a great first question to ask yourself if your sleep is off is, am I going to bed too late? And what do I need to do in order to get in bed earlier? Note that not all trackers are equal, and no tracker is 100 percent accurate, but they can still be quite helpful.
- **Evaluate whom you share a bed with.** Sleep is so important that if your partner has sleep apnea or restless legs, give sleeping solo a try. The same goes for pets—if your cat walks across your stomach in the middle of the night seventeen times, they might need to sleep in a different room. I had to start locking my kitty Amos out of my bedroom and Isabella's so that his nighttime adventures didn't wake us up. I know it's hard, but sleep is worth it.

I like to think of the daily habits that promote better sleep in terms of when they should occur. First, it makes it feel less like yet another to-do list. And second, it helps give your days a regular structure, which helps regulate your internal clock. And when your internal clock is well tuned, it will make it easier for you to fall asleep at bedtime and sleep through the night.

- **Noon:** Stop having any caffeinated drinks. And if you're very sensitive to caffeine (many of us don't metabolize it well), consider dropping it altogether. Caffeine can stay in your system for as long as six hours, so put plenty of time between caffeine's zone of influence and bedtime.

- **7 p.m.:** Finish your last bit of food, as the digestion process can be stimulating. (As discussed in Chapter 5, time-restricted eating is favorable for DNA methylation and insulin regulation.) You'll also want to finish up any strenuous exercise, as a workout too close to bedtime can rev your cortisol, which is a stimulant, and make it difficult to drift off. (For most of us, early morning exercise is best for deep sleep.) Again if you're more of a night owl or you're a shift worker and go to bed later, you can adjust this time to be later as needed, just know that the goal is to avoid food at least three hours before bedtime.

- **Three hours before bed:** Start to wrap up your screen time. If you partake in any screen time from here on out, use blue-light blocking glasses (although as I mentioned above, these are not a free pass to stare at your screens for hours every night). Make any shows or movies you watch of the calming variety—no intense thrillers or horror. For me, an intense thriller can be a recently published research paper on a topic near-and-dear to me, like epigenetics. I have to save those for another time, unfortunately.

- **Two hours before bed:** Have your last glass of liquid so that you are less likely to need to wake up and pee. And remember, you are foregoing alcohol altogether for at least the eight weeks of the Younger You Intensive.

- **Sixty minutes before bed:** Turn off all screens. Indulge in a pre-bedtime ritual. Take a bath, do a little light yoga or stretching.

- **Thirty minutes before bed:** Do your relaxation practice, such as the meditation on page 183.

- **Fifteen minutes before bed:** Brush your teeth, wash your face, and do any other personal care in the same order every night. The predictability of events will help cue the brain that sleep is coming.
- **Ten minutes before bed:** Turn on a white noise machine or app and/or an essential oil diffuser with lavender oil. Regular use will make this step a powerful cue to your body that it's time to sleep. Then read for a bit, take a few deep breaths, or give yourself a foot massage to further relax before shutting off the light.

BATHE YOUR WAY TO RELAXATION AND SLEEP

ONE THING THAT CAN SUPPORT YOUR EFFORTS BOTH TO RELAX AND TO SLEEP better are Epsom salt baths. Epsom salt is comprised of magnesium (a mineral that helps to relax your muscles, including the muscles of your GI tract, making it a helpful laxative, too) and sulphate (a form of sulfur and key detoxifier). Try taking a twenty-minute Epsom salt bath, with 2 cups or even more of salt, before bed three times per week to reduce stress and body aches and boost detoxification. In my clinic, we recommend Epsom salt from Ancient Minerals or SaltWorks.

· · · · ·

Troubleshooting Sleep Issues

I know many people depend on some form of sleep medication, but these medications take too big a toll on health in general, and DNA methylation in particular. Benadryl, Unisom, Tylenol PM, and Advil PM all share the same active ingredient—diphenhydramine, an antihistamine that has scary long-term effects. It's a clear contributor to dementia, with the risk increasing depending on dose and duration of use.[31] Being an anticholinergic drug, it depletes an important neurotransmitter called acetylcholine. Acetylcholine has a number of important roles, from activating muscles to regulating autonomic nervous system response. In the brain, it's involved in arousal, memory, motivation, and attention. Acetylcholine requires choline to synthesize it, and choline is an important methyl donor that's challenging to get enough of, hence our recommendation for eggs. So if we deplete acetylcholine, our body will work double time to make it, possibly stealing methyl donors from DNA methylation, or simply not making enough acetylcholine for the brain's high demands. For that matter, sleep medications including Ambien, Lunesta, and Sonata also deplete acetylcholine. If you are taking any of these, I recommend that you slowly taper down and stop.

There are many supplements that are supportive of a good night's sleep—I cover them in Chapter 8, so if you feel like you aren't able to sleep without some outside help and are ready to find an alternative to sleep meds, be sure to check them out.

There are some sleep-impeding issues that require a clinician's assistance, including hot flashes, sleep apnea, and nocturnal hypoglycemia. These are sleep dealbreakers and need to be remedied with professional guidance.

If you regularly wake up in the middle of the night, first, consult your physician to rule out any issues that might require medical help. Then, are you experiencing anxiety? I know I tend to wake up thinking about projects (or responding to a crying toddler). One of the most helpful interventions for me has been listening to a boring story, a long meditation, or a sleep "talk-down" podcast. There are literally thousands to choose from on YouTube. However, you want to keep your exposure both to blue lights and electromagnetic frequencies to a minimum in the middle of the night, so download them onto your phone rather than streaming them and use audio only.

I recognize that I've thrown a lot of options at you here, but know this: it's worth the time and energy it might take to find the right combination of practices, daily routines, and supplements that will help you get the sleep you need to restore yourself.

CONSCIOUSLY AVOIDING TOXINS

When I was at the clinical laboratory during the early years of my career, we developed a very sophisticated suite of tests for measuring body burden of a wide variety of toxins, based on the best available technology developed at the Centers for Disease Control. My department, the Medical Education

Department, was charged with diving into the science on these toxins and amassing the data that would be used to educate clinicians around the world about them. Over a period of months, our collective mood grew sour as we saw the proof mount that toxins are everywhere, they damage everything, and they are unavoidable. We decided to always include actionable steps whenever we educated people on the pervasive dangers of toxins; it's a philosophy I maintain today.

Before I get to those steps, though, let's take a look at toxins through the lens of DNA methylation and bio age.

It is difficult to overstate how problematic environmental toxins are to the genome and epigenome. Many environmental toxins damage DNA directly. And a far-reaching swath of toxins have been shown to negatively alter DNA methylation, including pesticides, fertilizers, inorganic arsenic, mold toxins, persistent organic pollutants, lead, mercury, cadmium, bisphenol A, phthalates, and more. They cause harm to DNA methylation in two primary ways: they disrupt the function of the enzymes that add and remove methyl groups to DNA, and they use up many of the precious resources that are needed for healthy DNA methylation, because eliminating toxins from the body can require copious amounts of our precious methyl donors.

Furthermore, we are learning through an emerging field of study known as toxicomethylomics that this damage to DNA methylation can accumulate in utero, and throughout life, via environmental exposures, often at much lower doses than we've previously understood, with the potential for long-range, far-reaching damage to gene expression.[32] Moshe Szyf summed up the ability of environment, diet, and lifestyle choices to create lasting changes in you and your offspring in a seminal 2011 paper on the topic of toxicomethylomics in which he said, "DNA function and health could be stably altered by exposure to environmental agents without changing the sequence, just by changing the state of DNA methylation."[33]

The fact that we are exposed to so many different toxins from so many different sources—water, food, air, personal-care products, cleaning products, fertilizers, and pesticides—means that even when we live very cleanly, we easily experience enough exposure to have an impact on our DNA methylation, and these changes may also be heritable: a 2004 study found that exposure of female rats to the pesticide methoxychlor—which was used as an alternative to DDT from 1948 to 2003—was associated with epigenetic mutations in four subsequent generations. Specifically, there was a significant increase in kidney disease, ovarian disease, and obesity in the offspring of the rats who were exposed. And remarkably, while we might intuitively think that the damage might be diluted over time, by the fourth generation, the offspring were actually more likely to have multiple diseases.[34] And that's just one particular toxin—we are exposed to multiple different toxins in varying amounts on any given day.

And now, let's look at what we can *do* about the toxic soup we are currently living in.

First, the good news: we know that some toxic exposure is actually a beneficial stressor, aka hormesis, aka "What doesn't kill you makes you stronger." As the body responds to a mild stressor, it kicks on your biotransformation system, which then releases a broad swath of antioxidant and anti-inflammatory molecules into circulation that provide benefit well beyond the toxic exposure itself. It's like saying you'll just pop the dishes in the dishwasher, but then decide to clean the whole kitchen once you get going. What are examples of toxin-induced hormesis? A hint of methylmercury, the form of mercury that is a common environmental contaminant and often bioaccumulates in fish, enhanced reproduction in ducks in one study;[35] and very-low-dose radiation in humans was shown to lower risk of cancer deaths (as compared to high- or normal-dose radiation exposure).[36] Jirtle found a similar result with his agouti mice, too: a hint of radiation to pregnant agouti mice kicked in DNA methylation, which turned off the negative agouti gene in offspring, acting like methyl donors.[37]

However, the science is clear—you can't hope that the hormetic effects of any environmental exposures you may experience will be enough to keep your DNA methylation in a good place. You need to avoid exposures to the very best of your ability, and you need to boost your body's detoxification—also known as *biotransformation*—functions.[38]

I'll cover simple but profound ways to reduce exposure in just a moment. First, I want to reassure you that the Younger You program is a boon to your systems of detoxification. The eating plan is jam-packed with foods that contain a class of compounds known as *xenohormetics*—these are polyphenols, most of which are also DNA methylation adaptogens, that kick in a host of protective mechanisms and were found by Dr. David Sinclair to demonstrate improved longevity in animal models.[39] Xenohormetics include sulforaphane (found in cruciferous vegetables), resveratrol (present in many berries, pistachios, almonds, and lentils), and curcumin (found in turmeric). Organic and wild-grown produce is extra-high in xenohormetics, because the plants don't have the protection of pesticides and need to develop these compounds to fight pests. (I'll state it more clearly below, but eating organic also reduces your toxin exposure in the first place.)

Other polyphenol-rich stars of the Younger You program have been shown to support the body's detoxification pathways, including almonds, apples, Brazil nuts, celery, citrus, coffee, dill, garlic, ginger, legumes (for vegetarians and vegans only on the Younger You Intensive, and everyone on the Everyday), olives, rosemary, Tartary buckwheat, and tomatoes.[40]

Polyphenols aren't the only protective compounds found in foods. A scientist who has inspired me for decades is Bernhard Hennig, PhD, of the University of Kentucky's nutritional sciences department, who says, "Consuming healthy diets that exhibit high levels of antioxidant and anti-inflammatory properties is a meaningful way to reduce the vulnerability to non-communicable diseases linked to environmental toxic insults."[41]

Dr. Hennig has focused a major amount of his research on looking at how nutrients mitigate the damage of toxins and has, for example, found that omega-3 fatty acids can lower the body's proinflammatory response to toxins like PCBs, thereby reducing the risk of heart disease and cancer associated with these toxins; and folate and other methyl donors can support the elimination of toxins like arsenic, lead, and mercury. Foods containing these nutrients are pillars of the Younger You program.

The lifestyle components of the Younger You formula also aid in detoxification: as I mentioned earlier in this chapter, exercise is another form of hormesis. It generates all sorts of oxidation in our mitochondria, which then cues the body to produce a wave of clean-up molecules that go above and beyond cleaning up just recent exposure—they process some stored toxins, too. Exercise also encourages detoxification via increased circulation of blood and lymph (the waste removal system of the body) as well as sweating.

Younger You also helps by getting you more deep sleep, which is when lymphatic cleaning occurs. And drinking half your body weight in ounces of clean, filtered water every day will help you excrete toxins through your urine, as well.

Beyond these fundamental pieces that will boost your ability to detox, there are many ways to further reduce your toxin exposure. From a diet perspective, these are the things to prioritize:

- Eat organic as much as possible. This is a DNA methylation two-fer, as eating organic directly reduces your pesticide exposure, and organic plants contain higher levels of toxin-protective nutrients. I know paying for organics can be expensive, prohibitively so for some. If this is you, know that any amount of organics you can afford will be beneficial to your DNA methylation. (I suggest following the Environmental Working Group's guidance on which produce is the most and least contaminated to decide what to spend extra for—you can find their Clean Fifteen and Dirty Dozen lists, which they update annually, at https://ewg.org.)

  If cost isn't an issue for you, and you're just digging in your heels (I have family members in this camp), know that the more people buy organic, the more the cost of organics will come down. For everyone, if you have any room for a couple of pots of herbs and tomatoes, or garden space, even better.

- For produce that you buy that isn't organic, use the following soaking method to reduce pesticide residue—this is a distant second option, but it's better than nothing at all. And peel it if possible, taking care to wash your knife between peeling and slicing to minimize contaminating the food, although for something like apples, the peel houses the nutrients so it's an imperfect solution.

  Soak your produce in a diluted white vinegar bath for twenty minutes. The longer you soak, the more completely you'll remove the pesticides. Although some will remain it will be significantly less than if you didn't rinse them. Here's the formula: four parts water to one part white vinegar.

- Avoid as much as possible all plastic food containers, including plastic water bottles. If you can't completely cut them out, definitely don't microwave food in them or leave plastic water bottles in your hot car and then drink the water, as heat will make some of the chemicals in the plastic leach into the food or water.

- Avoid nonstick cookware—not just pans but also waffle irons, rice cookers, electric griddles. The chemicals used to create the nonstick coating can leach into food if the surface gets scratched at all. If you must use nonstick cookware, make sure it's coated with Thermalon, which is silicon dioxide, and be sure to use wooden or silicon spoons and spatulas, not metal, as they are less likely to scratch.

- Learn to use more cooking methods that use lower temperatures—more braising, steaming, and low-heat roasting; less broiling, browning, and grilling at high enough heat to leave a char—as the burned bits of food contain pro-inflammatory and DNA-damaging advanced glycation end products (AGEs).

- Opt for glass water bottles and glass or Pyrex food storage containers, and buy food and water in glass instead of plastic or even metal cans (since many are still lined with the hormone-disrupting chemical bisphenol-A).

- Aluminum pans are also best avoided, as aluminum is a known neurotoxin and can leach from the pan into your food. Instead, look to stainless steel, glass/Pyrex, cast iron, or cast iron coated with ceramics (such as Le Creuset)—avoid cast iron pans if your iron levels are high, as they can increase the iron content of foods cooked in them.

Of course, we take in toxins via more than just food. Here are other important strategies to take for reducing overall toxin exposure (again, the Environmental Work Group, https://ewg.org, is a fabulous resource for helping you choose nontoxic products):

- Use natural cleaning products for your home and laundry.

- Avoid topical products, like lotions and sunscreens, that contain chemicals like phthalates, parabens, formaldehydes, and methylene glycol (a type of formaldehyde).

- If you have a vagina, choose your products with care. Nonorganic tampons can have chemicals and pesticides sprayed on them, which leaves a residue that gets introduced to your vagina, and the mucosal membranes there are very absorbant. Never use talc or baby powder in your underwear. Do not douche or put any deodorants or other fragrance-containing items in your vagina. Wear natural fiber underwear, use organic products (including lube), and consider a menstrual cup or period underwear to reduce waste and chemical exposure.
- If you have babies, consider the type of diaper you are using. Many contain plastics that come in contact with your baby's skin twenty-four hours a day, seven days a week. Consider cloth or nontoxic disposable diapers as an alternative.
- Take off your shoes inside the house so that you don't track toxic particulates into your home.
- Because synthetic fragrances are typically some of the most toxic chemicals, avoid any scented products (except those scented with essential oils), including air fresheners, odor-masking sprays, candles, cleaning products, and perfumes.
- Use nontoxic nail polish (or skip it altogether and just buff your nails until they shine).
- Use organic lawn and pest control in your yard, especially if you have kids or pets (who are themselves vulnerable to these toxins and can track them into the house).
- Choose mattresses and pillows made from natural materials—since you spend up to a third of your life in bed and since you detox during sleep.
- Don't carry your cellphone in your pocket or your bra or rest your laptop in your lap, as the radiation and electromagnetic fields emitted by these connected devices decrease dramatically with distance.
- Indoor air is nearly always more contaminated than outdoor air; we breathe far more air than we eat food or drink water. At the minimum, crack your windows. Also consider an air purifier(s) for your home—at least for your bedroom, which is where we tend to spend the most time in our homes, and where we do a lot of detoxifying work while we sleep.

- Get your water tested, as lead (from old pipes, both in your home and in the water system that carries water into your home) and other contaminants are frequently found in drinking water. For example, my well water is wildly high in iron, so I use a whole-house filtration system plus a point-of-use filter (at my kitchen sink) to manage it. (See page 432 for water-testing service recommendations.) Knowing which contaminants are in your water will help you determine what type of water filter to use; a good, basic option is to use a carbon filter, as I mention on page 111. You do have to replace the filter regularly, because when it is overloaded any contaminants it has previously trapped will flow right back into the water you're trying to purify.

THE IMPORTANCE OF COMMUNITY, RELATIONSHIP, AND TOUCH

If there's one element to our study that I wish we could have built in, it's community. Since it's difficult to "prescribe" in specific amounts (and we needed to be able to ensure a consistent experience) it's a challenge to build in community as a part of a randomized controlled trial. We had to sacrifice it for the sake of science, but there's no doubt about it, connection matters to bio age.

We theorize that the fact that our study participants talked with a live nutrition coach was a piece—and perhaps a significant piece—of their success. The Cleveland Clinic Center for Functional Medicine published a study in the *British Medical Journal* in 2021 that shows that the outcomes of their peer-supported group visits were significantly better (and way more affordable!) than one-on-one meetings with the Clinic's brilliant functional medicine physicians.[42] This really hits home the power of group support.

In our clinic, we run many different virtual nutrition programs, including for folks who are doing an elimination diet, for example. It's more efficient for our nutritionists to answer common questions to a group instead of over and over again to individuals, yes, but the true power is in the support and encouragement that travels among participants and between participants and their coaches. While, no, I don't see collective check-ups happening, I do believe that finding ways to have communal experiences is the future of functional medicine (and make this time-intensive model broadly affordable for all). And it's because of the power of connection.

When you are relating to someone else, whether that's a friend, a partner, a child, or a pet, you are reducing stress. A hormone significantly at play here is oxytocin.

The Importance of Oxytocin

Known as the love hormone or the cuddling hormone, oxytocin is an ancient peptide molecule that is released when you enjoy physical contact with a loved one (even a pet!). Since parenting is such a physical endeavor, having a child is an open invitation to bathe yourself and your baby in this wondrous neurochemical.

Because it plays a role in numerous vital physiological and psychological drives and functions, oxytocin

- Helps you cope with stress and recover from trauma
- Is anti-inflammatory and an antioxidant
- Improves glucose tolerance
- Lowers blood pressure
- Produces feelings of love and connection to others
- Creates a drive to reproduce, because it's released after orgasm
- Triggers your uterus to contract during childbirth
- Creates a good-feeling feedback loop that fosters a bond with your baby—the more you cuddle them and look each other in the eye, the more oxytocin you each produce, the more you want to keep taking care of them and the stronger your bond
- Helps you stop eating when you're full, or when you've had too much salt, or when in the presence of toxins

Oxytocin is so important that *not* getting enough of it, whether due to life circumstances or improper DNA methylation that shuts off oxytocin receptor genes, is harmful for humans of all ages, from infants to centenarians.

A sad truth is that oxytocin declines with age, and low levels are associated with many conditions seen in aging, including dementia, depression, hypertension, diabetes, wrinkles, and muscle loss.[43] Fortunately, it's easy—and important—to raise oxytocin. Adhering to the Younger You Intensive and Everyday principles can help—by supporting healthy methylation patterns of oxytocin receptor genes—as will many lifestyle practices (see list on page 203).

Of course, there's a U curve of benefit for oxytocin, too. Some research in humans suggests that there are negative impacts of oxytocin receptor genes that are either cranked up (i.e., excessively hypomethylated) or inhibited (excessively hypermethylated).

Too little oxytocin receptor gene action (thanks to hypermethylation) can usher in depression, including postpartum depression, disconnection, the social cognitive deficits seen in autism, and the rigid thinking present in anorexia. In other words, social, cognitive, and emotional function are all impaired. Excess oxytocin activity has been associated with anxiety, perinatal stress, autism, and mood disorders. Korean researchers found that a hypomethylated oxytocin receptor gene—which suggests that there is an above-average amount of oxytocin in play—is associated with obsessive compulsive disorder.[44] Another long-lasting result of impaired oxytocin receptors is that you become more likely to crave carbohydrates—especially sugar, which then paves the way for inflammation, diabetes, and obesity.[45]

Because this science is new and evolving, it affirms that the broad, safe diet and lifestyle choices that comprise the Younger You approach are a solid game plan, and that there's yet another reason to eat plenty of DNA methyl donors and methylation adaptogens, so that your DNA methylation is *just right.*[46]

The data are strong that your every interaction that involves loving touch, whether with your child(ren), your partner, and/or your pet, gives you regular doses of oxytocin, which then deliver long-lasting benefits for your (and your offspring's) epigenome. Even if your child isn't yours by blood, when you each get hits of oxytocin throughout the day, your DNA methylation—and thus your genetic expression—syncs up, even though you don't share actual DNA. Your ongoing, nurturing connection to one another becomes biologically embedded on your epigenome, creating a shared genetic expression. This idea is deeply moving to me as an adoptive mom.

Kids who don't get adequate amounts of physical affection and care have reduced tolerance for stress, a higher possibility for a lower IQ, a lack of social development, and a higher risk of obesity and diabetes later in life because of epigenetic changes. Kids who grow up in a low-contact household have different methylation patterns on their oxytocin receptor genes than kids who come from a high-contact home.[47] This likely plays a role in the well-established phenomenon that babies who aren't held enough fail to thrive—something we can now understand as being a result of imbalanced DNA methylation that prevents them from developing appropriately.

Of course, it's not just oxytocin receptor genes that are impacted by early loving touch—or lack thereof. A 2017 paper out of the University of British Columbia showed that the amount of hugging a child receives as an infant can influence epigenetic changes in at least five areas of their DNA, including those related to the immune system and metabolism.[48]

Luckily, it seems that whenever kids start to get more loving touch, they will experience benefits, although earlier is better. A 2011 study found that parentless children who were taken out of an orphanage and placed in foster homes before they turned two enjoyed "substantial" gains in cognitive function and social outcomes—much greater than children who stayed in the orphanage until later ages. This study also found low caregiver contact was associated with greater infant distress and a lower biological age at 4.5 years of age (in kids, a lower bio age means they're not developing appropriately). So lack of early contact can have significant long-term effects.[49]

For parents, the steady stream of oxytocin that parenting provides means a lower risk of dying from any cause. I know those tough, sometimes sleepless, days in parenting can make it feel like your kids are shaving years off your life, but science suggests the opposite is true: a 2012 Danish study that followed over twenty-one thousand women undergoing in vitro fertilization found that the women who went on to have children had a risk of dying from any cause that was a full four times lower than those women who didn't.[50] And a 2006 study analyzed life span in the Amish community and found that life span for both fathers and mothers extended in proportion to how many children they had—except for women, whose life span increases petered out if they had more than fourteen children.[51]

Josh Mitteldorf, a brilliant statistician who assisted in analyzing the data in our study, published a statistical analysis of the Centenarian Study in Boston that showed that women having children after forty were a whopping four times more likely to live to one hundred![52] The argument that women who conceive after forty are metabolically stronger isn't sufficiently strong to explain the full four-fold increase. Yes, likely these women are healthier, but the will to live and the deep ineffable connection to your offspring is also, likely, a big piece.

While having a child definitely gives you a strong will to live, which certainly has an impact on life span, it's the regular doses of oxytocin—big and small—that parenting provides that create healthier DNA methylation patterns, which then delay aging (which is, remember, the single biggest cause of chronic disease).

Of course, you don't have to have children to give yourself regular doses of oxytocin.

Simple Ways to Give Yourself an Oxytocin Boost (and Lower Stress)

In addition to cuddling with kids, partners, parents, and friends (anyone you feel safe with), there are many ways to give yourself a hit of oxytocin.

- **Pet a dog.** There are many reasons why dogs are a human's best friend—not least of which is that petting them triggers an oxytocin release, for you and your pooch.
- **Make eye contact.** You know how staring into a baby's eyes feels like it's recharging your energetic batteries? That's because it's bathing your cells in oxytocin. The same thing happens when you look anyone you're conversing with in the eye, no matter their age.
- **Take a warm bath or shower.** Oxytocin is released in response to warmth on your skin, so immersing yourself in warm water bathes your cells in oxytocin.
- **Have an orgasm.** Whether you're with someone else or on your own, having an orgasm creates a spike in oxytocin.[53]
- **Watch your favorite tearjerker.** A 2007 study found that watching an emotional video elicited an oxytocin spike and made participants more likely to be generous to a stranger.[54]

- **Listen to music.** I know the temptation to binge watch is real, but keeping the screens off and the tunes on can boost your oxytocin—and your relaxation. Better yet, sing along, as belting it out has been shown to boost the love hormone, too.[55]
- **Volunteer.** A 2013 study found that folks who regularly participated in charitable activities experienced fewer negative health consequences from stressful life events if they also had a specific genotype for their oxytocin receptors.[56]
- **Get a massage.** Part of the reason massages are so relaxing is that they trigger the release of oxytocin.[57]
- **Give a gift.** The adage that it's better to give than to receive probably isn't referring to the health benefits of giving, but giving a gift does raise oxytocin—so think about that the next time you're selecting a gift for someone else.
- **Share a meal.** Eating together is a great way to bond with others, and that sense of connection gets your oxytocin flowing.
- **Meditate while focusing on others.** A form of meditation known as loving-kindness, or *metta*, where you consciously send good wishes to another person, has been shown to boost oxytocin more than your basic mindfulness meditation. But there is plenty of research, including our own, to suggest that meditation leads to younger bio age, as well, so however you like to meditate, just do it.

To make sure you're getting plenty of connection in your life, aim to do at least one thing on this list to raise your oxytocin every day. And know that making time to have that phone call with a friend, or snuggle with your pet, or have sex with your partner (all things that can feel frivolous, especially when life is busy) is actually nourishing your epigenetics.

LIFESTYLE PRACTICES CHEAT SHEET

To sum up, here's a quick refresher on all the lifestyle pillars that will not only help you feel your best but also support your body's DNA methylation abilities.

Younger You Intensive

Exercise:

Thirty to sixty minutes of moderate-intensity exercise five times
a week as a baseline (this is what our study participants were
prescribed); adding in one or two sessions of HIIT a week (these
can be as short as seven minutes).

Relaxation:

Two ten-to-twenty-minute sessions of mediation per day, as described
on page 183.

Sleep:

At least seven hours a night.

Connection:

Use the Younger You digital program to access our community and
a nutritionist trained in the full program, or find a professional
nutritionist or a health-savvy friend with whom to have weekly
check-ins about how your Intensive experience is going—
troubleshoot problems, share wins, and get ideas. And of course, do
all the things suggested for the Younger You Everyday, below, to the
extent that you are able. (If you need to stay home more and avoid
social gatherings to stick to your eating plan, trust that impulse. You
can get back out there when you're feeling more rooted in the plan,
or the eight weeks are over—whichever comes first.)

Make time for friends and family; cuddle with loved ones and pets;
have sex.

Younger You Everyday

Exercise:

Moderate, at least three times a week (but preferably five—when you're
ready); work up to adding one or two bursts of intensity each week.

Relaxation:

Work up to meditating—or some other kind of relaxation practice—
for ten to twenty minutes, twice daily. You can start with just a few
minutes once per day if this is totally new to you, but keep adding

on until you get comfortable sitting for ten to twenty minutes at a time; then work up to doing it twice a day. Bonus points for Epsom salt baths three times a week.

Sleep:

At least seven hours a night.

Connection:

Make time for friends and family; cuddle with loved ones and pets; have sex.

There is just *one more* piece to explore when it comes to rounding out the full Younger You program—and that is ensuring that you are getting plenty of the nutrients needed for healthy DNA methylation. Although of course I strongly advocate for getting as many nutrients as possible through the diet, there are instances where a moderate dose of a well-chosen supplement is helpful for keeping DNA methylation humming. I'll guide you through what supplements to consider, how to choose the ones that are right for you, and a prudent dosage.

8

SUPPLEMENT SUPPORT

O F COURSE IN GENERAL I WANT YOU TO GET YOUR NUTRIENTS FROM whole foods wherever and whenever possible. As evidence, in our study, we only prescribed our participants a single-strain probiotic and an organic greens powder—the lion's share of nutrients came from food. After all, I spent most of Chapter 2 explaining why we don't want to rely on high-dose supplements to meet our need for methyl donors. *And yet.* If only medicine followed binary logic—supplements were always bad, and foods were always good. It just doesn't work that way. There is a time and place for everything, and that includes a few well-chosen, moderately dosed supplements.

Yes, you can get ample, yet safe, amounts of methyl donors from your diet. And yes, that is the optimal approach to take. But there may be nutrients that come packaged in foods that you just don't like, or don't eat for a reason. Say you have an allergy to eggs, for example: unless you're paying very close attention to alternative choline sources, you will not be likely to eat enough of them to cover your choline needs. Or, if you never eat salmon or other fatty fish, because you don't like it or are a vegetarian or vegan, you are probably not getting enough of the omega-3 essential fatty acids EPA and DHA that those foods contain. Or maybe you don't absorb some nutrients optimally (if you're on an acid-blocking medication, for example) or burn through others fast (I always, always need extra magnesium). In my clinical practice, using the broad nutrient testing that we use, it's the rare day that someone's levels are perfect from food alone.

In this chapter, I'm sharing the supplements I recommend in the following situations:

- You are following the Younger You Intensive; these are the supplements our study participants took, and therefore something everyone who follows the eight-week eating plan should consume.
- You are following the Younger You Intensive and are vegetarian or vegan; in addition to the supplements listed above, these are the supplements that will rectify any potential insufficiencies of DNA methylation–supportive nutrients due to your minimal intake or complete avoidance of animal-based foods.
- You want to support your overall health and shore up your epigenome even further; these include basic nutrients most people are deficient in, such as vitamin D and omega-3s, as well as key DNA methylation adaptogens that provide further epigenetic support.
- You want to preserve the methyl donors you already have—a more prudent strategy for boosting your level of methyl donors than supplementing with them directly, something we refer to in our clinic as "backdoor methylation."
- Other anti-aging supplements that I'm rather bullish on for myself, that you may want to consider also.
- In addition, I'll cover supplements that help you sleep, so that you can get your seven hours of sleep a night without having to rely on prescription sleep medications.

While I'm offering broad recommendations in this chapter, it's worth noting that we all have unique nutrient needs. That's why I recommend working with a clinician or nutritionist to ensure that your nutrient levels are in sufficient range. It's definitely worth seeking the extra care it takes to get your individualized nutrient needs assessed (something I do annually), vegan or not. I suspect you'll find it quite inspiring (and motivating) to see exactly what your body needs, rather than taking something and hoping for the best.

Note: if you are taking any prescription medication, check with your health-care provider for any contraindications, and while you're at it, ask them if your medications might cause an increased need for certain nutrients, too.

YOUNGER YOU INTENSIVE SUPPLEMENTS

As I mentioned earlier, there are only two supplements that our study participants took and that are technically part of the Younger You Intensive. Everyone who follows the Younger You Intensive should take at least these two, which I have listed first. And because liver is such a methylation super star—and because it's something not many people consistently eat two to three times a week—I also include a recommendation for a liver supplement that can help you tick this important box without actually buying, preparing, and eating liver.

- **Probiotics** (*Lactobacillus plantarum* 299V). In general, probiotics are great support for gut health. With regard to DNA methylation, there is some evidence that *Lactobacillus plantarum* 299V manufactures natural folate in the gut. Further evidence is that our study participants saw increased circulating methyl folate, although we can't say for sure that the probiotic alone did it. This strain has also been shown to reduce cortisol levels in human saliva—yet another lever it has to support healthy DNA methylation.[1] *L. plantarum* 299V is also generally well tolerated.

  Dosage: Aim to take 40 billion live CFUs per day (usually two capsules).

- **Greens powder with extra DNA methylation adaptogens.** We also used a proprietary greens powder that is flush with methyl donor and DNA methylation adaptogen nutrients, including powdered versions of various mushrooms, berries, flax seeds, turmeric, and beets. We use this product as a high-quality, super-clean, extra bit of plant-based insurance for our patients, too. It covers a lot of bases in one scoop. (See page 435 for specific recommendations.)

  You certainly don't need to use our specific blend. Any good greens powder will work well. Make sure it is organic and look for one that contains one or a blend of methyl donors and DNA methyl-ation adaptogens, such as those I just listed.

Dosage: Take one to two servings a day (as determined by the product label), either stirred into water, green or herbal tea, a Beet Bubbly (page 388), or mixed into the Basic Smoothie (page 289). Note that in our study, we prescribed our greens powder twice per day.

- **Liver supplements.** As I've covered, liver is a key way to get methyl do-nors in the diet and other DNA methylation supportive nutrients—it's like a methylation multivitamin in a food matrix. But . . . it's not some-thing that most people are likely to eat. If you are liver-averse, take a clean-sourced, nondefatted, freeze-dried liver supplement with third-party verification of the nutrients in it and the absence of pesticides and toxins. For a list of liver supplements I recommend, see page 433. And if you have high iron, consult with your provider before starting.

  Dosage: Up to 1,500 mg per day (which provides the nutrients found in about ½ ounce of bovine liver).

ADDITIONAL YOUNGER YOU INTENSIVE SUPPLEMENTS FOR VEGETARIANS AND VEGANS

To be clear, I am very supportive of plant-based diets—both forms of the Younger You eating plans are primarily plant-based! Yet, when I look at a diet that is excluseively plant-based, I have some concerns. As I covered in Chapter 5, there are a handful of nutrients that vegetarians and vegans tend to be deficient in. These include some of the vital amino acids—particularly the sulfur-containing methionine, cysteine, and taurine—the methyl donor vitamin B_{12}, choline, and the omega-3 fatty acid DHA.

Even vegans who are very health conscious are still at risk of these deficiencies. One of my vegan patients had a significant arrhythmia. Her labs showed that she was profoundly deficient in taurine and magnesium, two nutrients that are very important for heart health. When we corrected those, the arrhythmia resolved. She was an integrative physician—someone whom I expected to be very clued in to the health needs of vegans. If she had imbalanced taurine, it's very possible you do, too.

Below are the supplements I recommend every vegetarian and vegan take. I also suggest some that are included on the list of epigenome-friendly supplements that nearly everyone needs. I'll list them in both places, just so it's clear why they are particularly important for vegans and vegetarians (but that doesn't mean you need to double up on them!).

- **Organic protein powder that contains all nine essential amino acids.** In addition to just needing protein, vegans are vulnerable to deficiencies in the amino acids methionine and taurine. Taurine is a conditionally essential amino acid. That means your body requires taurine and *can* make it, but it requires methionine to do so. Vegans generally have to make all their own taurine, as the only foods that contain it are meat or dairy. Animal products are also the richest sources of methionine, although some plant foods do contain it. (See our list of food sources for methionine on page 416.) If you're a vegan you're likely not getting enough methionine to make sufficient amounts of taurine.

  Dosage: See page 436 in the Supplements section for the protein powders we recommend in our clinical practice. You can take them as directed on the label in a daily smoothie (such as the Basic Smoothie recipe, page 289).

- **An algae-based omega-3 supplement that contains both DHA and EPA.** Interestingly, it's all the algae that fish eat that makes fish such a good source of omega-3s; these supplements help you go straight to the source. And make sure you're eating plenty of plants that are rich in the omega-3 fatty acid alpha-linolenic acid (ALA), including flax seeds, chia seeds, walnuts, and hemp seeds. Your body has to convert ALA into the most important forms of omega-3s—EPA and DHA—and the conversion process is very inefficient for most of us. So it's helpful to eat a lot of ALA *and* take an algae supplement.

  Dosage:

  ALA: Shoot for about 3 to 5 grams of ALA per day, but I recommend using whole foods to get it. For ground flax seed (my top ALA source), that would be one to two tablespoons per day.

  EPA and DHA: Try to get at least 300 mg combined EPA and DHA daily, and possibly more if you are older, pregnant, or nursing,

or if you have an inflammatory condition such as heart disease, autoimmunity, or allergies. (Testing your levels of EPA, DHA, and ALA
is particularly useful.)

- **Vitamin B$_{12}$:** This important methyl donor, with few exceptions, is
  only found in animal protein. If you are vegetarian and eat eggs and
  dairy, you can still get some vitamin B$_{12}$. There are small amounts of
  B$_{12}$ in nori and shiitake mushrooms (although you'd need to eat 50
  grams of dried shiitakes a day to meet your daily requirements); nutritional yeast is also fortified with B$_{12}$.[2] Spirulina and chlorella appear to
  actually only contain biologically *inactive* B$_{12}$, so don't rely on them as
  sources of this vital nutrient. Unless you are dedicated to eating these
  foods on a daily basis, we generally recommend all our vegan patients,
  and most of our vegetarian patients, take a B$_{12}$ supplement. We recommend bioidentical forms (the same types that our body uses) of
  B$_{12}$, called methylcobalamin, adenosylcobalamin, and hydroxycobal-
  amin, rather than the synthetic form of B$_{12}$ called cyanocobalamin.
  The cyano form is still widely used in supplements, most likely due
  to its cheap price and stability; I don't think the cyano is harmful (it's
  way below a toxic dose of cyanide), but why go synthetic when you
  don't need to?[3] Listen, don't hesitate to get B$_{12}$ levels tested (and also,
  if you can, look at a surrogate marker of B$_{12}$ activity like homocysteine)
  to make sure you're getting enough. B$_{12}$ works with folate. If you're
  taking B$_{12}$, you want to be eating a lot of folate foods or might need a
  smidge of folate (around 400 ug/day) in your supplement, too.
  Dosage: 500 ug/day.

- **Vitamin D.** While vegan vitamin D is readily available as a supplement, levels are still generally found to be lower in vegetarians and
  vegans.[4] Thus, I recommend you make it a point to get extra vitamin
  D. See the box on page 218 for information on how to use mushrooms as a supercharged source of vitamin D$_2$, and a recipe for lactofermented mushrooms that ups the bioavailability of that vitamin D
  even more on page 313.
  Dosage: Anywhere from 2,000 IU to 10,000 IU per day—for most
  of us, 5,000 IU is the sweet spot.

- **Iron.** *If* you're diagnosed as deficient, I recommend supplementing with iron.

  Dosage: 40–80 mg of elemental iron **every other day** until your iron levels are restored, as research suggests our body is better able to use (and our guts better able to tolerate) a lower dose of iron taken every other day rather than a daily higher dose.[5] Improve absorption by taking your iron with 500 mg of vitamin C, or a vitamin C–rich snack (see the Nutrient Reference on page 407 for vitamin C foods).
- **Choline.** Our bodies make choline, but it is a labor-intensive and methyl-donor expensive journey. Thus, for most of us, and especially vegans and premenopausal or pregnant women, it's essential to get some additional choline through supplements.

  Dosage: 450–550 mg of choline bitartrate daily (on the higher end if you are pregnant or nursing).

EPIGENOME-FRIENDLY SUPPLEMENTS THAT NEARLY EVERYONE NEEDS

Regardless of whether you're following the Younger You Intensive or Younger You Everyday, these are the epi-nutrients that I think are essential for keeping your epigenome humming along that most of us don't get enough of. Despite all of the attention in the media, I see patients who are woefully low in vitamin D and omega-3 fatty acids, in particular, almost as a rule in the patients at our clinic (even in the sunny summer). Also included on this list are a couple of DNA methylation adaptogen superstars, including EGCG (the primary active constituent of green tea) and curcumin (found in turmeric). Of course, there are loads of DNA methylation adaptogens available as supplements (more are identified all the time—I write about new ones frequently on my website and include them in the Younger You app), and we all want to be taking in a nice variety of them all the time. If you are taking methyl donor supplements, you want to be consuming a load of DNA methylation adaptogens, too, so that they can direct DNA methylation to happen at the right spots—and not everyone enjoys drinking green tea or eating lots of turmeric every day.

Finally, this list includes important DNA demethylation supporters vitamin C, vitamin A, and iron. These nutrients support the active demethylator family of enzymes called TET (more on these enzymes on page 262 and 425), which actively remove errant methyl groups, allowing previously inhibited genes to be reactivated. As vitamin C is water soluble, and used in so many vital processes, nearly everyone could stand to have a little more of it on hand. Iron is only necessary if bloodwork shows you're deficient. And vitamin A levels can dip below sufficient if you are not eating liver (although I hope by this point in the book that you're starting to eat it regularly), or your thyroid function is impaired (as hypothyroidism slows down the conversion of certain carotenoids found in plants to vitamin A). As always, it's best to have your levels of all these nutrients checked so that you can determine whether you need the supplement at all, and if so, in what amounts.

- **Vitamin D.** Vitamin D is a workhorse nutrient responsible for the smooth sailing of many physiological processes, especially relating to normal immune function. We also know it's important in regulating many epigenetic mechanisms, including enzymes used in the DNA demethylation process.[6] Get your levels tested—I like to see levels between 50 and 70 ng/mL.

    Dosage: To maintain these levels, you need anywhere from 2,000 IU to 10,000 IU per day—for most of us, 5,000 IU is the sweet spot. This is significantly higher than the daily recommended intake of just 600–800 IU per day, which is fine if you can achieve optimal blood levels at this dosage. I have not seen this to be successful in my adult patients. Why? Maybe absorption is an issue. A top tip for D and any fat-soluble vitamin (like vitamins A, E, and K) is to take it with a little fat, such as a handful of nuts or nut butter, a little avocado, or even your omega-3 supplements!

- **Omega-3 fatty acids.** It's rare to consume enough of the longer-chain omega-3s, which are DHA and EPA. DHA in particular is suggested to support the methylation cycle (where we synthesize the universal methyl donor SAMe that works with DNA methylation). We're also particularly bullish on specialized pro-resolving lipid mediators (SPMs)—compounds our bodies make from omega-3s—that are important for many reasons, including their essential role in turning off inflammation and in brain health, pain relief, and more. While research is still forthcoming, given the number of SPMs we make in our bodies (including in our brains) and their wide role in health, I expect we'll see them as beneficial influencers on the epigenome, particularly as it pertains to inflammation.

Dosage: We routinely prescribe omega-3 supplements, around 2,000 mg per day for healthy adults of a blend of EPA and DHA. For patients dealing with inflammation we go up to 5,000 mg per day. SPMs are available in doses ranging from 500 to 1,000 mg. We recommend adding SPMs at 1,000 mg per day when inflammation of any form is an issue.

- **Folate and B$_{12}$.** While it's true that we should avoid overdoing folate and B$_{12}$ supplements (especially if you're older and/or you don't have a clear need for them or you've been diagnosed with cancer), you need sufficient amounts of these essential nutrients. While I recommend the always safe food-forward approach, sometimes it is appropriate to take extra folate and B$_{12}$ in supplement form. Reasons for taking folate and B$_{12}$ supplements include:
  - » Your blood levels of either or both nutrients are low.
  - » You have macrocytosis (your red blood cell size is large) or macrocytic anemia (your blood cells are large, and your hemoglobin and hematocrit are low).
  - » You have a medical condition that causes nutrient malabsorption.
  - » You are taking medications that increase demand for B vitamins including birth control pills, metformin, or acid blockers.
  - » Your functional medicine provider is recommending based on
    - – your lab tests and/or
    - – signs of significant deficiency that require more than you're ingesting in the Younger You Intensive—examples include peripheral neuropathy (pins and needles in your hands and/or feet, like my patient Paul whom I mentioned in Chapter 3 was experiencing) or difficult-to-treat depression.
  - » You are vegan.
  - » You are pregnant or trying to become pregnant and are advised by your health-care provider to take them.

Dosage: For folate, 400–1,000 ug per day and for B_{12}, 100–2,000 ug per day; both are according to your need (your health-care provider may prescribe differently, but this is a common range).

- **EGCG (Green Tea Extract).** If I haven't said it enough yet, I want to point out that many of the compounds showing themselves to be extraordinary DNA methylation adaptogens, like the green tea and curcumin discussed here, are nutrients that have been consumed the world over since time immemorial. That said, perhaps you do not particularly enjoy green tea (I confess, I don't love the tannins). If you aren't able or willing to drink strong green tea most days of the week, you can take green tea extract in capsules. I recommend the whole plant extract versus just EGCG alone because there are many other polyphenols in green tea that are likely important in health and DNA methylation. To ensure a quality product, make sure the extract is standardized to contain the primary constituent EGCG. Green tea extract (800 mg per day for four months) was shown in one study to be as potent as medication at reducing uterine fibroids; I've successfully prescribed it along with the Younger You Intensive to many of my female patients suffering with uterine fibroids and other conditions associated with estrogen imbalance, and it has helped them immensely.[7]

  Dosage: 500–600 mg standardized green tea extract daily (providing about 250–300 mg EGCG per day, the equivalent of about three cups of strong green tea) is considered safe and healthy.[8] Take higher amounts with clinician guidance.

- **Curcumin.** Like green tea, curcumin—the main active constituent in turmeric—has been used for millennia to bolster health. Also like green tea and the other DNA methylation adaptogen polyphenols, curcumin has pleiotropic activity: it's potently anti-aging, anti-inflammatory, antioxidant, anticancer, neuroprotective, GI protective, and antimicrobial to name some.[9] It regulates the epigenome via a variety of mechanisms, including, of course, DNA methylation. I use loads of curcumin in practice, as do my colleagues. I drink a hot mug of our extra-yummy Golden Turmeric Milk (page 386) almost every single day, and I take a little extra in capsule form for safe measure. It's difficult to overstate the importance of this rock star polyphenol.

Dosage: 500–1,000 mg per day. Take a product that is standardized for curcuminoids. Curcumin is not very bioavailable (i.e., it's tough to absorb); thus, good brands will address this issue, sometimes by including a smidge of black pepper (as piperine), as it aids in absorption. Also, curcumin is fat soluble, so take your capsules with a fat-containing meal or with your omega-3 fatty acid supplements to further improve absorption.

- **Vitamin C.** Refer to page 413 for a look at how vitamin C supports the epigenome. I tend to use l-ascorbic acid, because there's not a lot of data that the much more expensive forms are that much more effective. That said, if taking vitamin C tends to upset your stomach, look for a buffered form, and if you want a few extra DNA methylation adaptogens, many vitamin C products come with extra flavonoids.

  Dosage: 500–1,000 mg a day as baseline, more if you need extra antioxidant or immune support.

- **Vitamin A.** See page 412 for a rundown of the reasons why vitamin A is supportive of health in general and DNA methylation in particular. If you're not eating plenty of food sources of vitamin A on a daily basis (also listed on page 412), consider supplementing.

  Dosage: Take no more than 2,500 IU a day of retinol (a preformed version of vitamin A, meaning your body doesn't have to convert it), unless specifically prescribed a different dosage or form by your health-care provider.

- **Iron.** As discussed on page 412, iron is important in healthy methylation, but you don't want to supplement with it unless you have demonstrated need based on laboratory testing, or you are a vegan, or a low-meat-consuming premenopausal woman (i.e., women who still get regular periods). Pregnancy also increases iron requirements. Iron is one of those nutrients that is classically U curve: too little is bad—resulting in fatigue and anemia—and too much is also bad—iron is potently oxidative and damaging. A high percentage of premenopausal women get insufficient iron (even for meat eaters, it's common), but conversely, a high percentage of men (and to a lesser extent, postmenopausal women) can have too much iron. In our practice, we use a handful of tests, including iron, total iron binding capacity (TIBC), percent transferrin saturation (%TS), and ferritin to determine if iron is too low or too high. These reference ranges can change, depending on whether you are a man or woman, pre- or postmenopausal, but here are patterns to look for:

DISEASE	IRON	TIBC	%TS	FERRITIN
Iron Deficiency	Low	High	Low	Low
Iron Overload/ Excess	High	Low	High	High

We also look at a CBC to see how iron status might be affecting red blood cell indices.

Dosage: If you have your iron levels tested and they are low, I suggest an iron supplement with about 40–80 mg of iron **every other day** until your levels are where your care provider wants them. If you have too much iron and you are otherwise healthy, the best way to lower levels is to donate blood every few months. In fact, donating blood is a fairly common anti-aging strategy—that's how toxic excess iron is. But you don't want to overdo it and kick in anemia—something I've seen occur in overzealous anti-agers.

MAKE YOUR OWN VITAMIN D—USING MUSHROOMS (AND THE SUN)

HERE IS A REALLY COOL WAY TO ESSENTIALLY MAKE YOUR OWN VITAMIN D supplement—by exposing mushrooms to sunlight before eating them.

Mushrooms naturally contain vitamin D, which they make from sun exposure, just like we do. The form of D in mushrooms is D_2, which is a different form than the D_3 that most supplements contain. But humans are typically pretty good at activating D_2: a study conducted at Boston University Medical Center concluded that ingestion of mushrooms with 2,000 IU of vitamin D_2 was as effective as 2,000 IU of either D_2 or D_3 in supplement form.[10]

When you take the mushrooms that you've bought at the store or the farmers' market and set them out in the sun for at least fifteen minutes, and up to five hours, you dramatically increase the levels of vitamin D they contain. The exact amount of the increase depends on the variety of mushroom, the length of sun exposure, and the intensity of the sun's rays, but even a little can make a big impact.

Once they've had a chance to soak up the sun, you can cook mushrooms as you normally would. And to *really* amp up the benefits of mushrooms, see the recipe for Lactofermented Vitamin D Mushrooms on page 313, which deliver a healthy dose of friendly microbes that can shore up your microbiome, too.

Mushrooms may or may not be able to replace your vitamin D supplement. I often see patients who, despite high intake of vitamin D, still have inadequate levels circulating in their body. The only way to know for sure is to monitor your levels.

* * * * *

SUPPLEMENTS TO PRESERVE THE METHYL DONORS YOU ALREADY HAVE: AKA BACKDOOR METHYLATION

What happens if you are like my patients Paul or Sharon and you absolutely cannot tolerate or take B$_{12}$ and folate? If you're doing the full Intensive program, you may still need extra methyl donors. A somewhat sneaky approach (hence the "backdoor" name) to supporting DNA methylation is to take supplements of nutrients that require a lot of methyl donors to make. (Think of it like buying a premade cauliflower pizza crust versus making your own—it gets a lot more efficient to get dinner on the table.) Two supplements that help you do this:

- **Creatine:** Creatine phosphate is a molecule used in the body to rapidly recycle ATP, the body's main source of energy, in high-energy tissue, including skeletal muscles, heart muscle, and the brain. You synthesize and recycle creatine in the kidneys via a process that requires a *lot* of methyl donors (just think about all of the skeletal muscle you have—even if you're not a bodybuilder, added up together, skeletal muscles make up the largest organ in your body). For this reason, I sometimes prescribe creatine to spare those many methyl donors for use in other pathways, such as DNA methylation.

Folks who might benefit from creatine are those who don't tolerate B vitamins but need them, those with cognitive decline, muscle
loss (sarcopenia), fatigue, or individuals who require extra energy support. Athletes can also benefit from extra creatine.

Dosage: I generally start dosing at 3 grams and may increase up to 6
grams. (And see the Nutrient Reference on page 407 for food sources.)[11]

- **Choline and Betaine:** If you're not consuming enough eggs, you
might need extra choline. Choline is a conditionally essential nutrient and key methylation player involved in a variety of important
processes throughout the body, including in the muscle, brain, and
liver; cell membranes; and neurotransmitters such as acetylcholine.
While we can synthesize some choline, we do so very inefficiently:
it requires three methyl donor–dependent steps, making it a very
methyl donor–demanding process. We also need extra choline when
we get older for cognitive function and during pregnancy, as it's essential for a baby's cognitive development. Choline is eventually metabolized to betaine, another important methyl donor that can make
SAMe in the methylation cycle without the need of B_{12} and folate.

Dosage: 450–550 mg of choline bitartrate daily (on the higher
end if you are pregnant or nursing). Consider beet supplements for
a source of betaine, see page 434, or you can take three to six grams
of betaine itself.

Trimethylamine-N-oxide (TMAO), Choline, Betaine, and Heart Disease: Cause for Concern?

Because they are important methyl donor nutrients, sufficient intake of food sources of both choline and betaine are important parts
of the Younger You Intensive. These compounds (and also carni-
tine, from meat) can be converted by your gut microbiome to TMA
(trimethylamine), and then to TMAO (trimethylamine-N-oxide) by
your liver. In a 2020 study, higher circulating levels of TMAO were
associated with increased risk of major adverse cardiac events, although risk appears to be dictated in part by composition of the gut
microbiome (since the microbiome varies from person to person, we
don't all make the same amount of TMA).[12] The study findings were

challenged by other scientists for a few reasons, including the fact that participants who had some, but not a lot of, TMAO actually fared better than those with very low TMAO. The study was also challenged for not eliminating the impact of certain commonly prescribed drugs that are known to promote TMAO production, including statins, antibiotics, and proton pump inhibitors.[13] While scientists puzzle through whether these findings are significant, and how to best address high TMAO levels (likely by changing your gut microbiome and medications rather than eliminating vital nutrients, such as choline), your doctor can measure your levels of TMAO to see if you need to focus on shoring up your gut health and temporarily be mindful of your diet or supplement habits.[14]

· · · · ·

OTHER ANTI-AGING SUPPLEMENTS TO CONSIDER

While we created the Younger You Intensive as a stand-alone program, I believe that layering it into other anti-aging protocols could increase the benefit. Thus, I certainly don't shut the door when new science is published on the anti-aging benefits of supplements.

There are a number of supplements that either directly benefit DNA methylation and the epigenome or have some research on them as beneficial anti-aging compounds worthy of considering as adjunctive to the Younger You Intensive. I'm including those on my radar at the time of this writing, and be sure to visit our Younger You app and website (Younger YouProgram.com) for more supplement recommendations (and a discussion of the research), as this list is always evolving. How do you decide if you want to take these? I would recommend that you first do the full Intensive program as it's prescribed, and I'd strongly recommend you obtain an epigenetic bio age clock test at baseline, and when you're finished. After that, if you want to keep going down the anti-aging road, then consider trying a couple of these. Ideally, you'll take them for at least a couple of months, tracking how you feel with the MSQ every week or two, and even obtaining a periodic epigenetic DNAmAge test. I personally try to get my bio age assessed via a DNAmAge clock every six to twelve months. If you would like personalized guidance, refer to page 427 in the Resources for suggestions on finding a functional medicine provider.

- **Nicotinamide riboside (NR):** This form of niacin is readily converted into the form of niacin our body uses for energy synthesis in the mitochondria (NAD+). It's got a very nice body of research on it in animals and some in humans showing it to be potently neuroprotective and cardioprotective; it also repairs DNA and supports healthy metabolism and antiaging via a variety of mechanisms. A supplement company–funded research study suggests it might favorably influence epigenetic age when combined with an important DNA methylation adaptogen and antiaging polyphenol called pterostilbene (resveratrol's sibling, and a methylation adaptogen, it's found in blueberries [and some other berries] and almonds—see the Nutrient Reference).[15]

  Dosage: 150–600 mg

- **Alpha ketoglutarate (AKG):** AKG is an essential cofactor for active DNA demethylation via the TET family of enzymes. Thus, it's really important in helping hypermethylated genes to be turned back on, as well as cleaning up the epigenome during embryogenesis. AKG is also a key player in the production of energy in our mitochondria. We can make AKG in the body pretty easily, but it seems to drop in quantity as we age. There is compelling preclinical research on AKG as an anti-aging molecule that supports muscle, burning fat, and boosting mitochondrial activity.

  Dosage: 300–600 mg

SENOLYTIC ADAPTOGENS

SENOLYTIC COMPOUNDS ARE NUTRIENTS OR DRUGS THAT HALT THE AGING process by specifically inhibiting the accumulation of senescent cells (SC)—these are cells that stop dividing but don't get recycled, a sort of zombie of the cellular world. SCs accumulate as we age, doing considerable inflammatory damage themselves and also dumping toxic debris into circulation that contributes to the diseases of aging. Not surprising to me, a number of our fabulous DNA methylation adaptogens are also senoltyics, including:[16]

Curcumin

EGCG

Fisetin

Pterostibene

Quercetin

Resveratrol

(Refer to the lists that start on page 407 for food sources of each of these DNA methylation adaptogens.)

• • • • •

- **Fisetin.** In 2018, this DNA methylation adaptogen was shown to be beneficial as a senolytic agent in old mice and in human tissue, meaning, it made the mice immunologically younger and less inflamed.[17] Other animal studies show fisetin to be antioxidant, antitumerogenic, cardio- and neuroprotective and anti-inflammatory. A small study looking at inflammatory markers in colon cancer patients showed benefit at only 100 mg/day.[18] Stay tuned for larger human studies.

  Dosage: 100 mg

- **Hydroxymethylbutyrate (HMB):** HMB is recommended as an anti-aging compound good for building muscle and brain function.[19] HMB is one of our favorite supplements at the clinic: we have had success using it in people with poor muscle mass—including in cancer patients with tough-to-treat cachexia, children who are underweight, or folks just looking for more energy and muscle. I personally like HMB for biking or weight lifting; it appears to increase my endurance and strength.

  Dosage: 3,000 mg per day; if using for performance, best benefits might be seen with 1,500 mg before and 1,500 mg after exercise.

- **Luteolin** Luteolin is a polyphenol and DNA methylation adaptogen whose moment in the sun is just coming now. As more studies come forward, we are learning more and more about this polyphenol, which has already been shown to be anticancer, anti-inflammatory, antioxidant, antimicrobial, and a very useful antihistamine.[20] Along with quercetin, we use luteolin in practice with our allergy patients regularly. I suspect as research moves forward, we'll see that in addition to optimizing DNA methylation, luteolin has specific anti-aging mechanisms and is likely a senolytic agent.

Dosage: 500–1,000 mg

- **Quercetin:** As I mention above, quercetin is a great antihistamine that we prescribe with luteolin for our most allergic patients. Quercetin, as a senolytic agent, is also an anti-aging rock star. Next to resveratrol, it is probably the most studied polyphenol in aging research.

Dosage: 500–1,000 mg

- **Tartary buckwheat:** This form of buckwheat (*Fagopyrum tataricum*), native to the Himalayas, takes the term "superfood" to a new level—think of it as an epi-nutrient multivitamin. It's sometimes referred to as a pseudocereal, because it's used similarly to, but is not, a grain, nor is it closely related to wheat. It's a mega superfood, also known as a functional food, in part because it contains high levels of multiple flavonoid DNA methylation adaptogens, including quercetin, luteolin, rutin, hesperidin, diosimin, and another compound called 2-HOBA, which lowers blood pressure and rejuvenates immune function (all in therapeutic doses). Tartary buckwheat also contains the aforementioned HMB and is low-glycemic, fiber-rich, gluten-free (technically it's the seed of a fruit), and high in amino acids and healthy fats. Tartary buckwheat is now being grown (organically and regeneratively) in the United States, and you can take it either in capsule form or buy it as a flour to cook with. (You can find a recipe for almond butter muffins using Tartary buckwheat flour on page 304.)

Dosage: 2 caps twice per day

- **Medicinal mushrooms (reishi, shiitake, turkey tail, lion's mane, and chaga):** Packed with immune-rejuvenating beta glucan, we use medicinal mushrooms routinely for anything relating to immune resilience. We recommended them for COVID, for example; and we always use them for our cancer patients and cognitive decline patients. Mushrooms are dense with minerals, vitamin D, and some methyl donor nutrients—especially shiitake, which has a nice amount of folate. One study looking at reishi mushrooms in an animal model of Alzheimer's disease showed that they improved learning and memory, improved neuronal function, resolved brain atrophy, and upregulated DNA methylation enzymes in brain tissue.[21] When taking medicinal mushrooms, the only caveat is to make sure you're taking the "fruiting body," not grain-based mycelium, which should be clear on the label. If it isn't, look for another brand or call the company.

Dosage: 1,000–2,000 mg per day

SLEEP-SUPPORTING SUPPLEMENTS

Sleep is such a vital component of health and a cornerstone of both the Younger You Intensive and the Younger You Everyday. I discuss nonsupplement strategies for getting more sleep, as well as the reasons why you don't want to rely on sleep meds, in Chapter 7. If you need more help getting your zzzs, try these:

- **Melatonin:** Melatonin is a potent antioxidant and is considered a longevity agent. Start lower and see how you tolerate it; for some, melatonin causes strange dreams. For most, it's a very useful sleep-supporting supplement with a solid safety record.

  Dosage: 300 ug to 10 mg about twenty minutes before bedtime

- **Magnesium glycinate:** Magnesium is relaxing. Taking it as magnesium glycinate gives you the added benefit of the anxiolytic amino acid glycine. You can also try glycine alone—Metabolic Maintenance sells a three-gram stick of glycine powder that we love in our practice.

  Dosage: 200–600 mg at bedtime (I take about 600 mg most nights.)

- **L-theonine:** This is a main ingredient in green tea, but it's not stimulating. In fact, research shows it to promote relaxation and reduce anxiety. While you can use it at bedtime, you can take it during the day, too, and it won't make you drowsy.

Dosage: 100–200 mg, taken at bedtime (if you want to promote sleep; otherwise you can take it during the day whenever you're feeling, or anticipate feeling, anxious).

TAKEN TOGETHER WITH the eating plans and lifestyle practices outlined in Chapters 5, 6, and 7, these supplements round out the full Younger You diet and lifestyle. In the remaining chapters, I'll share how DNA methylation changes over the course of your life—and how and when to support it during each life stage. I'll also give you a glimpse into the future—your own personal future, the future of your family, and the future of the role of epigenetics on individual and public health.

PART 3

PUTTING THE "YOU" IN "YOUNGER YOU"

CUSTOMIZING THE YOUNGER YOU PLAN TO YOUR LIFE STAGE

D NA METHYLATION PLAYS SUCH A CRUCIAL ROLE IN HEALTH THAT everyone, at every age, at every level of health, with every genetic profile, stands to benefit from taking steps to support it. While the Younger You protocol as it's written is a potent umbrella policy that can improve health broadly, like a rising tide lifts all boats, it can become even more powerful when you tailor it to your particular life stage and, when possible, to your genetics.

In this chapter I'll walk you through the ages and stages where DNA methylation is amped up. I'll also cover the ailments and conditions that are halmarks of each of these time periods and that can be addressed by nurturing your DNA methylation. In the next chapters, we'll cover how to think about your genetic testing results, if you have them, the future of anti-aging science, and how to maintain the benefits of Younger You.

NURTURING DNA METHYLATION THROUGHOUT THE LIFE STAGES

When I first started researching the foods and lifestyle practices that positively influence DNA methylation, I was—and still am—focused on reversing, or at least slowing, biological aging in adults at midlife. But as I researched, I soon learned that the question really is, when *isn't* a good time to optimize DNA methylation?

I should point out that the research on DNA methylation during different life stages is very new. That being said, there are several periods during the lifecycle when your epigenome is more activated—so the efforts you make to take care of your DNA methylation have the potential to have a bigger impact. Some of these time periods happen very early on—if you are an adult, especially an adult in midlife or in your senior years, some of these moments will have already occurred.

As you read, keep this important point in mind: the single best time to start taking better care of your epigenome is now. In other words, don't spend any energy wishing you had done things differently in the past. Whether you are twenty-eight, fifty-eight, or ninety-eight, you can effect positive change quickly. (All the more reason to share what I cover here with the younger people in your life, whether they're your kids, grandkids, nieces and nephews, or friends' kids or grandkids. You get the picture.)

Infancy and Toddlerhood (Zero–Three)

In the earliest months of life, babies and toddlers are aging at a breakneck pace, and it's a beautiful thing to observe them transform physically and sprout new abilities before your eyes. If we, as parents and caretakers, can direct some attention toward the health of our children's epigenomes and good health in general, we are laying a sturdy foundation that could carry through not only our children's lives, but the lives of generations to come.

For this reason, if you are a breastfeeding mom, try to follow the nutrient intake goals of the Younger You Intensive (eggs, colorful and green veggies, beets, liver) while allowing yourself the expanded carbohydrate selection (legumes and whole grains) of the Younger You Everyday—I think of this as the Younger You Hybrid plan. Also be sure to eat organic as much as possible and to follow the guidelines I included on page 196 for minimizing toxin exposure. And if you quit smoking while you were pregnant, definitely don't start again. In fact, all parents (nonbreastfeeding moms and dads) and caregivers should follow these guidelines, as you are also big players in influencing your child(ren)'s epigenome.

As soon as babies are eating solid foods, it's time to introduce them to DNA methylation–supportive foods. Don't automatically assume they won't like beets, or spinach, or sunflower butter. (For more ideas, our list of DNA methylation–supportive nutrients and the foods that contain them, which starts on page 407, is packed with so many foods that you'll undoubtedly find several even the pickiest kids will eat.) Babies in particular tend to want whatever they see you eating, so let their watchful eyes inspire you to eat plenty of DNA methylation superfoods throughout the day. And even though you might be following the Younger You Intensive and avoiding legumes, beans, grains, and dairy, don't neglect to introduce your child to these whole foods, including those that can be allergenic, such as peanuts and wheat. Not only do infants need the energy that carbohydrates provide, but also very exciting research demonstrates that early food introduction and a broad menu can halt the development of food allergies.[1] (To that end, my daughter, Isabella, gets occasional organic dairy, has organic peanut butter on her bananas, and she definitely enjoys a slice of pizza as much as the next kid.)

Isabella's first solid food was a few bites of a coconut curry I was eating. After that, she dove headlong into eating everything I ate, including broccoli rabe, Brussels sprouts, beets, blueberries, and even a smidge of liver. Now that she is well into her toddler years, she's going to great lengths to pick anything green out of her foods, so I'm doing a little strategic blending of spinach and adding it in tomato sauce, or adding a greens powder or blending beets into a smoothie. (Luckily, purple is her favorite color.) You may have to be persistent—it can take several tries before a child decides they like a new food—or you may have to resort to being creative, but it's worth the effort to support healthy DNA methylation in your babies and toddlers.

Of course, nutrition isn't your only lever for balancing your child's DNA methylation: research suggests that physical affection—kissing them, snuggling them, giving them baths, and yes, even changing diapers!—actually alters their epigenome in a way that supports healthy neurological development, sufficient quantities of the feel-good hormone oxytocin (which I covered at length in Chapter 7), stress resilience, and even brain size; they also enjoy a decreased incidence of certain common childhood illnesses. Thus, a healthy physical connection reaps huge rewards in the development and maintenance of resilience for years to come, as well as in the lives of any potential offspring. I hope that hearing this helps reframe the idea that you're "not doing anything" by taking care of your baby all day. I know it can seem that way—by the time you bathe, dress, feed, and change the baby, it can feel like the entire day has gone by and you haven't "accomplished" anything, especially during the newborn period. But you are accomplishing extraordinary feats in terms of DNA methylation and the epigenome in general. When you give your baby ample loving touch, your baby will develop in a balanced, healthy way.

Animal research has demonstrated that physical touch by a caregiver—even if that caregiver is not the biological parent—has a marked beneficial influence on DNA methylation patterns in babies. Remember Dr. Moshe Szyf's study, covered in Chapter 7, that showed that baby rodents that are groomed (in other words, comforted) by their mothers during the first week of life biologically embed that experience in their DNA methylation and acquire a glucocorticoid (stress hormone) gene methylation pattern that isn't excessively sensitive; as a result, when they are full-grown, they tolerate stress better and are more trusting and more daring than rats not groomed by their mothers. Another insight from that study, which I didn't share in Chapter 7, is that if a baby rat was groomed by another rat—not their mom—they became less skittish, too.[2] That's right: in what I *know* will be a balm to the soul of all adoptive and foster parents, any loving caretaker can beneficially impact a child's genetic expression. If you are an adoptive, foster, or honorary parent to a child, you already knew that, didn't you? You could feel it, of course. But now you can know it intellectually, too: you and the child(ren) you provide consistent loving care to influence the most intimate recesses of each other's DNA.

All that caretaking you're providing is setting the pace of their biological clock to tick at the optimal rate. In other words, you're doing super-important work—not a waste of time by any measure.

Finally, in humans and animals, this time period of early childhood constitutes the most epigenetically sensitive and dynamic time period with regard to adverse childhood events (ACEs). During this particular time, significant gene modifications have been shown to happen via DNA methylation in response to the experience of a broad range of adversity, including poverty, family instability, caregiver pathophysiology, and abuse.[3] While we're still only starting to crack the nut of understanding the epigenetically sensitive time periods, and how to address them, it's already clear that babies and toddlers need connection and stability.

Younger You strategies for infancy and toddlerhood:

- If you and/or your partner quit smoking while you were pregnant, don't start again.
- If you are breastfeeding, follow the Younger You Hybrid—meeting the nutrient intake goals of the Younger You Intensive while also eating the legumes, grains, and minimal dairy allowed on the Younger You Everyday, for as long as you can, as you tolerate them.
- Once your baby is eating solid foods, introduce them to DNA methylation–supportive foods (don't assume that they won't like them, and if they don't at first, keep trying).
- Give your baby ample loving physical contact.

TREATING POSTPARTUM DEPRESSION BY TARGETING DNA METHYLATION

IMBALANCED DNA METHYLATION IS ASSOCIATED WITH POSTPARTUM DEpression, which one in seven women experience.[4] We know that the oxytocin receptor gene is significantly inhibited (via DNA methylation) in women with postpartum depression as opposed to postpartum women who don't develop it.[5] We also know that a history of PTSD—which has a potent impact on the DNA methylation on a number of genes including those associated with oxytocin, brain derived neurotropic factor (BDNF), and the glucocorticoid receptor NR3C1 genes—can play a role in postpartum depression, too.[6]

Thus, if you find yourself feeling low during or after pregnancy, load up on epi-nutrients by using the Younger You formula, whether you follow the Intensive or the Everyday version.

Exercise, meditation, and an anti-inflammatory diet are all generally beneficial for mood disorders for reasons beyond methylation, but it's likely that some of the reason why they are helpful is that they're influencing positive DNA methylation changes. Any aspects of that formula you can muster—and you may need to lean on supplements for a while and be guided by a professional educated in our program (see the Resources section for guidance on finding one, including the nutrition team available through the Younger You digital program)—will help give you the energy and the wherewithal to keep adding more pieces. And as you do, you'll be taking great care of your child's genetic expression as well as your own.

You needn't be the birth mother to experience postpartum depression. I had a tough transition to motherhood after I adopted my daughter and experienced postadoption depression. The extreme sleep deprivation and steep learning curve of early parenthood, all without a partner, was as hard as everything I've ever done, all rolled into one intense period. Isabella's pediatrician assured me it wasn't as hard as learning medical biochemistry, but as much as I adore and trust him, I beg to differ. Recommitting to all things DNA methylation–related helped—especially loving on Isabella and soaking in the oxytocin that contact provided.

I know that PPD can make taking care of the baby feel onerous—have your partner or trusted caregiver do as much as possible, reach out for additional help in whatever form is available to you, and don't hesitate to seek professional care from your doctor and/or a therapist or psychiatrist. There is no shame in needing support during what can be an overwhelming time; you deserve it and so does your baby.

・ ・ ・ ・ ・

Middle Childhood (Four–Seven)

This time period doesn't yet have much research to support it as a particularly epigenetically active time, although I suspect that we'll come to see that many aspects of development—from periods of extra brain plasticity to growth spurts—are governed by epigenetic changes. Kids at this age do appear to be more epigenetically resilient than babies and toddlers. For example, in contrast to the epigenetic sensitivity to trauma displayed by infants and toddlers, research thus far shows that kids in middle childhood show DNA methylation changes only for the most severe adversity exposures, such as sexual or physical abuse. Stay tuned for sophisticated "epigenomic maps" across the life span that will help guide us to how we might best support these sensitivity periods with nutrition, lifestyle, learning, community, and connection.[7]

In the meantime, adopt the following tactics.

Younger You strategies for middle childhood:

- Keep feeding your kids as many DNA methylation–supportive foods as you can.
- Help them establish healthy sleep patterns and movement habits.
- Continue cuddling them (as at some point in the not-too-distant future, they won't be as interested in being physically close to you).
- Keep them intellectually stimulated and challenged.

Late Childhood (Eight–Thirteen)

This is what's known as the slow-growth period, where it seems at a glance as if not much is happening—children have morphed from babies into kids, a status they hold on to until, seemingly overnight, they shoot up and become adolescents.

However, this is a very sensitive period for boys, as their sperm is developing in these years before puberty. (Girls have a similarly intense epigenetic window, but it comes later.) In fact, the Överkalix study that I mentioned in Chapter 2 demonstrated that the years between ages nine and twelve in boys is one of the most significant time periods for epigenetic inheritance that occurs outside of pregnancy: boys who had either excess or lower amounts of food during this period appeared to create lasting epigenetic changes to their sperm that were impactful to their own health and the health of their future offspring, especially influencing heart disease, diabetes, and longevity.[8] Another study looking at toxin exposures during the slow-growth period likewise showed epigenetic changes to sperm that resulted in lower counts and motility later in life; the same changes were not noted to boys exposed to the same toxin during puberty.[9]

Why? For boys, it turns out the development in this period really isn't so slow. For them spermatogenesis is highly active, and all of that newly assembled DNA is being marked with methylation groups.[10] For all kids of all genders, the hypothalamus-pituitary-adrenal axis, which regulates the body's response to stress, is waking up, and the body is preparing for sexual maturation.

A confounding factor is that these are the years when, for many kids, it can be hard to get them to eat the DNA methylation–supportive foods because they are enamored of the typical American diet—the pizza, mac and cheese, chicken nuggets, and very few vegetables that they see their friends eating. Kate, who works in my office, covers a lot of her tweens' methylation superfoods bases with either smoothies (she adds probiotic powder, greens powder, berries, and seeds) or eggs for breakfast, crudités with hummus (or our Herbed Beet Yogurt Dip, page 328) for dipping, and a nightly salad with a lot of chopped vegetables and greens served with organic ranch dressing, which, while not at the top of any methylation superfood lists, does often have a magical sway over kids. If it (along with the mighty ketchup) helps kids get the methyl donors and DNA methylation adaptogens they need during a particularly epigenetically vital time, so be it. She also finds that setting out sliced fruit or veggies before dinner—when kids are often their hungriest—means they will gobble them up, even when they would overlook the same food packed into a lunchbox, for example.

Younger You strategies for late childhood:

- Do what it takes to get DNA methylation–supportive foods into your kids'—especially boys'—regular diet: smoothies, eggs, cut-up fruits and veggies, and a salad, using whatever sauces or dressings make it so that kids will eat them.

- Prioritize their sleep—kids this age should get between nine and eleven hours per night—and their movement, as these two pieces are every bit as important for DNA methylation for kids as they are for adults.

Adolescence (Fourteen–Twenty-four)

Puberty and sexual maturation are also a sensitive time period for epigenetic activity, and perhaps more so in girls, given that oocytes—which are cells that can go on to develop into eggs—are finishing their development now. Thus, supporting the best genetic expression patterns as possible in girls is an important goal. However, we don't want to exclude the boys: physiologically, for both sexes, lots of changes are happening, and anytime we are developing and bringing new systems online (think: new cells, new DNA, new DNA methylation) it's a vital time for eating DNA methylation–friendly foods.

In adolescence, hormones swoop in, triggering physiologic changes so that we become physically capable of reproducing. And our brain isn't fully developed until our midtwenties, meaning this epigenetically potent time lasts for nearly a decade. One study looked at hundreds of thousands of DNA methylation sites in boys and girls in pre- and postadolescence and found the adolescent transition to be associated with changes in fifteen thousand DNA methylation sites! These were associated with immune system development and cell growth. Other factors associated with DNA methylation changes included BMI in the slow-growth period, smoking, and the use of nonsteroidal anti-inflammatory drugs (pain-relieving medication) during this time.[11]

As many teens and college students experience a lot of school-related and social stresses, the teen years and early twenties are an excellent time to establish a meditation habit or other relaxation practice, like yoga or breathing. The many meditation apps can make this more accessible and appealing to young adults—refer back to page 181 for a list of them.

Sleep is also vital at this time, and only about 8 percent of adolescents actually get the sleep they need.[12] We know sleep deprivation changes DNA methylation patterns for the negative, both in the brain and body.[13] Research also shows that when a pattern of poor sleep continues in teenagers (think video games, TikTok, homework) they tend to eat more carbs, eat more food in general, and have more belly fat. Less sleep also increases depression in teens.

It's important to know that staying up late and then sleeping in is not just your teen being willful: fluctuating hormones drive that tendency to stay up late and sleep in, and school schedules generally squash that impulse (although some schools are moving toward delaying start times). Teens can also have erratic levels of melatonin, the chief sleep hormone. Thus, a melatonin supplement can be a helpful sleep support for them— refer back to page 225 for more on this and other supplements to support sleep, and page 187 for lifestyle strategies that can also help teens get more zzzzzs. And the structure that we, as parents, enact around bedtimes, study times, and screen time is essential.

It's also important to tend to brain health now, since it is still developing until the midtwenties. The brain is about 70 percent fat, making omega-3 fatty acids—and especially DHA—essential for healthy brain function. Fortunately, salmon isn't a difficult fish to eat for most kids, and it's loaded with good fats. (Just follow the shopping guidelines for salmon I shared on page 151.) Researchers suspect that epigenetics might be a key mechanism that drives the benefits of omega-3 supplementation, including those exerted on brain development as well as warding off the development of metabolic syndrome in childhood.[14] Much remains to be understood, especially with regard to kids and teens, but the science is strong enough to recognize omega-3s as an important class of fatty acids to get both through food intake and, when necessary, supplementation.

Because adolescence is often when we first begin drinking alcohol, many times in binge drinking patterns, it's worth reiterating that alcohol inhibits all forms of methylation and the absorption of folate.[15] So chronic alcohol use is going to ultimately wreak havoc on all types of methylation, including DNA methylation. If you are the young adult reading this, every drink you *don't* have will help support your DNA methylation. And when you do drink, consume some extra methyl-donor foods that day and the day after—such as greens, eggs, beets, and liver. If you are the parent of an adolescent or young adult, share this information with your kids, and it may be a new way into a conversation about imbibing responsibly.

For anything hormone-related, such as migraines that start in puberty or occur in tandem with the premenstrual phase of the cycle, painful periods, or premenstrual syndrome (PMS) or premenstrual dysphoric disorder (PMDD), the Younger You Intensive or Everyday will be helpful with balancing and detoxing hormones thanks to their high content of cruciferous veggies (which contain the compound DIM that helps the body process estrogen) and lack of pro-inflammatory foods. Exercise and stress management are also both documented to be helpful in PMS and PMDD. And it is extra-important that you avoid toxins as much as you can, as many of them are "endocrine disruptors," which means they can aggressively disrupt our own hormonal system and drive not just PMS and PMDD, but also, with both early exposure and years of exposure, cancer. This link between cancer and endocrine-disrupting chemicals is driven in part by hypermethylation (and inhibition) of tumor-suppressor genes, such as BRCA in breast cancer. All the more reason to eat plenty of DNA methylation adaptogens, which clean up hypermethylation and allow for the re-expression of those inhibited genes. All the toxin-avoiding advice I shared on pages 192–199 applies here.

Younger You strategies for adolescence:

- Introduce your teen to relaxation practices, such as meditation, yoga, and breathing, to help them manage their stress.
- Encourage them to exercise regularly.
- Consider magnesium or a melatonin supplement to help aid them in getting the sleep they need, and refer back to the sleep strategies I shared starting on page 187 to see which could help your teen get the sleep they need.
- Enact boundaries around screen time, especially at night.
- Talk to your teens about alcohol's potentially lasting, negative effects on their brain DNA methylation patterns.
- Prioritize omega-3-rich foods, such as salmon, and consider a supplement for them if needed (refer back to page 214).
- Encourage them to eat plenty of cruciferous vegetables and avoid personal care products and home-cleaning products that have the potential to contain endocrine-disrupting chemicals to help promote hormonal balance.

Peak Adulthood (Twenty-five–Forty-five)

This is a wide swath of life that encompasses our peak. This highest height means, in some (not all—I discuss the benefits of growing older in Chapter 11) ways, it's all downhill from here. Part of this is recognized as evolutionary. Billions of years ago, bacteria and fungi were the only life forms, and some were immortal—rather than dying, they split in two, in a process called *fission*. Once organisms evolved enough to allow genetic material to be handed down and new individuals to be created, the older individuals became dispensable and therefore susceptible to aging and, eventually, death.[16]

For humans, after we've passed sexual development (in men, testosterone begins a very slow decline at twenty; fertility in women starts to drop after thirty[17]) and the brain has finished developing (anywhere from age twenty until forty-five, depending on the measure[18]), we're at the top of the mountain.

Maybe during this time you've got a bit of a break with regard to DNA methylation patterns. You might get away with a few late-night fast-food binges and partying into the wee hours, but truth is, just as you are peaking and enjoying your arrival, there is only one way to go—and we want to go as elegantly, slowly, and gracefully as possible. Thus, if you are in this age range and want to stay there biologically for the long haul, now is a prime time for nurturing your DNA methylation—protecting your assets, as it were. Because by the time most people start to think about anti-aging strategies—around the midforties—the rearranging of DNA methylation patterns associated with aging have already started to pick up steam.

Now is the time to turn the volume on your aging journey down and set the stage to stay healthy, happy, and very high functioning throughout the rest of your life (in keeping with James Fries's "compression of morbidity" that I mentioned in the Introduction).

This also changes, regardless of your gender, the minute you start to think about having children, whether you'd like to conceive in six months or as far away as two years. You absolutely want your DNA methylation to be its best before you pass any of your epigenetic marks on to your offspring.

Younger You strategies for this life stage:

- Make the Younger You Dynamic Dozen foods a regular part of your rotation, and complete the Younger You Intensive a minimum of once per year to keep your DNA methylation primed.
- Adopt as many of the Younger You lifestyle practices as you can—get your seven hours of sleep; start a relaxation practice; and make time for moderate movement no matter how busy you are with work and family.

Pre-conception

Following some version of the Younger You program all of the time is smart, but there are a few times when it moves beyond smart to essential, and trying to conceive is one of them—for both women and men. If you can nudge your genetic expression into tip-top shape, you'll be handing a pristine-as-possible imprint to your offspring. That's because your diet and lifestyle choices affect the germ cells that you pass on to your child, which will, in turn, impact the germ cells that your children will pass on to *their* offspring (aka your grandchildren), and likely, generations beyond that, too.

Because your epigenetic status has such a direct impact on your descendants, ideally you (meaning both the mother- and father-to-be) will follow the Younger You Hybrid: combine the nutrient targets of the Intensive (greens, liver, eggs, fish, beets, DNA methylation adaptogens, and superfoods) with the legumes and whole grains of the Everyday. If you want dairy or sugar occasionally, and you tolerate them, that's OK. An important exception is if you or your partner has a demonstrated carbohydrate intolerance such as insulin resistance, polycystic ovary syndrome (PCOS), or diabetes. If that's the case, stick with the Intensive and keep carb intake lower during pre-conception.

For everyone, when you're trying to conceive, as with pregnancy, I would skip alcohol because it inhibits methylation across the board, including DNA methylation.

If you are inclined, work with a functional medicine practitioner to take a full medical history and suite of labs so that you can be sure you are hitting all of your nutrient targets and that your inflammation, blood sugar, and toxin exposures are all in a healthy range. I have done many of these pre-conception workups on my patients over the years—they are informative and rewarding. Your practitioner can further individualize the Younger You program for your needs.

Even small DNA methylation–friendly improvements to your diet in this pre-conception time can have a big impact: a 2020 study found that men who ate 60 grams (about two ounces) daily of mixed nuts (a blend of almonds, walnuts, and hazelnuts; all rich in methyl donors) without changing any other aspect of their standard Western diet for fourteen weeks experienced beneficial DNA methylation changes, and their sperm count, as well as the size, motility, and viability of their sperm, improved.[19] That's pretty impressive for one small tweak, and yet another illustration of the power of the epi-nutrients contained within food and the epigenome's responsiveness to those epi-nutrients.

Conversely, now is an important time to clean up your intake of toxins, tobacco, and marijuana: research has shown that a man's exposure to both nicotine and tetrahydrocannabinol (THC, the psychoactive compound in marijuana) can negatively change DNA methylation in sperm on seven genes that play a role in neurodevelopment, many of which are associated with autism.[20] In a recent animal study, the herbicide glyphosate (the active ingredient in Roundup) was "shown to promote the epigenetic transgenerational inheritance of pathology and disease in subsequent great-grand offspring [three generations!]."[21] If you're not eating organic yet, now is the time.

Younger You strategies for pre-conception:

- Follow the Younger You Hybrid—unless you have PCOS or diabetes, then follow the Younger You Intensive—as much as possible.
- Skip alcohol as much as you possibly can.
- Consider working with a functional medicine practitioner to do a thorough assessment of your current health and nutrient status.
- Reduce your exposure to toxins, nicotine, and THC as much as possible—eat organic, stop using marijuana, and follow the suggestions starting on page 192 to lower your toxin exposure.

Pregnancy

Once you conceive, the window for influencing your baby's epigenome, in what's called "gestational programming," is open wide. You can see how important it is to support DNA methylation in the earliest trimester when you look at the outcomes of the children whose mothers were pregnant with them during the Dutch Hunger Winter: the babies of the women who were in their first trimester of pregnancy experienced more and longer-lasting negative impacts to their health outcomes (as did their children) than those born to women whose pregnancies were further along.

In earliest stage of embryogenesis, there's an all-important demethylation process that happens on the DNA that's been donated from the egg and the sperm. Essentially, the DNA donated by the egg and the sperm is scrubbed clean of methyl groups. Or *almost* clean, as about 30 percent of epigenetic marks remain after the demethylation process is complete. It's this remaining 30 percent that contains some of the experience of the previous generations, which is sometimes referred to as the "imprintome" because it carries the imprint of our parents' epigenome. It's here that our past generations' nutrients, life experiences, stressors, and toxin exposures influence our epigenome.

As with pre-conception, I recommend following a Younger You Hybrid plan—hit the daily/weekly nutrient targets of the Younger You Intensive, but include the legumes and well-chosen grains and occasional dairy of the Younger You Everyday. In general, you want to be eating heartily, as pregnancy is a calorically demanding time: a full-term pregnancy requires about 77,000 calories![22] It's a good thing there is no calorie counting on the Younger You program; you can eat until you are satiated and nourished.

An important deviation from both the Younger You Intensive and Everyday for pregnant women is that you want to eat more protein—15 percent more in the second trimester and a whopping 25 percent more by the third trimester. And these numbers increase for twins and triplets. But in general, for a single pregnancy, you want to be at a *minimum* of 1.1 grams of protein per kilogram of body weight from week sixteen through delivery. This is at least 70 grams/day for a 140-pound woman, and it will rise as you and the baby put on weight. Protein during pregnancy should be about 15–25 percent of total food intake, increasing intake as time progresses. (Note that the Younger You plan is 15–20 percent protein, so you'll be above our requirements as your pregnancy progresses. This is, of course, correct to do.)

During the earliest part of the first trimester, vitamins C and A and iron are hugely important for epigenetic programming, as they support the enzymes responsible for demethylation. While you want to get as many nutrients as you can through food, in my experience, almost all pregnant women need supplemental iron—refer back to page 217 for guidance on how to do it.

Equally important: as the DNA is scrubbed clean, shiny new methylation marks are being placed down. This is part of the process that tells the embryo's stem cells what to be when they grow up—whether they'll be a skin cell, a nerve cell, a muscle cell, or a brain cell, etc. And determining that fate requires a lavish sprinkling of methyl donors—which means plenty of folate, vitamin B_{12}, betaine, and choline. (You likely have questions about folate and folic acid, since it is often advised as a key prenatal supplement. I'll talk about that in just a bit.)

PRENATAL SUPPLEMENT RECOMMENDATIONS

THESE VALUES ARE GENERAL RECOMMENDATIONS; DOSES CAN BE ADJUSTED based on individual needs. For instance, if blood testing shows that you have an extra requirement for iron, zinc, vitamin D, EPA and DHA, or B vitamins, and/or the presence of the MTHFR gene variant (see page 266), your supplement program may be adjusted accordingly. Work with a functional medicine practitioner to get these levels dialed in for you and your particular physiology (see the Resources section for finding a practitioner well-versed in DNA methylation).

Vitamin A mixed carotenoids	5000 IU	Methylcobalamin	800 µg	Chromium (Chromium niacinate)	200 µg
Vitamin C	250 mg	Biotin	100 µg	Molybdenum (molybdenum glycinate)	25 µg
Vitamin D₃	2000 IU	Pantothenic acid (d-calcium pantothenate)	25 mg	Omega-3 fatty acids	620 mg
Vitamin E (mixed)	110 IU	Iron (iron bisglycinate)	25 mg	EPA	400 mg
				DHA	200 mg
Thiamine (mononitrate)	5 mg	Iodine (potassium iodide)	150 µg	Other Omega-3	20 mg
Riboflavin (5 phosphate)		Zinc (zinc citrate)	25 mg		
Niacinamide	25 mg	Selenium (L. seleniumethionine)	100 µg	L-carnitine 1000 mg (L-carnitine tartrate)	1000 mg
B₆ (Pyridoxal 5 phosphate)	15 mg	Copper (copper gluconate)	1.5 mg	Probiotic blend: Lactobacillus acidophilus Bifidobacterium lectis,	60 B CFU
L-5-Methylfolate	1000 µg	Manganese (manganese gluconate)	5 mg	Lactobacillus plantarum, Lactobacillus salivarius, Streptococcus thermophilus	

Abbreviations: CFU, colony-forming unit; DHA, docosahexaenoic acid; EPA, eicosapentaenoic acid; µg, micrograms.

Source: GrowBaby Health[23]

Both the Centers for Disease Control (CDC) and the World Health Organization (WHO) recommend pregnant women take a minimum of 400 ug of folate, either as synthetic folic acid or naturally occurring folate, in addition to consuming a diet high in folate-rich and folic acid–fortified foods.[24] And if there is a family history of neural tube defects, the WHO and CDC recommendation jumps ten-fold, to 4,000 ug per day for the first trimester. Meanwhile, the National Institutes of Health (NIH) recommends 600 ug folate daily, including folic acid from fortified foods.[25]

There has been no upper limit of daily folate intake set for pregnancy, although the NIH states that adults nineteen years and older should not exceed 1,000 ug/day. Yet, potential issues in offspring exposed to excess folate/folic acid in utero in animal and human studies include asthma, metabolic syndrome, obesity, and autism.[26] Because of these findings, the Society for Endocrinology recognizes that an upper limit recommendation for pregnant women—especially in the first trimester—is urgently needed.

Where does that leave us? When I look at the CDC, WHO, and NIH recommendations, in combination with the remarkable birth outcome data from GrowBaby Health that I include in this section, I make the following recommendations:

1. Whenever possible, supplemental folate should be natural folate, not synthetic folic acid.
2. Avoid or minimize eating fortified foods during pregnancy for ease of tracking total folate/folic acid intake (these can include nut milks and some veggie burgers that contain grains—read labels on everything you eat that has a label).
3. Total supplemental folate (including the folic acid found in fortified foods, but *not* including natural folate found in whole foods such as greens, mushrooms, liver, etc.) should be, at minimum, 400 ug, and should not exceed 1,000 ug, unless specified by your health-care provider.

As always, but even more so now, you want to stay in the sweet spot of a *just right* amount of folate as well as fellow primary methyl donor, vitamin B_{12}. In 2016, Johns Hopkins released findings that pregnant women who took either very high amounts or very low amounts of (or no) vitamin B_{12} and folate gave birth to offspring with a significantly increased risk of autism. For the very high folate group, fortification plus supplementation was likely a factor. This study validated how essential these nutrients are *in the right amounts*, as those pregnant women who took a moderate course of supplements (three to five times per week) gave birth to children with a decreased risk of autism. Choosing your prenatal supplement well and being mindful of not overconsuming folic acid–fortified foods will help you stay in that zone of not too little and not too much.

And if you consume soy frequently, which if you're vegetarian or vegan, you probably do, you want to be extra vigilant about avoiding folic acid–fortified grains or nondairy milks when you are pregnant—particularly if you are supplementing with folate as part of your prenatal vitamins. Why? Another big finding to come out of Dr. Jirtle's work with agouti mice, which I covered in Chapter 2, was that when they gave the pregnant mice genistein—an important isoflavone in soy, and a potent DNA methylation adaptogen—alone, without other methyl-donor nutrients, it increased DNA methylation in offspring, which is a role that generally only methyl donors play. As a result, the mice gave birth to pups that were trim, healthy, and brown. It's not entirely clear yet why genistein acted like a methyl donor in the study; it's suspected that it may have helped reposition the gene to more readily receive the methyl groups in circulation.[27] In the genistein study, Jirtle and his colleagues speculate that excess consumption of methyl donor compounds through all these supplemental sources could lead to unforeseen epigenetic consequences, such as hypermethylating important genes that we really want to stay on.

And if you're eating a lot of soy *and* a lot of refined grains—nearly all of which are fortified with folic acid, including anything made from wheat, of course, but also white rice, some oatmeal, and corn meal—and taking a prenatal vitamin—which is likely to have folate in it—your levels of methyl donors can get overly high. In general, good sources of soy are a healthy addition to any diet (as I discussed on page 137), including in pregnancy, but you want to keep it to less than two servings per day. The

American College of Obstetricians and Gynecologists agree — moderate soy consumption during pregnancy is safe.[28]

PRIORITIZING DNA METHYLATION ENHANCES BIRTH OUTCOMES

THE GOOD NEWS IS THAT TAKING SPECIAL CARE OF YOUR DNA METHYLAtion has the potential to significantly improve birth outcomes. One Oregon clinic—GrowBaby Health, an integrated medicine and nutrition program for women who are seeking to get pregnant founded by nutritionist Emily Rydbom, CN, BCHN, CNP, and her parents, Dr. Leslie Stone and Dr. Michael Stone—is doing remarkable work in the field of methylation assessment and support during pre-conception, pregnancy, and the postnatal period. The GrowBaby team incorporated many components of the Younger You Intensive into the Grow-Baby (GB) methylation core eating plan that they use with about 25 percent of their patients (particularly those with a variant of the MTHFR gene, which, as you'll learn more about later in Chapter 10, can reduce the body's ability to methylate—as you can imagine, addressing this during pregnancy is wildly important). And the results they are getting with it are nothing short of extraordinary.

During the years of 2011 to 2017, GrowBaby worked with 410 pregnant women who experienced the following birth outcomes.[29] When you compare these numbers to the outcomes of all pregnant women in the United States, you can clearly see what a tremendous impact prioritizing healthy DNA methylation, lifestyle, and general nutrition can have on infant health.

	GROW BABY	U.S.
Preterm birth	0%	11.5%
Small for gestational age	1.5%	11.5%
Gestational diabetes	0.2%	9.2%
Pregnancy-induced hypertension	0.7%	6.7%

In addition, the babies born to those 410 women had no incidence of autism or immunity challenges, atopic dermatitis, or asthma. This is remarkable. The GrowBaby approach is accessible medicine—it is covered by insurance and Medicare—and is being considered by hospitals around the country.

Any functional medicine practitioner who works in obstetrics is seeking to improve methylation—as folate is such an important nutrient for a healthy baby and a key player in the methylation cycle—but GrowBaby has taken it to the next level by prescribing a methylation-supportive diet, including both methyl donors and DNA methylation adaptogens, that also prioritizes stress reduction, sleep, exercise, and community. And it's working, suggesting that even though some of your kids' epigenetic realities are influenced by your parents' choices—and, therefore, seemingly out of your control—you actually have a lot of leeway in correcting for any epigenetic challenges you may have inherited.

· · · · ·

Younger You strategies for pregnancy:

- Continue with the Younger You Hybrid from when you were trying to conceive.
- If you consume it, limit your consumption of organic, preferably fermented, soy to two servings per day.
- Read labels carefully (especially on grain-based foods, veggie burgers, and nondairy milks) to ensure that your total supplemental folate consumption—from both your prenatal vitamin and fortified foods—stays under 1,000 ug per day (unless otherwise directed by your health-care provider).
- Get your iron levels tested and supplement, if necessary, following the information on page 217, or as instructed by your health-care provider.
- Increase your protein intake according to the guidelines I shared on page 242.
- Follow the supplement recommendations on page 243.

Perimenopause and Menopause

If you menstruate, you begin your transition toward menopause typically sometime in your midforties, although it can happen in the late thirties for some women and mid to late fifties for others. Your estrogen levels start fluctuating erratically and you will likely notice some changes to your menstrual cycle—your periods may get longer or shorter, heavier or lighter, and you'll likely start missing cycles altogether. Declining estrogen levels are associated with other impacts that include disruptions to sleep, changes to libido, mood swings, irritability, forgetfulness, an increased risk of depression, vaginal dryness, a little urinary incontinence (perhaps you start to pee a little bit when you sneeze or laugh), a decrease in bone density, an increase in abdominal adipose, and a loss of muscle mass. This period typically lasts around four years. Once you have gone a full calendar year with no menstrual cycles, you are officially out of perimenopause and in menopause.

As I type this list of impacts, I can't help but think: *really, evolution?* Did our transition really need to be accompanied by such a rough collection of experiences? It's true that some women have few if any noticeable impacts of perimenopause. No matter what your experience, the Younger You protocol is supportive in so many ways that can help smooth the waters of your passage. Also, no matter what your particular transition is like, it's important to note that perimenopause is also a spiritual journey into a time of deeper reflection and self-possession—and not just a prank of evolution.

Now that you know how involved DNA methylation is in every system of the body, you probably won't be surprised to hear that the transition to menopause is accompanied by dramatic changes in your epigenome. In simple terms, menopause, and the perimenopausal journey that leads to it, turns the volume up on aging in women, and the earlier it happens, the higher your biological age tends to be.[30] This is on top of the typical changes to DNA methylation that come with aging, which I'll cover next. It's a major double-whammy that explains why it can feel like your body is suddenly someone else's.

If you are a woman already in your forties, or rapidly approaching them, the Younger You Intensive is a powerful antidote to the negative changes to DNA methylation that are ramping up now. It's protective and preventative against further imbalance, but it is also restorative. Even without its focus on foods rich in DNA methylation–supportive nutrients, the Younger You Intensive remedies the largest driver of a negative menopausal experience: the pro-inflammatory trifecta of the standard American diet, a lack of exercise, and high stress.

If you are perimenopausal or menopausal, there are DNA methylation adaptogens that have some gentle phytoestrogenic activity, meaning they can replace some of the function of your lost estrogen in a healthy way, so you'll want to increase your consumption of those foods that contain them. They include soy (remember to keep it organic and preferably fermented, such as tempeh or miso), flax seeds and maca powder (both of which you purchase ground and add to smoothies), red clover, and green tea.

Another challenge for women in their midlife years is that they are often taking care of kids and aging parents just as their careers are at their height. It's a foot-long stress sandwich, and as we've covered, stress acts like gasoline on the fire of aging. In addition to the eating strategies of the Younger You Intensive, exercise and relaxation practices are just hugely important for you now, and well beyond the eight weeks that the Intensive lasts. The older you are, the more exercise has to offer you, so don't let your age convince you that you can take it easy now. And remember that the busier you are, the more you stand to benefit from relaxation practices. Don't wait to find the time. Make it. (Refer back to page 184 for guidance on how to do just that.)

Because sleep can become impaired during perimenopause and menopause, the sleep tips I shared starting on page 187 are extra vital for you now, too. As I covered in Chapter 7, you only need to aim for seven hours of sleep per night as a baseline. I hope that thinking of sleep as anti-aging will help you prioritize it, even if it requires letting some things go in order to do so—things like answering every single email or making sure every dish is done before you go to bed. Your health is more important than the tidiness of your inbox or your kitchen.

Younger You strategies for perimenopause and menopause:

- Follow the Younger You Intensive for a minimum of eight weeks.
- Lean on DNA methylation adaptogens and include those with phytoestrogenic properties, including (organic and preferably fermented) soy (unless you are following the Younger You Intensive

and are *not* vegetarian or vegan; then omit for those eight weeks), red clover, ground flax seed, maca powder, and green tea.

- Commit to regular exercise and relaxation.
- Follow the tips starting on page 187 to get at least seven hours of sleep per night.

Midlife and Beyond (Midforties On)

When I interviewed David Sinclair, Harvard professor of genetics and author of *Lifespan*, on my podcast, he shared that middle adulthood (starting in the forties) is just as impactful of an epigenetic time as embryogenesis. Although this time around, most of the DNA methylation changes, frankly, suck.

In both sexes, pro-inflammatory genes become hypomethylated and get ramped up, tumor-suppressor genes become progressively more silenced, genes that code for antioxidant and detoxification enzymes such as glutathione transferase (which also happens to be an important tumor-suppressor gene!) get turned off, and genes that promote cancer (known as oncogenes) are turned on. Even our beautiful stem cells stop renewing and replenishing, instead becoming inflamed and less productive. The methylation cycle itself gets wonky, a state that correlates to a rise in homocysteine, which is associated with heart disease and Alzheimer's when at high levels. It's like we embark on a journey of gradually dying. (Looking at this list, it's easy to accept the theory that aging is a preprogrammed event that I discussed in Chapter 1, and not the random wear-and-tear espoused in the theory of aging as "epigenetic drift.")

That's why it's in the years of middle life to old age that we are at the highest risk of developing the chronic diseases that are ubiquitous in society: heart disease, cancer, dementia, diabetes, osteoporosis, and Parkinson's disease. And why chronological and biological age are the highest risk factors for complications and even death from COVID-19.[31] It's also why we selected middle-aged men as our study population, because we knew they'd be on this journey of disordered methylation and we wanted to see if we could improve what had already been started (as mentioned earlier, we didn't include women because our study was too small to stratify the population for pre-, peri-, and postmenopausal changes—but we will absolutely include women in the larger study that we are currently designing!). That answer was a clear yes. Which leads to the good news in all this for those of us who are in the second half of our lives: it's never too late to have a positive effect on your DNA methylation.

Exercise is super-duper mega-important for the over-fifty set, as the older you are, the more effective it appears to get. It acts like a DNA methylation adaptogen and has been shown to turn tumor-suppressor genes that had been hypermethylated and turned off back on more effectively, more powerfully than when you're younger. If you aren't currently exercising and don't have plans to change that, you do so at your peril. While you don't need to be the weekend warrior who pushes themselves to the max on occasional outings, it is possible to find a movement habit that respects the changes that have happened in your body. If you have a specific issue, like knee pain or asthma, or have mobility issues, a disability, or a general concern about overdoing it, get assessed by your physician, an exercise therapist, or a chiropractor to get guidance on choosing forms of exercise that are appropriate for your particular body.

Once you are over fifty, if you've never done so, it's worth combining the Younger You Intensive with a short-term elimination diet (especially if your score on the MSQ form on page 83 isn't in the optimal range). That's because over your life span your gut changes—your microbiome and intestinal permeability are influenced by the medications you've taken, foods you've eaten, toxins you've been exposed to, and the stress you've experienced. All of these factors can prompt the development of new, adult-onset sensitivities, intolerances, or allergies to foods. These are inflammatory reactions that can wreak big havoc in your life with symptoms like heartburn, digestive issues, rashes, headaches, joint pain, and more. They can push the aging process forward, too.

As I covered on page 113, the Intensive is free of the most common food irritants, like gluten and dairy, but it does include eggs, finned fish, shellfish, tree nuts, sesame, and the nightshade vegetables, all of which can be sources of food allergies, intolerances, and sensitivities. Consider avoiding all of these foods that I just mentioned as you do the Younger You Intensive. Basically, eat your seven cups of vegetables, your beets, your seeds, your liver, and your clean animal protein for a minimum of four weeks, then walk yourself through a careful reintroduction period when you test your reaction to the potentially problematic foods that are included on the Intensive, such as tree nuts, tomatoes, and eggs.

⬤ HOW TO TEST YOUR REACTIONS TO SPECIFIC FOODS

TO REINTRODUCE POTENTIAL ALLERGENS, CHOOSE ONE OF THE FOODS YOU'VE eliminated and eat two servings of it in one day—then carefully monitor your symptoms (using the MSQ form on page 83 daily) for seventy-two hours. If you notice anything like headaches, runny nose, diarrhea, gas, constipation, rash, joint pain, or fatigue, it's indicative of a reaction to that food, and it's best for you to continue to keep it out of your diet for a longer time, and then periodically rechallenge it every six weeks or so. After each seventy-two-hour period, you can test a new food, gauging your reaction each time and deducing which foods agree with you, and which don't. If you discover that you are reactive to multiple different foods, work with a health-care provider who is well versed in food reactions to guide you in doing the underlying healing work that will help you get back to eating a broad diet, as you don't want to remain on a highly restricted diet long term.

To do a comprehensive elimination diet, omit the following common allergen foods from your diet for a period of twenty-one days.

COMMON ALLERGENS

Eggs*	Sesame*
Dairy**	Shellfish*
Finned fish*	Soy**
Nightshades*	Tree nuts*
Peanuts**	Wheat

* Foods allowed on the Younger You Intensive
** Foods allowed on the Younger You Everyday (except for soy, which is also allowed on the Younger You Intensive for vegetarians and vegans)

⬤ ⬤ ⬤ ⬤ ⬤

Linda, one of my patients, is a woman in her late seventies who was struggling with severe pain from osteoarthritis in her knee. Hoping to avoid a full knee replacement, Linda followed the Younger You Intensive/elimination diet combo. On the program, she lost a quick ten pounds and her pain level lowered significantly, from a nine on a one-to-ten scale to a six. During her testing phase, she also discovered that she's reactive to tomatoes, which came as a big surprise because it was a new reaction. After she finished the Intensive she continued to test a broad range of foods and found out she was profoundly sensitive to gluten, dairy, and sugar. This may sound like bad news, but Linda's reduction in joint pain, weight loss, and improved energy makes going without those foods easy to do. (She also discovered that she loves liver pâté, beets and beet greens, and kale chips, so she has some new favorite foods to experiment with.)

My only caveat in doing an elimination diet is if you have any tendency toward disordered eating, work with a nutritionist to guide you so that you don't eliminate too many foods, calories, or sources of nutrients.

Finally, once you are over sixty, you also want to eat more protein to help compensate for the loss in muscle mass that is a hallmark of aging. Refer back to page 96 for guidance.

Younger You strategies for midlife and beyond:

- Find an exercise routine that you enjoy and you can stick to and that includes resistance work, as we tend to lose muscle as we age; if you have to consult with a fitness professional or physical therapist, the bio age reversal benefits that regular movement offers are worth the investment.
- If you've not recently done so, consider following an elimination diet to identify any specific foods that may be causing digestive or inflammatory issues.
- If you're over age sixty, be sure to up your daily protein intake per the guidelines on page 96.

10

TAILORING YOUR YOUNGER YOU PLAN TO YOUR GENES

NO MATTER WHAT GENETIC HAND YOU HAVE BEEN DEALT, NOURISHing your DNA methylation can mitigate the risks and help you find your level of optimal health, as Melissa's story exemplifies so well.

As a twenty-eight-year-old New Yorker with a career in the fashion industry, Melissa prided herself on being able to power through twelve-hour workdays—even those times when she was jet-lagged after flying back from Paris Fashion Week. A lifelong athlete and dancer, Melissa worked out for at least an hour every day. She was also a vegetarian who never smoked and rarely drank anything other than water. Her resilience kept her healthy even when her coworkers got sick. In addition, Melissa was newly engaged. Life was great.

Melissa took her dedication to living a healthy life so seriously that she also performed a daily breast self-examination; a ritual she'd performed since she was eighteen. Breast cancer ran in her mother's side of the family—despite being healthy overall, Melissa's mother had been diagnosed with stage 1 breast cancer at thirty-six. And Melissa's grandmother had been diagnosed with breast cancer at age twenty-nine; ovarian cancer took her life just before her fortieth birthday.

Melissa's awareness of her increased risk fueled her devotion to exercising, eating well, and monitoring her breast health. Yet one jet-lagged morning, Melissa found a lump during her daily breast exam. She got an appointment with her gynecologist for later that same day.

Melissa's Ob/Gyn confidently told her she was too young to have breast cancer, regardless of her family history. Melissa wanted to believe her, but couldn't shake the feeling that something was wrong. So she sought a second opinion. When this doctor said Melissa's mini-lump had no tumor-like characteristics, and that there was only a 1 percent chance it was cancerous because she was so young and healthy, Melissa wanted to believe her, too. Just to confirm what she already knew to be a correct diagnosis, the doctor did a needle biopsy and sent Melissa home.

About a week later, Melissa got the call that everyone dreads. The tiny bump was malignant. Worse yet, her young age meant that her cancer was highly aggressive and reoccurrence was likely. That meant she'd need chemo and radiation—although not a bilateral mastectomy. The treatments would cause her to lose her hair, the skin on her breast to harden (making any future reconstruction extremely difficult), and one or both of her arms to potentially swell indefinitely. On top of that, the treatment was expected to bring post-treatment menopause and all of its symptoms, with only a 25 percent chance of ever getting pregnant. They also recommended genetic testing and, if Melissa had the BRCA 1 or 2 gene, that she should have an elective oophorectomy (removal of her ovaries) before she turned forty in order to ensure the best odds of survival.

Melissa contacted a work colleague who, she remembered, had been diagnosed with breast cancer in her midthirties. That colleague detailed the treatment plan she had followed—surgery, a staggered chemotherapy protocol, and IV therapy. Her protocol also included dietary interventions, supplement regimens, and relaxation practices. Melissa booked an appointment with her friend's oncologist, and it changed everything.

This oncologist devised a treatment plan that included surgery and an open-ended chemotherapy course that they would develop collaboratively. Melissa would work with a nutritionist to create a dietary plan focused on detoxification, immune support, and genetic expression. This sounded especially appealing to Melissa as she had since learned that she had the BRCA1 gene mutation. The plan included intermittent fasting (to protect healthy cells but kill fast-growing tumor cells); an antioxidant-rich diet that consisted of nine to ten cups of colorful, low-glycemic fruits and vegetables each day; regular intake of bioactive food components such as genistein, curcumin, choline, and sulforaphane (which we now recognize as DNA methylation adaptogens); and a daily sleep journal to record time spent not just sleeping but also resting. Ultimately, the goal of Melissa's treatment plan was to reset her future genetic expression away from cancer and toward health, and its pillars very closely resembled the Younger You Intensive.

No other provider had mentioned diet, nutrients, or relaxation to Melissa. And while the idea of favorably influencing genetic expression (rather than being a victim of "bad genes") was new to her, it also made sense to treat the root cause, and not just target the tissues.

After four rounds of strong, but staggered chemotherapy, an elective bilateral mastectomy, new daily routines that included a plant-based diet with small amounts of organic animal protein, an emphasis on stress reduction, at least eight hours of daily sleep, plus meditation and acupressure, Melissa no longer had signs of any health issues and was pronounced cancer-free. What she did have was

- Menstrual regularity throughout the entire course of treatment without a single sign of menopause
- An absence of swelling, discomfort, or physical restriction in both arms
- Enough energy and resilience to continue working full time without restriction and remain active
- A head of hair that grew back quickly and surgical scars that are now barely detectable
- The opportunity to plan her wedding without fear or trepidation
- And last, but certainly not least, a renewed trust in herself, her instincts, and her body

Now, over twenty years later, Melissa has two children and a master's degree in clinical nutrition, and she is currently one of the functional nutrition residents in my clinic (in fact, she developed many of the vegan recipes in this book).

I love Melissa's story for many reasons—that she survived an early-onset and aggressive cancer, of course. But also that she was an early adopter of diet and lifestyle practices aimed at improving genetic expression, and that they helped her get rid of cancer *and* have kept her cancer-free in the decades since. And not least, Melissa's story proves that even a genetic mutation like BRCA1 doesn't have to dictate your fate.

In this section I'll talk through how to approach genetic variations and mutations (there's a difference), including perhaps the best-known genetic mutation of all—the one that occurs on the BRCA genes so closely associated with significantly increased risk of hormone-related cancers. I hope to dispel some of the mystery and fear you may have encountered after receiving your own genetic testing, or if you're facing disease with a genetic component.

WHAT INFLUENCES THE RISK OF BREAST CANCER MORE— GENES OR ENVIRONMENT?

Many of us have Angelina Jolie to thank for raising our awareness of the BRCA gene. The actress, who had a strong family history of cancer—her mother died young of ovarian cancer—opted to have a preventative double mastectomy in 2013 after identifying that she carried the BRCA1 genetic mutation.

Deriving its name from "breast cancer," BRCA is a very important tumor-suppressor gene. When it's mutated, the likelihood of developing hormone-sensitive cancers rises exponentially. Indeed, if you have a BRCA mutation, your lifetime risk of developing breast cancer is 82 percent. Which I can certainly understand feel like insurmountable odds, regardless of your health choices.

However, BRCA isn't anywhere near the most common cause of breast cancer. In fact, only about 10 percent of breast cancer incidences are considered hereditary. And of those 10 percent, only about 25 percent are associated with mutations like BRCA1 or BRCA2.[1]

Also, when you look into the history of the BRCA mutations and cancer risk, you find that before 1940, the risk of developing breast cancer was 24 percent with the BRCA mutation, not 82 percent, as it is today.[2] Clearly, something has changed. And that something is the environment, including toxic exposures, diet, and stress. Specifically, your environment affects your epigenetics, and your epigenetics then influences how your genes are expressed—whether toward or away from cancer.

Dr. Mary-Claire King, the scientist who discovered the BRCA mutations, recognized the environmental influence on cancer risk. She specifically cited adolescent obesity, lack of exercise, and early age of menarche as factors in the rise of BRCA-associated cancers—all things that have been on the rise since the 1940s.[3]

However, you don't need to be born with the BRCA1 or BRCA2 mutations to have this gene contribute to your risk of cancer. Even genes without mutations can be inappropriately methylated, and therefore *act* like a mutated gene without actually being mutated. For example, a number of studies show that the all-important BRCA1 and BRCA2 genes can be hypermethylated and shut off.[4] Science has also shown that mothers can pass on a hypermethylated BRCA1 gene to their daughters.[5]

● THE FUTURE OF PREDICTING BREAST AND OVARIAN CANCER RISK

DID YOU KNOW THAT THERE ARE MORE THAN FIVE HUNDRED KNOWN BRCA mutations that are of "unknown clinical significance," which means we don't know whether the mutation increases cancer risk or not?[6] A 2020 study argues that routine, broad genetic testing for mutations on BRCA and other tumor-suppressor genes could prevent up to an estimated 2,666 cases of breast cancer per million women, and up to 449 ovarian cases per million women.[7]

Beyond mutations, assessing the methylation patterns on BRCA genes will become quite useful for determining risk. In time, careful, broad assessments of DNA methylation patterns will help guide breast and ovarian cancer prevention and treatment, too—catching unfavorable changes and reversing them well before disease is present.[8] If we look for the gene mutations *plus* the DNA methylation patterns, how many more cancers could be prevented?

· · · · ·

Once you have cancer, we know that it hijacks epigenetic machinery for its own nefarious aims (namely, rampant growth). Tests of the DNA methylation patterns present in breast cancer tumor cells shows that tumors are *older*, epigenetically, than the surrounding, normal tissue. Specifically, genes that inhibit the cancer are turned off, and genes that allow cancer to grow unchecked are on—which, unfortunately, is the same pattern we see in aging in general.[9]

This is all to say it needn't be a BRCA1 or BRCA2 gene mutation that increases your risk of cancer. In fact, more likely, it's your epigenetics, and how it is affecting whether those genes are turned on or turned off. The typical pattern associated with cancer is hypermethylation of tumor-suppressor genes, which essentially turns those all-important protector genes off. The trick, then, is to reverse that hypermethylation via demethylation.

There are so-called dirty demethylating drugs that can serve this purpose, but so far, most of them demethylate indiscriminately, and can have much broader effects than simply turning tumor-suppressor genes back on. They are kind of like bringing a gun to a knife fight. Also, we have such a strong, safe option available to us, and that is consuming ample amounts of DNA methylation adaptogens, as Melissa did.

These polyphenolic epi-nutrients appear to be super important for keeping the BRCA genes well functioning: Two in vitro studies have shown that exposure to toxins does indeed contribute to the silencing of BRCA1 via hypermethylation, and that resveratrol—the antioxidant present in red and purple grapes, red wine, blueberries, cranberries, and more—reversed the effect.[10] Other studies show that, in addition to resveratrol, the flavanols EGCG (from green tea) and genistein (from soy) also reverse hypermethylation of BRCA1.[11] Another component of soy is the isoflavone daidzein, which is transformed by your gut microbes into equol. And equol has been shown to not only demethylate BRCA1 and BRCA2 genes, and thus promote re-expression of these genes, but also upregulate production of the all-important, protective proteins that the BRCA1 and BRCA2 genes code for.[12] (About 70 percent of people don't have the microbiome to make equol—although those ingesting a highly polyphenol-rich, plant-based diet, including soy, are much more likely to have the right microbiome to produce it, another reason to follow the Younger You program.[13]) In other in vitro studies, quercetin and curcumin together epigenetically enhanced BRCA1 expression via multiple mechanisms.[14] These effective phytochemicals are all parts of the Younger You Intensive and Everyday plans.

In addition, every one of us has a lot of other tumor-suppressor genes. Luckily, many of them, including BRCA 1 or 2, have been shown to have their genetic expression favorably altered by certain nutrients; I call any gene for which this is true a nutrient-responsive gene. So even if you have a BRCA 1 or 2 genetic mutation, you can support your other nutrient-responsive tumor-suppressor genes by taking care of your DNA methylation with the Younger You approach, and it can help *all* of your important anticancer genes function their best. (And know that we are researching how the Younger You diet and lifestyle practices influence specific nutrient-responsive genes in humans, so our understanding will only continue to evolve. See drkarafitzgerald.com to stay tuned for details of this important and interesting work.)

NUTRIENT-RESPONSIVE TUMOR-SUPPRESSOR GENES

When it comes to preventing and treating cancer, tending to DNA methylation using the Younger You Intensive is likely to be an important strategy, as changes in DNA methylation underlie cancer initiation, promotion, and progression, particularly on tumor-suppressor genes (TSG), which are frequently hypermethylated (and thus turned off) in cancer.

Below are the nutrient-responsive tumor-suppressor genes that have the most research linking their DNA methylation status to cancer, as well as the specific nutrients—all of them DNA methylation adaptogens—that have been shown in in vitro studies to help balance their DNA methylation. Importantly, as you glance at these nutrients, they will be familiar to you. Not only from this book, but because many of these polyphenols have long histories of being used by traditional systems of medicine for a broad array of uses, including reducing inflammation, providing antioxidant support, and treating conditions including cancer, heart disease, and allergies. Likely, the way these are exerting their influence in such a broad range of conditions is in big part due to their ability to augment epigenetic expression and DNA methylation in particular.

Naturally, I support following the Younger You Intensive or Everyday as I think it's the most comprehensive and upstream approach to fostering healthy DNA methylation patterns on your nutrient-responsive genes.

However, if you've gotten genetic or epigenetic testing results that show that you have a mutation, a single nucleotide polymorphism (or SNP, discussed below), or imbalanced DNA methylation on any of these genes, you can focus on prioritizing the nutrients that have been shown by research to support that particular gene's expression. To find a list of foods that contain each of these nutrients, refer to the Nutrient Reference on page 407.

NUTRIENT-RESPONSIVE GENE	STANDS FOR	NOTES	NUTRIENTS
BRCA1 **BRCA2**	Breast Cancer Gene 1 Breast Cancer Gene 2	BRCA is a tumor-suppressor gene that also repairs DNA and regulates estrogen production. Many mutations have been identified in BRCA genes, of both known and unknown significance—the most well-known are associated with an increased risk of hormone-related cancers, including ovarian and breast.[15] BRCA hypermethylation (which inhibits the gene from working) has also been associated with numerous cancers including: breast (male and female), ovarian, prostate, pancreatic, melanoma, Fanconi's anemia, stomach, bladder, and lung cancers.[16]	resveratrol EGCG curcumin quercetin genistein daidzein/equol sulphoraphane kaempferol[17]
GSTP1	Glutathione S Transferase P1	The GST family of enzymes act as antioxidants. Because they are important players in the detoxification of many carcinogenic and cytotoxic compounds, they contribute to cancer prevention by inhibiting DNA damage. GSTP1 has been found to be hypermethylated in prostate, breast, liver, and lung cancer; measuring methylation status of GSTP1 could be an effective biomarker for diagnosis and monitoring of certain cancers.[18] Other glutathione detox genes, including GSTM1 and GPX3, are also associated with cancer prevention and may be hypermethylated and inhibited in cancer.[19]	EGCG lycopene curcumin daidzein (equol) genistein myricetin ellagic acid hesperidin apigenin

continues

continued

RARß2	Retinoic Acid Receptor- ß2	Retinoic acid is derived from vitamin A and is involved in cell growth and differentiation. There are four types of RARß; of these, RARß2 is considered to suppress cancer growth. RARß2 may be hypermethylated in prostate, breast, cervical, head and neck, non-small cell lung, bladder, and brain cancers. Assessment of DNA methylation status of RARß may be useful for early detection, prognosis, and drug response.[20]	EGCG myricetin daidzein (equol) genistein
MGMT	O-6-methylguanine DNA methyltransferase	The enzyme this gene codes for is involved in DNA repair—specifically, it prevents mismatching and errors during DNA replication. MGMT has been found to be hypermethylated in prostate, testicular, breast, ovarian, cervical, brain, and colon cancers and lymphoma.[21] One exception is glioblastoma, where MGMT hypermethylation predicts better survival.[22] We don't yet understand why this is; yet these findings reinforce seeking to balance and optimize DNA methylation through diet and lifestyle so that when you need more, you get more, and where you need less, you get less.	EGCG genistein kaempferol olive leaf extract[23]
TET1 TET2	Ten-eleven translocation enzymes	TET enzymes are needed for demethylation of all genes, including tumor-suppressor genes, from embryogenesis on into adulthood. TET enzyme genes are inhibited in nearly all cancers.[24]	vitamin C vitamin A vitamin D alpha ketoglutarate sulforaphane

DNMT	DNA-N-Methyltransferase	The DNMT family of enzymes methylate DNA both during, and outside of, cellular replication. Tumors can hijack DNMT enzymes, using them to hypermethylate tumor-suppressor genes and other important genes like NRF2 (see below).[25]	EGCG luteolin sulforaphane genistein curcumin resveratrol apigenin myricetin fisetin ellagic acid pterostilbene vitamin E vitamin A selenium
NRF2	Nuclear factor erythroid 2-related factor 2	NRF2 increases production of anti-inflammatory/antioxidant molecules to protect against toxins and oxidative damage. It is downregulated in many chronic diseases, including heart disease, neurodegenerative disease, diabetes, autoimmunity, and cancer, and has been found to be hypermethylated in liver, prostate, colorectal, breast, bladder, stomach, and ovarian cancer.	sulforaphane EGCG curcumin apigenin
OPCML	Opioid-binding protein/cell adhesion molecule	This newly discovered tumor-suppressor gene plays an important role in regulating opioid receptors and promoting cell differentiation. Hypermethylation of OPCML has been identified in breast, ovarian, colon, liver, lung, gastric, lymphoma, esophageal, nasopharyngeal, cervical, and prostate cancers.[26]	luteolin

Now that you hold in your hands a playbook for keeping your DNA methylation balanced and younger, you know how to exert a powerful protective influence on your genes and your risk for disease. Even cancer.

When you start making new choices, bathing your cells in the ingredients for optimal DNA methylation and lowering the volume on outside influences—such as pesticides, chemicals, and stress—that impair DNA methylation, you start to clean up the epigenetic marks on your nutrient-responsive genes and pass those improved patterns on to your own daughter cells, essentially creating a younger, healthier, less-prone-to-cancer version of yourself.

Two Instances of Cures: The Power of Nutrients to Influence Genetic Expression

THERE ARE TWO CASES I ENCOUNTERED THAT SHOWED ME THE PROFOUND ability of nutrients to treat conditions with genetic roots—they were moments when I truly grasped the power of nutrition.

One boy, whose physician I consulted with for years, had an extremely rare genetic condition that confined him to a wheelchair and gave him a life expectancy of five years. The affected gene codes for a protein involved in bone synthesis; when this gene is mutated, it leads to far-reaching deformities in all bones that result in short stature, curved spine, joint damage, and more. The boy's clinician used blood and urine tests to evaluate his essential nutrients, and we designed a specific nutrition program that included all the vitamins and minerals his body needed (in the doses he needed, all administered through a feeding tube, which his condition necessitated). Not surprisingly, his protocol included a rich complement of methyl donors and DNA methylation adaptogens. He went on to graduate from high school, believed to be the oldest living male with this condition. Now, we cannot say for certain it's the dietary program he followed, but it makes sense that optimal nutrition helped him function better than following the standard American diet.

Another story was of a teenaged girl who developed severe epilepsy and whose laboratory tests revealed a genetic defect in a protein that requires the B vitamin biotin as its coenzyme. It wasn't wholly the genetic defect's fault, as she had been healthy up until her teens. Who knows what changed? Our gut microbiome makes biotin—perhaps she had one too many antibiotics that damaged her gut and impaired her biotin production, until one day the biotin shortage was significant enough that, along with the gene variant in a biotin-dependent enzyme, her seizures ensued. We can't know for sure. Nevertheless, she was prescribed a higher-dose biotin supplement (along with gut work and a nutrient-dense diet that was the precursor to Younger You) to boost her biotin levels, and her seizures stopped.

· · · · ·

PUTTING YOUR GENETIC TESTING RESULTS IN PERSPECTIVE

Throughout my years in clinical practice, I've frequently had patients arrive in my office who have had direct-to-consumer genetic testing done and are distressed about the information they've received about the state of their genes, particularly about their single nucleotide polymorphisms, otherwise known as SNPs (pronounced "snips") or genetic variants. Extremely common, SNPs are the simplest of all genetic mutations.

Something important to keep in mind as you attempt to understand the results of your genetic testing is that genetic variants, especially when considered one at a time, are rarely that impactful. In fact, scientists are quite open about the high expectations for—and subsequent disappointment at the failure of—SNP testing to pave the way for understanding disease. That said, newer research is focused on looking at the influence of many related SNPs (each contributing just a small effect) leading to a net increased risk—or not—of a given disease such as diabetes or cardiovascular disease. This new line of inquiry is called polygenic risk profiling.[27] While I think this area could evolve into a useful way to use SNP data, without considering epigenetics, any insight polygenic risk profiling will provide will be muddy at best.

Every one of us has about four million SNPs, the vast majority of which make no difference in our physical function or health. After all, humanity has made it this far with them! The truth is SNPs generally only become significant if they are negatively influenced by an environmental trigger.

But I don't want to dismiss all single SNPs wholesale. There are a few studies that suggest that SNPs can interact with epigenetics in a meaningful way. Take the MTHFR gene, which codes for the enzyme methylenetetrahydrofolate reductase, a fundamental player in the methylation cycle. The MTHFR C677T variant is one of the most common SNPs and perhaps the best known. (It is the variant I mentioned at the start of Chapter 2, in Rhonda's story.) When this variant is present, it is generally considered to slow down the methylation cycle for all biochemical methylation, including DNA methylation, meaning it's associated with hypomethylation. Some very preliminary research also suggests that the MTHFR C677T variant might accelerate bio age, and supplementation might restore it.[28] We will be looking at the MTHFR variants in our next study participants to see if the preliminary observation holds up, and how these participants respond to the Younger You Intensive. Stay tuned for more data.

Just because you have a SNP—or a mutation, for that matter—it doesn't mean that it's impacting you physiologically. You'll need some thoughtful inquiry to determine whether the genetic hand you've been dealt is something you need to be concerned about. For example, if you have an MTHFR SNP (outside of being pregnant, when you probably want to give yourself and the growing baby extra support), you can gauge if it's having a negative impact on your biochemical methylation by seeing if your homocysteine is high—something that's easy to assess with a simple lab test. If it *is* high, that implies that you're probably not methylating your folate enough to recycle homocysteine. And if it's *not* high, then that suggests you're likely fine. Even if you do have an elevated homocysteine level, it's hardly due to just the SNP itself. There are lots of other things to take into consideration, as well, such as, are you eating enough methyl donors? How is your gut health (where we make folate)? Are you exercising? And what's your stress level like?

The major takeaway on genes, mutations, and SNPs is that your environment—which includes your diet and lifestyle, including your toxin exposures—is the biggest player in whether your genetics has a negative impact on your health or not. And no matter what your particular genetic profile is, you really want to take exquisite care of your DNA methylation and epigenome over the long term.

We'll talk about how to make your epigenetic and biological age improvements lasting in the next chapter—as well as how this exciting new area of our understanding might change our collective health in the not-so-distant future. I'll also cover some of the cutting-edge developments that our unfolding understanding of aging and epigenetics is making possible.

11

FUTURE YOU

O UR BURGEONING UNDERSTANDING OF GENETIC AND EPIGENETICS, including DNA methylation—in other words, the omics revolution—is ushering the fields of science and medicine in a period of intense change that is as significant as the Industrial Revolution was to manufacturing and commerce and finance. It's incredibly exciting—and, truth be told, a little scary.

As devoted as I am to science, I also know that it's an important endeavor to periodically weigh where our ever-expanding knowledge might be leading us so that we can decide if the future we're creating is one we actually want to inhabit. We are in the throes of leaping forward, but I don't think we're quite able to see over the ledge to exactly where some of these advances will take us. Because of the accelerated pace of possibility, there are important questions to be asked, such as, what are the practical, medical, and ethical ramifications of winding our clocks back? And how far do we truly want to take it?

In this chapter, I'll take a look at a few ideas for what's on the horizon for anti-aging in general and DNA methylation applications in particular, and how it all relates to you, so that you can make choices now that help create a future you want to inhabit. I'll also cover how to lock in the benefits of the Younger You program so that you stay vital and vibrant for the long term.

THE POWER OF KNOWING YOUR BIO AGE

The ability for health-conscious individuals to be able to test their biological age is rapidly approaching. It will be such a change from when we first embarked on our study: then, each epigenetic test cost us over $1,000, and we needed to collect each specimen in special tubes, deep freeze them, then ship them overnight on dry ice from the Helfgott Research Institute in Oregon, who gathered the specimens, to Yale in Connecticut, who analyzed them—not exactly affordable or accessible. As I write this, the same bio age testing technology that we used is on the verge of being available to individuals and clinicians, and significantly less expensive.

In addition to measuring bio age, we'll likely be regularly using DNA methylation assessments to sensitively predict risk of disease. This is a wave that has already started to reach the shore, but it has by no means crested: There are currently DNA methylation assessments that are used to predict risk of colon cancer (the Cologuard at-home colon cancer screening test I mentioned on page 43) and to predict whether a particular drug will be useful in brain cancer treatment. In addition to assessing risk or guiding treatment in other forms of cancer—including breast and ovarian, as I discussed on page 258—these coming DNA methylation tests may help shed insight on dementia, heart disease, autoimmune disease, allergic diseases, COVID, or other infectious diseases. I am giddy with excitement that these important, health-saving, life-expanding tools are already here or are close by. (I myself am working on researching and developing a test that looks at a host of DNA methylation patterns, including a variety of bio age clocks and what we think are nutrient-responsive genes, and collaborating with Dr. Dale Bredesen to look at methylation patterns in important Alzheimer-associated genes.)

My area of interest is preventative, actionable medicine, thus I see these tests as guiding us in individualized interventions to reverse bio age, ward off chronic disease, and optimize health. The epigenetic testing *may* deliver on the promise that we all expected from genetic testing by showing us where our weaknesses and strengths lie in terms of the diseases and conditions we are more susceptible to. Beyond that, it will help us identify the causes of many conditions and help develop—and assess the effectiveness of—customized treatment plans. Eventually, we'll be able to perform this test in utero, too.

Looking slightly farther ahead, we'll likely be able to see our bio age in real time thanks to a wearable device: as someone who has tracked my sleep, movement, heart rate and heart rate variability, and glucose levels via wearable monitors, I can attest that objectively seeing how your choices create a measurable impact on your well-being is very motivating. That may sound like I'm hooked up to a jumble of wires, but it's just a simple ring around my finger and a small disc on the back of my arm.

We know that certain epigenetic marks change in real time in response to current exposures. Throughout these pages, I've mentioned studies where changes to DNA methylation have been demonstrated after very short-term experiences, including four hours of exposure to traffic pollution; a single high-sugar meal; one session of meditation or exercise; or one poor night of sleep. So imagine when we have the technology—perhaps a device similar to the continuous glucose monitor on my arm—that can tell you in real time whether your DNAmAge is ticking forward or backward based on how you're living your life. I assure you, someone, somewhere is thinking about how to develop this technology.

The ultimate goal of affordable bio age testing and wearable biological age–tracking devices is to put your health into your hands and take it back from Big Pharma, insurance, and the medical complex—all those profiting in trillions and trillions of U.S. dollars by keeping us propped up on drugs and profoundly unwell for our final sixteen-plus years of life. It's an important advancement toward the vision my team and I adopted years ago: "The widespread adoption of a health-care model that reverses the global epidemic of chronic disease and supports the development of vibrant longevity."

With regard to longevity, we are at a wildly exciting time. On one hand, we are actively moving forward with safe and accessible diet and lifestyle practices that slow or reverse aging. But on the other hand there are other areas of research into epigenetics and genetics that go far beyond this approach—and while I'm very curious (and excited) about them, as you'll see, they also raise their own profound concerns.

CURRENT AND FUTURE ANTI-AGING STRATEGIES

At least since the start of the 1500s, when Juan Ponce de León sailed from Spain to Florida in search of the fountain of youth, we've been actively seeking external sources of longevity. Now that our scientific understanding of aging is leapfrogging ahead, there is no shortage of cutting-edge approaches coming down the pike.

One such strategy that uses existing technology in new ways is the practice of taking certain medications for their anti-aging properties, even though these drugs were developed and are prescribed for different uses. At the top of the list is rapamycin, a molecule produced by bacteria that forms the basis of a drug used with organ transplant patients because it suppresses the immune system and therefore makes the body less likely to reject the new organ.

Given its origins, it's no wonder that rapamycin is, in anti-aging circles, given almost mystical properties: it was discovered in 1964 in the soil of Easter Island (native name: Rapa Nui), home to the moai statues of huge stone heads facing out to sea. The molecule itself was identified in the mid-1970s. It wasn't until the mid-1980s that Dr. Suren Sehgal, a pharmaceutical researcher, discovered the molecule's immunosuppressive properties.[1] Then it took until 1999 for rapamycin to receive FDA approval as an immunosuppressant for patients receiving organ transplants.

After its release, researchers kept looking for other benefits of this intriguing molecule. By the mid-2000s, studies had found that rapamycin extended life expectancy in yeast and worms. A 2009 study found that it significantly lengthened the life span of mice—by 28 percent in males and 38 percent in females. Although these were animal studies and not human studies, that was all the evidence early adopters of anti-aging remedies needed to start taking it themselves; either securing it from the rare doctor in America (a 2019 article in *Men's Health* claimed there was then only one[2]) who was willing to prescribe it for aging or buying it through questionable online sources.

We now know that rapamycin works to delay aging by suppressing a cellular pathway known as the mammalian target of rapamycin complex 1 (mTOR), which regulates cell growth. When mTOR is inhibited, it suppresses cellular growth, including the production of old, pro-inflammatory senescent cells, which in turn slows down aging. This is also one of the pathways that caloric restriction suppresses (see Chapter 3). Because mTOR1 is activated by eating, activation is also altered by fasting mimicking, and time-restricted eating (also discussed in Chapter 3).

I understand how tantalizing the thought of a pill that extends life is. But rapamycin is immunosuppressive; it has a dangerous potential to make you more vulnerable to infection. Early adopters are trying it and reporting it is safe for them, but I recommend some caution until we know more. In fact, there are anecdotal reports of more frequent infections, such as skin and kidney infections, that rapidly become dangerous if they aren't treated quickly with antibiotics. Paradoxically, rapamycin can also contribute to insulin resistance and high blood glucose, which generally leads to diabetes (and the associated diseases of aging). However, a number of scientists, including Mikhail Blagosklonny, argue that the mechanisms driving rapamycin-induced insulin resistance are not actually detrimental and may be life extending, as is the case in animal research.[3] Clearly, we need to keep an eye on this complex molecule.

In the meantime, the FDA, which gave the drug its most severe "black box" warning when prescribed for transplant patients, lists the following possible side effects:[4]

- Increased susceptibility to infection
- Increased risk of skin cancer and lymphoma
- Impaired or delayed wound healing
- Increased serum cholesterol and triglycerides
- Deterioration of kidney function
- Interstitial lung disease
- Fluid retention

It's difficult to study longevity in humans because we live for such a long time, so there is no evidence to suggest a safe and effective dosage of rapamycin when used to extend life. Deciding how much to take for longevity purposes remains a guess. Biohackers are experimenting with doses less than 6 mg per week, and some are doing this just a few weeks of the year. The dosage prescribed for organ transplant recipients is about

5 mg per day, continuing indefinitely; this is the dosage that triggered the warnings about infection and cancer. But still; if extended health span is the goal, one needs to ask, are these risks truly worth it? For some of us, it's an unequivocal yes. For others, it's a "no way," especially when there are dietary practices and natural compounds found in food that may also inhibit the production and accumulation of old, pro-inflammatory cells.

Another wildly popular medication taken for possible life extension (and often also taken by those on rapamycin) is metformin, the diabetes drug that Fahy included in his TRIIM study, which I covered in Chapter 1, and that is the most commonly prescribed medication worldwide for type 2 diabetes because it very effectively lowers blood sugar. It also has been shown to inhibit mTOR and beneficially affect the microbiome, making it capable of producing more short-chain fatty acids that reduce inflammation and support weight loss. In animals, metformin potently extends life span and health span; in humans, it reduces age-related diseases beyond type 2 diabetes, including cancer and neurodegenerative diseases like Alzheimer's.[5] It's no wonder we're interested in it.

While metformin is pretty well tolerated, both as a treatment for diabetes and as an anti-aging strategy, it also has its side effects. Documented less-than-desirable accompaniments of metformin include vitamin B_{12} deficiency (which, paradoxically, negatively impacts DNA methylation); GI issues such as diarrhea or constipation, nausea, and vomiting (a dealbreaker issue for many); and an increased risk of lactic acidosis (which can lead to coma and even death). While living with GI issues has its own undesirability, what concerns me is the admittedly rare increased risk of lactic acidosis, which is caused by metformin impairing function of mitochondria, the organelles that metabolize macronutrients into energy, via a protein called complex 1.[6]

Lactic acid is produced when cellular respiration (the molecular process of creating energy from oxygen that occurs within the mitochondria) is inhibited. While it's totally normal to make some lactic acid when you're using extra energy—like during a workout, after which that buildup of lactic acid will make your muscles feel sore—if you are making a lot without reason, it's a clue that something's going wrong within the mitochondria. When you see very high levels of lactic acid being excreted in the urine or circulating in the blood, it can be a full-tilt emergency known as lactic acidosis, or, if it's in a subclinical range, it suggests that the mitochondria are struggling. It's essential that our mitochondria be in great health as we age so we want to tread lightly regarding interventions that might impair function.

While diabetics are known to biologically age more rapidly than their nondiabetic counterparts, and metformin may be playing a role in mitigating the accelerated aging that accompanies diabetes, science is not at all clear on metformin's benefits to healthy, nondiabetic individuals in terms of life span and health span.[7] To that end, a 2019 study showed that older, basically healthy people prescribed both an aerobic exercise program and metformin displayed problems with skeletal muscle mitochondrial respiration, cardiorespiratory fitness, and insulin sensitivity.[8] This suggests that metformin may reduce the benefits of exercise in healthy people. If the choice is between exercise and metformin, I recommend exercise! This and other studies seem to suggest that metformin's use may be best limited to those with a chronic condition like diabetes or cancer and avoided if you are healthy.

Testosterone has been the subject of a major marketing campaign for men, with claims that supplementing with the male sex hormone can increase energy, boost mental sharpness, and restore sexual function. It's pretty compelling stuff, and can be true in some cases, until you consider that testosterone may also increase risk of cardiovascular problems, including heart attack, stroke, and death from heart disease, and these risks are more pronounced the older the men are. The risk is so significant that researchers in a 2010 study looking at the effects of testosterone replacement in older men (who, admittedly, had higher rates of chronic disease) pulled the plug on the study when the participants had a noticeable uptick in heart problems.[9]

Some men who take testosterone also experience acne, irregular breathing while sleeping, and a tendency toward high red blood cell counts, which can increase the risk of clotting. Also, once you supplement with testosterone, the body stops producing it, making it hard to wean off. And perhaps most troubling is the fact that testosterone is a growth promoter. It ramps up mTOR, which rapamycin, metformin, and caloric restriction all inhibit. Anything that pushes growth forward carries a risk of also pushing forward cancer, because cancer is growth gone wild.

Testosterone is undeniably important, but testosterone replacement comes with some risks. Like many other compounds we've discussed, the benefits of testosterone have a U curve: too little isn't good, but neither is too much. A study of over three thousand men found that older men with midrange testosterone levels tend to live longer and experience fewer bone fractures.[10] That means that whether or not testosterone replacement is useful depends on where your levels currently are.

A NATURAL APPROACH TO BOOSTING TESTOSTERONE

IN MY PRACTICE, WE SEE TESTOSTERONE DROP IN MEN AS THEY GET OLDER, but a lot of times what's happening is that testosterone is getting converted to estrogen in men—and women—who have high blood sugar and accompanying inflammation. For men, that looks like gynecomastia (visible or larger breasts on men), erectile dysfunction, muscle loss, and a belly. For women, it can mean increased estrogen-driven conditions like fibroids, PMS, endometriosis, muscle loss, and loss of libido. In both, it can also play a role in cognitive impairment and depression. When patients present with high blood sugar, inflammation, low testosterone, and elevated estrogen, our first step is to place them on the Younger You Intensive program. It can rapidly drop blood sugar and inflammation, thereby turning the dial on the brutal testosterone steal way down.

· · · · ·

One of the most mind-bending area of epigenetics and anti-aging involves proteins known as Yamanaka factors. Shinya Yamanaka, a stem cell researcher and professor at Kyoto University and University of California, San Francisco, along with Sir John Gurdon, an evolutionary biologist at Cambridge University, were awarded the Nobel Prize for Medicine in 2012 for their separate work that showed that mature cells can be reprogrammed to become unidentified stem calls, or what are known as induced pluripotent stem cells. This is turning the clock back as far as you can possibly go: manipulating epigenetics via DNA methylation and demethylation to the point where stem cells return to the state they were in when you were just an embryo.[11]

This dramatic age reversal is orchestrated by proteins now known as Yamanaka factors. Your body naturally makes these proteins—they are present in high amounts during embryogenesis—but Yamanaka discovered a way to synthesize them outside of the body and introduce them back into cells in vitro. It's an astounding discovery, and we still don't exactly know how it will play out. The possible implications include the ability to make new organs, manufacture new red blood cells, and repair tissues. And, yes, to shave years off biological clocks.

In fact, a landmark study has just been published by Harvard Medical School scientists, including biologist and professor of genetics David Sinclair. In a study published in *Nature*, the team shared how they reversed vision loss due to a glaucoma-like condition by using Yamanaka factors to turn back the epigenetic age of damaged nerve cells in the eyes of mice.[12] Essentially, the administration of three of the four Yamanaka factors made the nerve cells younger, and they regained their function, leading the researchers to conclude, "old tissues retain a faithful record of youthful epigenetic information that can be accessed for functional age reversal." It's exciting, and a little trippy—a combination that elicited some expressions of concern from other longevity researchers.

"At the beginning of this project, many of our colleagues said our approach would fail or would be too dangerous to ever be used," lead study author Yuancheng Lu said in a news release about the study. "Our results suggest this method is safe and could potentially revolutionize the treatment of the eye and many other organs affected by aging."[13] It could even extend to our entire being: if what we believe is true—that aging and death are preprogrammed in the DNA—there may come a time when we can reverse it with some type of a Yamanaka factor cocktail or similar-acting compounds and march ourselves back to a biological childhood.[14]

It's not quite as simple as it sounds, though. While the thought of being able to reverse glaucoma-related vision loss and other age-related diseases is undoubtedly tantalizing, research also shows that Yamanaka factors could also promote the formation of cancer.[15,16]

There's also Clustered Regularly Interspaced Short Palindromic Repeat (CRISPR) technology (also known as "genetic scissors"), which lets us essentially rewrite our genes. The scientists involved in this discovery,

Emmanuelle Charpentier and Jennifer Doudna, were awarded the Nobel in 2020—an indication of how big a deal both these discoveries are.[17] That said, CRISPR was almost immediately misused, skating us right onto the ethical thin ice: remember how we watched in horror as the news unfolded of the 2018 birth of CRISPR-edited twins? As I write this in 2021, further experiments on embryos reveal deep failure—the loss of an entire chromosome in an attempt to edit out a mutation associated with blindness.[18] "If our results had been known two years ago, I doubt that anyone would have gone ahead" and tried it on embryos intended for pregnancy, said biologist Dieter Egli, who led the study.[19]

Despite this profound failing, CRISPR technology is already being used in livestock and crops and holds promise for reversing age-related diseases.[20] In rodents, inactivation of genes associated with aging is happening now, with early outcomes demonstrating rejuvenation.[21] And a small 2021 human trial showed CRISPR effectively cleared amyloid in the deadly genetic disease called amyloidosis.[22] While CRISPR raises loads of ethical and medical questions, I am absolutely paying attention. From curing a lethal genetic disease to safely rebuilding an old, torn meniscus, thereby revitalizing a knee joint and (perhaps) removing some of the obstacles of aging, the possibilities of CRISPR (and Yamanaka factors) are staggering.

There is also a compound that was developed by Harold Katcher, the academic director for the natural sciences at the University of Maryland and a member of the team who identified BRCA1 as a breast cancer gene, that is aptly named "Harold's Elixir" (also known as E5). In 2020, Katcher's proprietary blend was shown to halve bio age (in fact, Steve Horvath did the calculations in the study) in mice. It also lowered inflammatory markers, lipids, and blood glucose and increased antioxidants.[23] As mind-boggling and potentially exciting as the promise of Harold's Elixir, or any longevity concoction, is, you have to remember that humans are not rodents. The test of success for mice is successfully running a maze. We have a lot more complexity in our lives, inside and out, than rodents. We also live a long time. The real proof that any longevity-promoting interventions are safe and work will come only decades after early adopters jump in with both feet.

In these heady discussions of what's possible now and in the near future in terms of anti-aging, I like to keep things grounded in current reality. Even if you have the desire, the access, and the means (because they won't be cheap or covered by insurance any time soon) to engage in more aggressive biohacking, be it rapamycin, metformin, a CRISPR-based intervention, Harold's Elixir, or any of the other myriad interventions currently being investigated, there are always risks that you're simply not going to find with a diet, exercise, and lifestyle program.

In fact, if there is one aspect of health that gains clarity with each new discovery, even during this time of accelerated scientific understanding, it's how essential diet and lifestyle practices are to fundamental health. Our genome and epigenome evolved by responding to the potent, complex input of whole foods, movement, sleep, and community. Over the last century, we learned what happens when we try to "improve" upon natural food sources—processed foods, artificial flavors, fortification, and other forms of food technology landed us right in a huge health crisis. Let's not make the mistake of thinking we can outsmart Mother Nature again. Rather, let's work with her. (Let's also remember that Mother Nature has arranged for us to live 80 to 100 years under the best of circumstances. If you are aiming beyond that range and are willing to run the risk, exotic interventions will almost certainly be needed.)

While there may be developments in the near or distant future that have the potential to help us live better, longer, many profound tools are available now. Some of those tools—like food—only require a trip to the grocery store, farmers' market, or even a backyard plot or patio container to procure. And some—like meditation, cuddling, sleep, and movement—require nothing at all except the willingness to do them. Add in the knowledge of how to put these tools together into a program designed to fine-tune your DNA methylation and, thus, your biological age, and you have everything you need to become a younger you. And since you've come to the end of this book on that very subject, you are ready to go. In fact, I hope you have already started and are at least a few days into your first Younger You protocol—whether it's the Intensive or the Everyday—by now. Know that for every choice you make that benefits your DNA methylation, you are making immediate changes that, with consistency, can become lasting.

LOCKING IN YOUR EPIGENETIC BENEFITS

Our bodies are continually renewing, which means our cells are always dividing. Depending on the tissue, cellular turnover happens quickly—in the GI tract, for example, cells turn over around every three days. And when those cells renew, so do their methylation marks. That means you can likely begin to change the course of your genetic expression at any moment.

The only hitch is, you have to keep doing the things that favor balanced DNA methylation, or else the stress or the crappy food will creep back in and start influencing new epigenetic marks. Making as many Younger You foods and lifestyle practices a regular part of your life as you can is how you can lock in the epigenetic benefits you create.

The truth is, the Younger You principles are a marriage, not a fling. It's up to each of us to continually renew our commitment to taking care of our genetic expression by implementing these diet and lifestyle tweaks.

Over the long term, implement as much of the Younger You Everyday that you can. And ideally you'd complete the full eight weeks of the Younger You Intensive at least once a year. You may find that the program makes you feel so much better that you're motivated to keep it up.

That being said, I know that life happens. For those times when you veer off the path, whether you decide to have a few drinks to celebrate something exciting or help take the edge off a particularly tough time, or you fall prey to a high load of stress after losing a job or a loved one, or you just gradually fall back into old eating patterns—all you ever have to do is start again. And if you don't have the wherewithal to get back to a formal Younger You program at this particular point in time, use whichever of the many tools that support DNA methylation you can manage to help offset any negative effects—go to bed earlier, double down on green tea, cuddle extra with your partner or your kid or your pet, or opt to have a vegetable-packed salad instead of picking up fast food. Any step you take will help you keep some momentum going.

On the other hand, if you find yourself becoming overly anxious about following the program impeccably, and as a result your nutrient choices (and lifestyle habits) become more and more restrictive, causing you to feel bad if you "don't get it right," you might be moving toward orthorexia. In my personal and clinical experience, I see both men and women succumbing to disordered eating, and I believe there has been an uptick in both groups, but for perhaps different reasons. For some men, we see extreme nutrient biohacking, like water-only fasting, severe time-restriction, or very limited keto plans, especially as these tactics are—with some validity—tacked to longevity and survival. In women, we saw an uptick in disordered eating (both too little and too much) with the COVID-19 pandemic; when it seemed that the world was veering out of control, food became a focus. If there are times when you need to be gentler and less rigid with your eating choices, prioritize the lifestyle practices that support healthy DNA methylation (and remember to keep your exercise moderate). It will keep your seat warm for when you're ready to get back to making healthier food choices, as well as assist you in maintaining some of the positive changes you've already created as a result of your time spent following the Younger You Intensive or Everyday plans.

● Signs Associated with a Vulnerability to Orthorexia

- o Obsession with wellness, health, biohacking, and/or longevity
- o Feeling guilty or unwell anytime you diverge from your chosen eating plan
- o Forbidding any foods that aren't perfectly aligned with the eating plan
- o Avoiding restaurants
- o Limiting social commitments or hobbies because so much time is devoted to shopping for and preparing food

• • • • •

LET'S NOT FORGET THE BENEFITS OF AGING

We tend to think of aging categorically as a raw deal; an unavoidable accumulation of indignities and infirmities—loss of energy, aches and pains, thinning hair, sagging skin, memory loss. And worse—heart disease, susceptibility to infection, cancer, dementia.

Of course it's OK to want to preserve our youth and slow our rate of aging so that we don't have to lose our faculties, our strength, our independence, our resilience, and our lives prematurely. But let's also not overlook the perks of aging. Although I can't point to research that backs up my point—because I am not aware of it being conducted yet—it's my strong suspicion that as we age, we biologically embed a more nuanced sense of morality and a deeper wisdom into our DNA methylation patterns.

I think of it this way: when I practiced Zen in my twenties, Zen master Seungsahn described us students engaged in practice as dirty potatoes cooking in a big pot. The experience of bumping up against each other in the pot enabled a deep cleaning. Our rough edges were smoothed in the experience of Zen practice (and living together in community), but of course he was also talking about life in general, beyond the walls of the Zen center. And so it goes with age: our rough spots come up against many opportunities to soften and deepen. How is this experience captured biochemically? I have no doubt it's in large part mediated by changes to DNA methylation. After all, the biological embedding of trauma happens in part via DNA methylation; doesn't it stand to reason that likewise the biological embedding of maturity, love, forgiveness, and wisdom happen in much the same way?

Which begs the question, if you take a Yamanaka blend in search of regaining your physical prime, or clip out a couple of age-driving genes in the equivalent of a CRISPR facelift, does the biological embedding of maturation get wiped away, too? When we launched our Younger You program, Tom, a physician friend of mine, texted and said in his refreshingly direct fashion, "I am not interested in being younger. I am very interested in aging gracefully. For me (probably only me) the name *Younger You* is a big turn off. I am an elder of my tribe. I am not chasing vanity, or trying to be something I am not. But I hope to stay active, physically and mentally, for some years to come." I love what he says. I appreciate it. And I suggest that this maturity he's appreciating is mapped out somewhere on his epigenome. Conversely, when I ask my friends who are deep longevity scientists and/or avid biohackers, they confess that they don't much discuss the positive side of aging—nor the potential for its loss—in their longevity-seeking circles.

Aubrey de Grey, a controversial figure in the field of gerontology, be-lieves firmly that aging as we know it will soon be a vestige of the past, and that the human who will be the first to live to one thousand is alive today. He believes we will essentially be able to decide our bio age, whether it's twenty or forty, and strongly resists what he terms our society's "pro-aging" trance.[24]

Let me be clear: I don't judge anti-aging enthusiasts. I am one! I know how tempting it is to want to do anything to reduce risk of disease and reverse aging. Remember, I became a mother at age fifty. I long to be younger with every fiber of my being because I want to be present—physically, mentally, emotionally—for as many years of my daughter's life as possible. But the truth is, every external intervention has a down-side to it, and significant inhibition or reversal of aging—as appears to one day be possible with Yamanaka factors, CRISPR technology, or Har-old's Elixir—is an occasion for treading lightly with both eyes fully open. What happens if (or should I say "when"?) unintended and negative consequences arise, are the changes irreversible? Not only that, but how does prioritizing youth over all else jibe with the biological embedding of wisdom?

I don't know that I need to be the one that lives to one thousand. And I definitely don't care to revert to being a teenager, or even relive my twen-ties. I won't be first in line to gobble down an untested eternity potion, although I'll be paying close attention to the people who do it. Color me boring, but like my friend Tom, I want to enjoy my years of being a cleaner potato, as my meditation teacher referenced. I want to be able to age in a way that empowers me to act on and share the insight I manage to accu-mulate, and live well until the end.

On the other hand, I definitely don't want to be propped up in a nurs-ing home, giving Isabella's hard-earned inheritance to the corporations making trillions off of extending life span without health. Neither do I want to spend all my time and energy focused on managing the symptoms, conditions, and loss of function that currently eat up the sixteen-plus years of the average American's life. After all, it's not possible to implement and share the wisdom you've acquired if you're trapped in a downward spiral of health that gets progressively worse. Personally, I'd rather spend those years furthering my research, pursuing hobbies old and new, and spending time with my loved ones—and I want you to have the same option to decide what you want to do with your time and energy.

I want an aging journey that's about adding instead of subtracting; something that a passage from Robin Wall Kimmerer's amazing book *Braiding Sweetgrass* sums up nicely. In it, she's describing her years-long effort to reclaim a pond on her property from the weeds and algae that had overtaken it. (Emphasis mine.)

> Like many an old farm pond, mine was the victim of eutrophication, the natural process of nutrient enrichments that comes with age. Generations of algae and lily pads and fallen leaves and autumn's apples falling into the pond built up the sediments, layering the once clean gravel at the bottom in a sheet of mulch. All those nutrients fueled the growth of new plants, which fueled the growth of more new plants, in an accelerating cycle. This is the way for many ponds—the bottom gradually fills in until the pond becomes a marsh and maybe someday a meadow and then a forest. *Ponds grow old, and though I will too, I like the ecological idea of aging as progressive enrichment, rather than progressive loss.*

Let's aim for progressive enrichment, shall we?

THE RECIPES

THE MAJORITY OF THESE RECIPES ARE APPROPRIATE FOR THE Younger You Intensive, although I've also included some that are only suited for the Younger You Everyday.

Of course, you can eat Intensive recipes when you are following the Everyday—and they are so tasty that I'm guessing you'll want to add them to your daily rotation! But unless you're a vegetarian or a vegan and you need to eat some legumes in order to meet your daily protein requirements while on the Younger You Intensive (refer back to page 99 for details), skip the Everyday recipes while you are on the Intensive.

I've coded each recipe so that you can see at a glance which phase of the program the recipe is appropriate for, as well as whether it's keto-friendly, paleo-friendly, vegan, or vegetarian. All recipes are gluten-free and dairy-free.

Remember that some foods are both methyl donor *and* DNA methylation adaptogens, as different compounds within a food can play different, and multiple, roles in the body. So don't let the fact that one food appears on two different lists confuse you (or think that we've made a mistake!).

RECIPE KEY:

K   *keto-friendly*
KL   *keto-leaning (low carb, but not necessarily*
          adherent to a strict keto diet)
P   *paleo-friendly*
V   *vegan*
VGT *vegetarian*
YYI   *Younger You Intensive*
YYE   *Younger You Everyday*

Breakfast

Basic Smoothie (YYI)
Sunberry Smoothie Bowl (YYE)
Rainbow Breakfast Bowl (YYE)
Berry Muesli (YYI)
Matcha Coconut Crunch (YYI)
Cranberry Apple Cinnamon Oatmeal (YYE)
Salmon and Spinach Omelet (YYI)
Green Eggs and Shiitake Ham (YYI)
Baked Eggs Two Ways (YYI)
Veggie-Wrap Breakfast Burrito (YYI)
Savory Onion and Chard Muffins (YYI)
Zucchini Banana Muffins (YYE)
Almond and Tartary Buckwheat Muffins (YYI)
Blueberry Beet Scones (YYI)
Chocolate Avocado Banana Bread (YYE)

Light Dishes (Salads, Sides, Dips, and Dressings)

Mix-and-Match Rainbow Salad (YYI)
Herbal Epigenetic Dressing (YYI)
Tangy Citrus Dill Dressing (YYI)
Turmeric-Pickled Daikon (YYI)
Lactofermented Vitamin D Mushrooms (YYI)
Red Cabbage, Beet, and Pomegranate Slaw (YYI)
Warm Salmon and Roasted Cauliflower Salad (YYI)

Colorful Quinoa Lentil Salad (YYE)

Quinoa Tabbouleh (YYE)

Spiced Butternut Squash and Red Lentil Soup (YYE)

"Everything" Seed Crackers (YYI)

Rosemary and Sea Salt Crackers (YYI)

Nut and Seed "Everything" Bread (YYI)

Luscious Liver Pâté (YYI)

Baked Spinach and Artichoke Dip (YYI)

Herbed Beet Yogurt Dip (YYI)

Garlic and Rosemary Sunflower Seed Butter (YYI)

Roasted Mushroom Tapenade (YYI)

Cabbage Steaks with Pomegranate and Creamy Drizzle (YYI)

Fragrant Spiced Rice (YYE)

Baked Golden Tempeh (YYI for vegans and vegetarians, otherwise YYE)

Main Courses

Mix-and-Match Stir-Fry (YYI)

Spiced Salmon Cakes with Vegetable Fries (YYI)

Rosemary Chicken with Tomato, Avocado, and Bacon (YYI)

Creamy Garlicky Chicken with Cauliflower Rice (YYI)

Creamy Coconut Curry with Chicken and Vegetables (YYI)

Red Lentil and Tempeh Curry (YYE)

Epigenetic Chili (YYI for vegans and vegetarians, otherwise YYE)

Mediterranean Stuffed Pork Tenderloin with Green Beans (YYI)

Not Your Mama's Burger with Kohlrabi Mash (YYI)

Simple Pan-Fried Steak with "Creamed" Greens (YYI)

Pan-Fried Cauliflower Steak with Creamy Lemon Garlic Greens (YYI)

DNA Methylation Minestrone (YYI)

Wild Mushroom Ragout (YYI)

Lemon Garlic Broccoli Rabe and White Bean Stew (YYI for vegans and vegetarians, otherwise YYE)

Broccoli Pesto with Pasta (YYE)

Turkey Meatballs (YYI)

Veggie Balls in Marinara Sauce (YYI for vegans and vegetarians, otherwise YYE)

Crispy Garlicky Tempeh with Cauliflower Rice
   (YYI for vegans and vegetarians, otherwise YYE)
Cauliflower-Crust Pizza (YYI)

Snacks and Sweets

Spicy Buffalo Cauliflower "Popcorn" (YYI)
Oven-Baked Beet Chips (YYI)
Rosemary, Garlic, and Lemon Olives (YYI)
Cinnamon Nut Crunch (YYI)
No-Bake Golden Energy Balls (YYI)
Blueberry Gummy Squares (YYI)
Matcha Gummies (YYI)
Raspberry Cacao Truffles (YYI)
No-Bake Sunbutter Chocolate Squares (YYI)
No-Bake Chocolate Almond Cups (YYE)
Individual Coconut Cacao Chia Puddings (YYE)
Rosemary Lemon Tart (YYI)
Sunberry Sorbet (YYE)

Beverages

Energy Boost Green Smoothie (YYI)
Vegan Megaboost Shot (YYI)
Golden Turmeric Milk (YYI)
Matcha Latte (YYI)
Beet Bubbly (YYI)
Iced Oolong Tea with Orange and Rosemary (YYI)
Calming Herbal Tonic (YYI)
Exercise Recovery Drink (YYE)
Fire Cider (YYI)

BREAKFAST • • • • • • • •

BASIC SMOOTHIE

YYI | K, P, V (if not using honey), **VGT**

1 serving   *Prep time: 6 minutes*

Smoothies are a great, easy, and delicious way to get a lot of your methyl donors and DNA methylation adaptogens in one fell swoop—and you only need to clean the blender! Vary these ingredients as you like, or based on what you have on hand.

Methyl donors: green leafy vegetables (spinach, kale, Swiss chard), berries, avocado, seeds (sunflower, pumpkin, flax, chia, hemp), shredded coconut

DNA methylation adaptogens: green leafy vegetables (that are also cruciferous, such as collard greens, Swiss chard, kale), berries, avocado, coconut oil, seeds (sunflower, chia), lemon, lime, shredded coconut

- 8–10 ounces unsweetened nut or seed milk (e.g., coconut, hemp, flax, almond, cashew)
- 2 cups green leafy vegetables (e.g., spinach, kale, collards, Swiss chard)
- ½ cup berries (e.g., blueberries, raspberries, blackberries, strawberries)
- 2 tablespoons protein powder (make sure it's plant-based if you are vegetarian or vegan)
- ¼ avocado or 1 tablespoon MCT oil
- 1–2 tablespoons seeds (e.g., sunflower, pumpkin, flax, chia, hemp)
- 1–2 tablespoons dried shredded coconut, unsweetened

1. Blend all ingredients in a high-speed blender until smooth.

TIPS/VARIATIONS

Add extra nondairy milk or water to desired consistency.

Include 1 teaspoon matcha powder for extra adaptogen support.

Add lime or lemon for additional tanginess and adaptogen support.

Make it a fun challenge to create a rainbow with colorful vegetables and fruits.

Add 3 to 5 drops liquid stevia or monk fruit (or 1 teaspoon honey, if you're on the Younger You Everyday) for additional sweetness.

Smoothies are a superb way to hide supplements (and cut down on capsules): consider adding liquid fish oil, probiotic powder, and/ or a greens powder.

NUTRIENTS

(calculated using almond milk, spinach, blueberries, collagen protein, MCT oil, 1 tablespoon pumpkin seeds, 1 tablespoon shredded coconut)

Fat: 55.8%	Calories: 351.5 kcal	Fiber: 4.8 g
Carb: 19.1%	Fat: 23.5 g	Sugar: 9.9 g
Protein: 25.1%	Carbohydrates: 18.1 g	Protein: 23.7 g

SUNBERRY SMOOTHIE BOWL

YYE | P, VGT, V

1 serving   *Prep time: 20 minutes*

So simple, so delicious, so packed full of YY nutrients—and an easy way to get beets into your day! Because it contains so much fruit, it's not appropriate to the Younger You Intensive (which limits you to two ½-cup servings of fruit per day), but is a great way to support your DNA methylation once you're on the Everyday.

Methyl donors: beets, banana, flax seeds, sunflower seeds

DNA methylation adaptogens: berries, beets, bananas, lemon, kiwi, sunflower seeds, mint

FOR THE BASE:

1 cup raspberries, fresh or frozen

½ cup cooked beets, fresh or frozen (about 1 medium beet)

½ banana

1 tablespoon ground flax seeds

Juice of 1 lemon

¼ teaspoon monk fruit or stevia powder (optional)

FOR THE TOPPINGS:

½ banana, sliced

¼ cup raspberries

¼ cup blueberries

1 kiwi, peeled and diced

2 tablespoons sunflower seeds, finely chopped

Sprig of mint

1. Blend all the base ingredients in a high-speed blender until completely smooth.
2. Pour the smoothie base into your serving bowl.
3. Arrange the toppings on top of your smoothie base and serve.

NUTRIENTS

Fat: 24.1%	Calories: 536.2 kcal	Fiber: 26.3 g
Carb: 67.9%	Fat: 15.4 g	Sugar: 53.4 g
Protein: 8%	Carbohydrates: 100.1 g	Protein: 13 g

RAINBOW BREAKFAST BOWL

YYE | P, V, VGT

1 serving   *Prep time: 6 minutes*

This smoothie bowl is almost too pretty to eat! And it's positively loaded with methylation donor foods and adaptogens. Although all these fruits are typically available year round, this is a dish that's best in summer when fruits are at their freshest.

Methyl donors: banana, apple, mango, pumpkin seeds, flax seeds

DNA methylation adaptogens: bananas, blueberries, strawberries, mango, kiwi, apple, pumpkin seeds

FOR THE PUREED BASE:

½ small banana

¼ cup frozen or fresh blueberries

½ apple, cored and diced
¼ cup almond milk

FOR THE TOPPINGS:
1 kiwi, peeled and sliced
¼ cup strawberries, sliced
¼ cup blueberries
¼ cup diced mango
½ small banana, sliced
¼ cup chopped pumpkin seeds
1 tablespoon ground flax seeds

1. Add the base ingredients to a food processor and blitz until smooth. Add a little extra almond milk, if needed, to help keep it at a creamy consistency.
2. Pour the pureed base into a bowl and arrange the toppings to your liking.

NUTRIENTS

Fat: 35.2%
Carb: 54.8%
Protein: 10%

Calories: 500.3 kcal
Fat: 21 g
Carbohydrates: 73.8 g

Fiber: 15.4 g
Sugar: 43.9 g
Protein: 14.4 g

BERRY MUESLI

YYI | P, V, VGT

2 servings   *Prep time: 2 minutes*

This no-cook option is great for busy mornings when you don't have much time, and lazy mornings when you just want something easy. It also helps you meet your daily seed requirement first thing in the morning. This fact also makes it pretty calorically dense, meaning it will fill you up for a long time, so it's also good for days when you'll be on the go or in back-to-back meetings without easy access to food.

Using a food processor lets you adjust the consistency to your liking, but if you don't have one, you can dice the apple and toss it with the other ingredients right in the bowl, top with almond milk and berries, and voilà—breakfast!

Methyl donors: apple, sunflower seeds, pumpkin seeds, shredded coconut

DNA methylation adaptogens: apple, sunflower seeds, pumpkin seeds, shredded coconut, berries

> 1 medium Granny Smith apple, cored and quartered
> ⅓ cup sunflower seeds
> ⅓ cup pumpkin seeds
> ¼ cup dried shredded coconut, unsweetened
> Pinch of salt
> ¼ cup almond milk
> Handful of fresh berries

1. Add the apple, seeds, coconut, and salt to a food processor and pulse until finely chopped.
2. Transfer to a bowl, pour the milk over it, and top with fresh berries. Enjoy immediately.

NUTRIENTS

Fat: 63.7%	Calories: 376.2 kcal	Fiber: 7.7 g
Carb: 25.2%	Fat: 28.6 g	Sugar: 11.3 g
Protein: 11.1%	Carbohydrates: 23.7 g	Protein: 12 g

MATCHA COCONUT CRUNCH

YYI | K, P, V, VGT

10 servings
(1 serving = ½ cup)   Prep time: 10 minutes   Cook time: 12–15 minutes

We call this "green granola" in my house, where it never lasts long. Ever versatile, it makes a great snack and travels well. You can sprinkle it on top of unsweetened coconut milk yogurt or pour almond milk over it to eat it like a cereal. Top with a handful of your favorite berries to add even more taste (and more DNA methylation adaptogens). If you're snacking, you can eat it right out of a small container with your hands.

Methyl donors: maple syrup, sunflower seeds, pumpkin seeds, almonds, walnuts, shredded coconut

DNA methylation adaptogens: sunflower seeds, pumpkin seeds, matcha powder, almonds, walnuts, coconut oil, shredded coconut

> 1 cup sunflower seeds
> 1 cup pumpkin seeds

1 cup almonds, sliced or roughly chopped

1 cup walnuts, roughly chopped

1½ cups dried shredded coconut, unsweetened

½ teaspoon salt

3 tablespoons matcha powder

2 tablespoons coconut oil

2 tablespoons water

½ teaspoon stevia or monk fruit powder (or 1 tablespoon maple syrup if you're on the Everyday)

1. Preheat the oven to 300°F and line a large baking sheet with parchment paper.
2. In a large bowl, combine the seeds, nuts, coconut, salt, and matcha. Mix well.
3. In a small saucepan, melt the coconut oil until completely liquid (unless it's over 78 degrees in your kitchen, in which case the coconut oil will likely already be liquid). Add the water and sweetener and stir through.
4. Add the melted coconut oil mixture to the dry mix and toss several times to evenly distribute. Hands work great for this!
5. Spread the mixture onto your baking sheet and press it down so that the surface is even.
6. Bake for 12 to 15 minutes or until the nuts and seeds are toasted and turning a light golden brown.
7. Remove from the oven and allow to cool before serving.
8. Keeps in an airtight container for several weeks.

NUTRIENTS

Fat: 75.5%	Calories: 408.8 kcal	Fiber: 6.1 g
Carb: 13.9%	Fat: 36.6 g	Sugar: 3.4 g
Protein: 10.7%	Carbohydrates: 14 g	Protein: 12.4 g

CRANBERRY APPLE CINNAMON OATMEAL

YYE | VGT, V

2 servings   Prep time: 5 minutes   Cook time: 20 minutes
(not including presoak time for the oats)

This flavorful oatmeal is like eating fall in a bowl. While all the ingredients are health promoting, it is on the hearty side—I recommend saving it for days when you'll be on the go so that you can burn off some of the carbs. (It will give you long-lasting energy, so go on that hike or big bike ride!)

For more specific information on soaking, see page 402.

Methyl donors: rolled oats, apple, walnuts, maple syrup

DNA methylation adaptogens: extra-virgin olive oil, coconut oil, apple, cranberry, cinnamon, walnut

> 1 teaspoon extra-virgin olive oil or coconut oil
>
> 1 cup steel-cut oats or thick-cut rolled oats, soaked overnight
>
> 2 cups water
>
> 1 apple, diced
>
> ½ cup fresh cranberries (if using dried cranberries, use only ¼ cup)
>
> Dash of cinnamon, to taste
>
> Pinch of salt
>
> ¼ cup walnuts
>
> ½ to 1 teaspoon maple syrup or raw honey, optional

1. Heat the oil in a pot for a couple of minutes. Add the oats to the oil and stir to coat. Toasting the oats like this gives them more flavor and helps prevent the oatmeal from getting clumpy.
2. Add the water and cover the pot. Allow to boil and then simmer on low for 5 to 7 minutes.
3. Add apples, cranberries, cinnamon, and salt and stir the oatmeal well. Continue to simmer on low-medium heat for another 5 to 10 minutes, stirring occasionally.
4. Remove from heat when the liquid is absorbed and it has reached the consistency you like. Top with walnuts and maple syrup and serve.

NUTRIENTS:

Fat: 27.9%	Calories: 477.6 kcal	Fiber: 12.7 g
Carb: 62.8%	Fat: 15.8 g	Sugar: 14.6 g
Protein: 9.3%	Carbohydrates: 75.4 g	Protein: 12.8 g

SALMON AND SPINACH OMELET

YYI | K, P

1 serving   Prep time: 15 minutes   Cook time: 8 minutes

This recipe results in a fancy-tasting breakfast that is very easy to cook. It's also a great vehicle for the DNA methylation adaptogen superstar turmeric.

Methyl donors: eggs, spinach, turmeric, salmon

DNA methylation adaptogens: eggs, spinach, extra-virgin olive oil, turmeric, salmon

Splash of extra-virgin olive oil
1 cup baby spinach, washed and well packed
2 eggs
¼ teaspoon turmeric
Pinch of salt
Freshly ground black pepper, to taste
2 slices smoked salmon, diced, about ¼ cup

1. Set a small sauté pan over medium heat.
2. Add the oil and spinach leaves and stir until just wilted.
3. Meanwhile, whisk the eggs, turmeric, salt, and pepper in a medium bowl.
4. When the spinach is soft, add the egg mixture to the pan.
5. As it starts to cook, gently push the outer parts of the omelet in toward the center with a spatula, allowing the raw mixture to spread back out to the edges of the pan.
6. Once the omelet is cooked through (no visible raw egg remains on the surface), about 4 to 6 minutes, sprinkle the smoked salmon over one half of the omelet.
7. Carefully fold the omelet in half with your spatula.
8. Slide onto a plate and serve immediately.

NUTRIENTS

Fat: 67.6%	Calories: 355.7 kcal	Fiber: 0.9 g
Carb: 2.9%	Fat: 26.9 g	Sugar: 1.3 g
Protein: 29.6%	Carbohydrates: 2.8 g	Protein: 24.7 g

GREEN EGGS AND SHIITAKE HAM

YYI | K, P, VGT

2 servings   Prep time: 10 minutes   Cook time: 15 minutes

Every single ingredient in this savory breakfast dish actively supports healthy DNA methylation, making it a great thing to eat any time you've gotten off track in your Younger You efforts. The bright yellow of the turmeric and deep green of the collards makes it a feast for your eyes, too.

> *Tip:* To de-stem collard greens, fold the leaf in half lengthwise, lay it on the counter, and use a sharp knife to slice through both halves of the leaf to cut away the stem as far up as you can.

Methyl donors: eggs, collard greens, turmeric

DNA methylation adaptogens: eggs, extra-virgin olive oil, collard greens, shiitake mushrooms, turmeric

> 1 tablespoon extra-virgin olive oil
> 2 large collard green leaves, de-stemmed, chopped, and washed
> ½ cup sliced shiitake mushrooms (stems removed)
> 4 eggs
> 1 teaspoon turmeric
> ¼ teaspoon salt
> ¼ teaspoon black pepper

1. In a sauté pan over medium heat, wilt the collard greens in the olive oil until completely soft, about 5 minutes.
2. Pour greens and any cooking liquid from the pan into a small bowl and set aside.
3. Return the pan to the heat and add a splash more olive oil; sauté the mushrooms until soft and slightly browned, about 5 to 7 minutes.
4. While the mushrooms cook, whisk the eggs, turmeric, salt, and pepper in a medium mixing bowl.
5. Add the collard greens to the bowl and stir to combine—everything will start to look a little green.
6. Add the egg mixture to the pan with the mushrooms and cook, stirring slowly and scraping cooked parts off the bottom of the pan as you go.

7. Once the egg mixture is cooked through, about 4 to 6 minutes, transfer to two serving plates and enjoy in good company!

NUTRIENTS

Fat: 67.3%	Calories: 235.3 kcal	Fiber: 2 g
Carb: 7.8%	Fat: 17.7 g	Sugar: 1.7 g
Protein: 24.9%	Carbohydrates: 5.1 g	Protein: 14 g

BAKED EGGS TWO WAYS

YYI | K, P, VGT (option 1)

1 serving   *Prep time: 5 minutes*   *Cook time: 18–20 minutes*

Eggs are wonderful because they're so simple to prepare, but when you are eating five to ten of them each week, the basic preparations (like scrambling, frying, or hard-boiling) can get a little ho-hum. This recipe gives you two options for making a flavor-packed breakfast (or brunch, or dinner) that's absolutely packed with DNA methylation–supportive nutrients. No more "eggs again?" blues!

Methyl donors: eggs, tomato, rosemary, garlic, onion, chives, chicken liver
DNA methylation adaptogens: eggs, tomato, rosemary, shiitake
    mushrooms, garlic, onion, red pepper flakes, chives, extra-virgin olive oil

BASE OPTION 1:
    ½ cup shiitake mushrooms
    2 cloves garlic, minced
    Splash of extra-virgin olive oil
    Pinch of red pepper flakes

BASE OPTION 2:
    2 chicken livers, rinsed and patted dry, then chopped
    1 small onion, sliced
    1 tablespoon chives, chopped
    Splash of extra-virgin olive oil

    1 tablespoon tomato paste
    2 eggs
    ¼ teaspoon fresh rosemary

Pinch of salt

Freshly ground black pepper, to taste

1. Preheat oven to 375°F. Grease a single-serving ovenproof dish such as a large ramekin or small baking dish.
2. Make the base in a small sauté pan over medium heat.
   - **Option 1:** Sauté the mushrooms and garlic in the olive oil over medium-low heat until softened, about 5 to 7 minutes. Stir in the red pepper flakes.
   - **Option 2:** Sauté the chicken livers and onions in the olive oil over medium-low heat until the liver is cooked through, about seven minutes. Stir in the chives.
3. Stir the tomato paste into your base.
4. Layer your base into the bottom of the greased single-serving ovenproof dish.
5. Crack two eggs on top of the base, being careful not to break the yolks.
6. Bake in the oven for 8 to 10 minutes, until the whites are set but the yolks are still a little runny.
7. Top with the fresh rosemary, salt, and pepper and serve immediately.

OPTION 1 NUTRIENTS

Fat: 70.5%	Calories: 309 kcal	Fiber: 1.7 g
Carb: 10.2%	Fat: 24.4 g	Sugar: 4 g
Protein: 19.3%	Carbohydrates: 8.7 g	Protein: 14.5 g

OPTION 2 NUTRIENTS

Fat: 57.9%	Calories: 464.1 kcal	Fiber: 1.8 g
Carb: 9.5%	Fat: 30 g	Sugar: 6.1 g
Protein: 32.6%	Carbohydrates: 11.7 g	Protein: 35.7 g

VEGGIE-WRAP BREAKFAST BURRITO

YYI | P, V, VGT

1 serving   *Prep time: 10 minutes*   *Cook time: 10 minutes*

This eat-with-your-hands burrito is a tasty—and unique—blend of flavors that will add some novelty to your breakfast rotation. And it is positively jam-packed with methylation-supporting foods! If you double the filling ingredients, the extra will keep in the fridge for up to three days, and then you'll only need to reheat it and wrap it in another collard green leaf for a quick breakfast on another day.

Methyl donors: collard greens, onion, garlic, carrot, sunflower seeds, apple, cumin, ginger, tahini, avocado

DNA methylation adaptogens: collard greens, extra-virgin olive oil, onion, garlic, carrot, sunflower seeds, apple, tahini, cumin, avocado

FOR THE WRAPPING:

> 1 collard green leaf, washed and any tough stems carefully removed with a sharp knife, leaving as much of the leaf intact as possible

FOR THE FILLING:

> 1 tablespoon extra-virgin olive oil
>
> ½ onion, diced
>
> 1 carrot, peeled and grated
>
> 1 clove garlic, minced
>
> ¼ cup sunflower seeds, roughly chopped (a mortar and pestle works well for this)
>
> 1 apple, skin on, cored and diced small
>
> ½ teaspoon cumin
>
> ¼ teaspoon ginger
>
> ¼ teaspoon salt
>
> Freshly ground black pepper, to taste
>
> 2 teaspoons tahini
>
> ¼ avocado, sliced

1. Heat a medium sauté pan over medium heat.
2. Add the olive oil and onion and cook for 3 to 4 minutes, stirring occasionally.
3. Add the carrot and garlic and cook 3 to 4 minutes more, until carrot starts to soften.
4. Add the sunflower seeds, apple, cumin, ginger, salt, and pepper. Add 1 tablespoon of water to moisten, if needed.
5. Turn the heat down to low and cook the mixture, stirring slowly, for 5 more minutes.
6. Take off the heat and stir the tahini through the mixture.
7. To assemble your burrito, take the collard green leaf and lay it out flat. This will serve as your wrap. If you have a cut down the middle from removing the stem, overlap the edges to hide the seam.

8. Place the mixture in the center of the leaf and shape the mixture into a log. Lay the avocado slides on top.
9. Roll up the leaf around the filling, folding the edges of the leaf over into the middle as you roll.
10. Slice your roll in half on the diagonal and serve.

NUTRIENTS

Fat: 66.6%	Calories: 546.9 kcal	Fiber: 11.3 g
Carb: 26.4%	Fat: 42.8 g	Sugar: 18.3 g
Protein: 7%	Carbohydrates: 38.6 g	Protein: 11.4 g

SAVORY ONION AND CHARD MUFFINS

YYI | KL, P, VGT

4 servings
(1 serving = 2 muffins)   Prep time: 15 minutes   Cook time: 25 minutes

For those of you who *don't* like sweet in the morning, these give you the portability of a muffin without the cloying sweetness. Their airy texture makes them a cross between a muffin and a frittata. And their crunchy topping means they still give you something to sink your teeth into with a satisfying mouthfeel. Bake these on a Sunday afternoon and you'll have breakfast at the ready for most of the next week.

Methyl donors: almond flour, rosemary, eggs, red onion, Swiss chard, pumpkin seeds, garlic

DNA methylation adaptogens: almond flour, rosemary, eggs, extra-virgin olive oil, red onion, Swiss chard, pumpkin seeds, garlic, red pepper flakes

FOR THE BASE:

1½ cups almond flour

⅓ cup tapioca flour

1 teaspoon baking powder

½ teaspoon baking soda

1 tablespoon dried rosemary

½ teaspoon salt

2 eggs

⅓ cup extra-virgin olive oil

½ cup nondairy milk, unsweetened

1 red onion, finely chopped

½ cup Swiss chard, measured after de-stemming and finely chopping

FOR THE TOPPING:

¼ cup pumpkin seeds, finely chopped

¼ teaspoon garlic powder

½ teaspoon salt

½ teaspoon red pepper flakes

A splash more extra-virgin olive oil

1. Preheat the oven to 350°F. Grease a muffin tin or line with paper liners. (You need to prep 8 muffin compartments in total.)
2. In a medium mixing bowl, thoroughly combine the almond flour, tapioca flour, baking powder, baking soda, rosemary, and salt.
3. In a separate bowl, whisk the eggs and then add the olive oil, nondairy milk, onion, and Swiss chard. Stir to combine.
4. Add the wet mixture to the dry mixture and stir through.
5. Spoon the mixture into the prepared muffin tin, filling each muffin cup about two-thirds full.
6. Now make the topping: combine the topping ingredients together and distribute evenly on top of each unbaked muffin.
7. Bake for 25 minutes until lightly golden. Test for doneness with a toothpick—muffins are done when it comes out clean.
8. Transfer to a rack to cool. Remove from the muffin tin once cool enough to handle and continue to cool on the rack.

Note: The muffins can be stored in an airtight container in the refrigerator for one week. They also freeze well and can be revived in a few minutes in a toaster oven or a few seconds in a microwave.

NUTRIENTS

Fat: 75%	Calories: 374.9 kcal	Fiber: 3.8 g
Carb: 15.5%	Fat: 32.6 g	Sugar: 2.5 g
Protein: 9.5%	Carbohydrates: 14.6 g	Protein: 9.8 g

ZUCCHINI BANANA MUFFINS

YYE | V, VGT

12 servings   *Prep time: 15 minutes*   *Cook time: 20–30 minutes*
(1 serving = 2 muffins)

This recipe comes in extra handy at the end of summer when gardens and farmers' markets are overflowing with zucchini. But it's always a good time for healthy muffins! You can store leftovers in the fridge or the freezer and then defrost them individually.

Methyl donors: banana, applesauce, nutmeg, clove
Methylation adaptogens: banana, zucchini, applesauce, extra-virgin olive oil, lemon, cinnamon, nutmeg, clove

- 1 banana, overripe and mashed well
- 2 cups grated zucchini
- ¾ cup applesauce
- ¼ cup extra-virgin olive oil
- 1 tablespoon lemon juice
- 1½ teaspoons real vanilla extract
- 3 cups gluten-free flour (I like Namaste's flour blend, available at Costco)
- ⅓ cup unrefined organic sugar
- 1½ teaspoons baking soda
- 1 teaspoon baking powder
- 1 teaspoon cinnamon
- Pinch of nutmeg
- Pinch of ground clove
- 1 teaspoon salt

1. Preheat the oven to 350°F. Line two twelve-cup muffin tins with cupcake liners or grease well with olive oil.
2. Combine all wet ingredients in a medium mixing bowl (banana, zucchini, applesauce, olive oil, lemon juice, and vanilla).
3. Separately, thoroughly combine the dry ingredients in a large mixing bowl (flour, sugar, baking soda, baking powder, cinnamon, nutmeg, cloves, and salt).

4. Add the wet ingredients to the dry and stir well. Scoop about ¼ to ⅓ cup of the mixture into each muffin cup. Bake for 20 to 30 minutes until just beginning to brown and a toothpick inserted comes out clean.
5. Let cool completely on a wire rack before storing.

Note: These can be frozen if needed and defrosted individually.

NUTRIENTS:

Fat: 23.7%	Calories: 191.2 kcal	Fiber: 1.7 g
Carbs: 72.5%	Fat: 5.2 g	Sugar: 9 g
Protein: 3.1%	Carbs: 34.8 g	Protein: 1.8 g

ALMOND AND TARTARY BUCKWHEAT MUFFINS

YYI | KL, VGT

6 servings
(1 serving = 2 muffins)
Prep time: 15 minutes   Cook time: 20–25 minutes

Muffins are such a great, tasty, and portable way to get your DNA methylation–supportive nutrients, and these pack an extra punch thanks to the Tartary buckwheat flour they contain. Thanks to Barb Schiltz, MS, RN, CN, of the Big Bold Health FoodLab, who developed and contributed this recipe.

Methyl donors: Tartary buckwheat, almond flour, egg

DNA methylation adaptogens: Tartary buckwheat, almond flour, egg, coconut oil

1 cup Tartary buckwheat flour
1 cup almond flour or almond meal
2 teaspoons baking powder
¼ teaspoon salt
⅓ cup coconut oil, melted
⅓ cup water
⅓ cup Lakanto monk fruit syrup, room temperature
3 eggs, room temperature, beaten
¾ to 1 cup fresh or frozen blueberries or raspberries
Almond butter, for serving, optional

1. Preheat the oven to 350°F. Line a twelve-cup muffin tin with cupcake liners or grease well with olive oil.
2. Mix dry ingredients together well in a medium-size bowl and set aside.
3. In another medium-size bowl, mix oil, water, and monk fruit syrup together, then add beaten eggs and mix.
4. Add wet ingredients to dry ingredients. Stir thoroughly.
5. Fold in berries and spoon batter into muffin cups (fill about two-thirds full) and bake for 20 to 25 minutes. Prior to enjoying your muffins, consider drizzling almond butter on them for an extra kick of healthy fats and protein!

NUTRIENTS

Fat: 53.1%	Calories: 362.2 kcal	Fiber: 2.7 g
Carbs: 35.4%	Fat: 22.0 g	Sugar: 3.2 g
Protein: 12.3%	Carbs: 32.1 g	Protein: 11.2 g

BLUEBERRY BEET SCONES

YYI | P, VGT, [V]

4 servings
(1 serving = 2 scones)   *Prep time: 15 minutes*   *Cook time: 20 minutes*

These tasty (and purple!) scones come together quickly and can satisfy an urge for something sweet without grains and with a heaping helping of methylation-supportive nutrients. If you can't find beet juice, blend a roasted beet with water to thin it out to a liquid consistency. Or, use the cooled cooking liquid after boiling your beets—while the nutrient content hasn't been verified by research, I suspect it has benefit. And if you *can* find beet juice but balk at the price, know that it makes a great DNA methylation adaptogen–rich addition to a glass of sparkling water or in our Beet Bubbly (page 388).

> *Tip:* This recipe can be made vegan by replacing the egg with 1 flax egg—combine 1 tablespoon ground flax seeds with 2½ tablespoons water and let sit for 5 minutes before adding to the recipe along with the wet ingredients.

Methyl donors: almond flour, arrowroot powder, egg, beets

DNA methylation adaptogens: almond flour, eggs, coconut oil, beets, blueberries

DRY INGREDIENTS:

> 1¼ cups almond flour
>
> ¼ cup coconut flour
>
> ¼ cup arrowroot powder
>
> 1 teaspoon baking powder
>
> ¼ teaspoon salt
>
> 1 teaspoon monk fruit sweetener or stevia powder (or 1 tablespoon honey if you are following the Younger You Everyday)

WET INGREDIENTS:

> 1 teaspoon real vanilla extract (or the inside scrapings of one vanilla pod)
>
> 1 egg
>
> 2 tablespoons coconut oil, melted
>
> ¼ cup beet juice, room temperature or slightly warm

LAST-MINUTE ADD:

> ½ cup blueberries, room temperature

1. Preheat the oven to 350°F. Line a baking sheet with parchment paper.
2. Mix the dry ingredients in a medium mixing bowl until thoroughly combined (a whisk works well at this stage).
3. In a smaller bowl, mix the wet ingredients together until well combined.
4. Add the wet mixture to the dry mixture and stir with a spoon until there are no more dry patches and everything is pink.
5. Add the blueberries and gently fold through.
6. Using your hands, first form the mixture into a ball and then press down into a disc shape on your lined baking sheet. You should get a disc that is around 6 to 7 inches diameter and about 1 inch thick.
7. Cut the disc into eight wedges and separate them from each other slightly.
8. Bake for around 20 minutes or until lightly golden.
9. Once done, transfer to a cooling rack and let cool completely before enjoying.

> *Note:* Once cooled, these can be stored in an airtight container for up to 3 days.

NUTRIENTS

Fat: 60.8%	Calories: 378.6 kcal	Fiber: 7.6 g
Carb: 28.6%	Fat: 26.8 g	Sugar: 9.9 g
Protein: 10%	Carbohydrates: 27.5 g	Protein: 10.4 g

CHOCOLATE AVOCADO BANANA BREAD

YYE | P, VGT

10 servings   Prep time: 10 minutes   Cook time: 45–55 minutes
(1 serving = 1 slice)

This grain-free banana bread includes avocado and almond butter to make it extra creamy and delicious. While of course you can eat this at the start of your day, or for a midmorning snack, Isabella and I love it as a delicious dessert.

Methyl donors: avocado, banana, almond butter, eggs, coconut flour, cocoa, pumpkin seeds

DNA methylation adaptogens: avocado, banana, almond butter, almond flour, eggs, coconut oil, cinnamon, cocoa, pumpkin seeds

   ½ medium avocado, mashed
   3 ripe bananas, mashed
   ½ cup almond butter
   ¼ cup + 2½ tablespoons coconut oil, melted
   4 eggs
   ½ cup coconut flour
   1 teaspoon cinnamon
   1 teaspoon baking soda
   ⅛ teaspoon salt
   ½ cup dairy-free stevia-sweetened dark chocolate chips
   ¼ cup pumpkin seeds

1. Preheat the oven to 350°F.
2. Combine avocado, banana, almond butter, coconut oil, and eggs in a large bowl and mix until blended.
3. In a separate bowl combine flour, cinnamon, baking soda, and salt and stir to mix.
4. Add dry ingredients into wet ingredients and mix well. Stir in the chocolate chips and pumpkin seeds. Pour into a lined loaf pan and bake for 45 to 55 minutes. Cool completely before slicing; serve warm.

   Note: The bread can be stored in the refrigerator for up to 5 days or in the freezer for up to 3 months.

NUTRIENTS

Fat: 67%	Calories: 304 kcal	Fiber: 6.2 g
Carb: 23.4%	Fat: 23.4 g	Sugar: 5.5 g
Protein: 9.6%	Carbohydrates: 20 g	Protein: 7.7 g

LIGHT DISHES • • • • • • •

MIX-AND-MATCH RAINBOW SALAD

YYI | KL, P, VGT, V

1–2 servings   *Prep time: 15 minutes*   *Cook time: 10–20 minutes*
(for protein of choice, although less if you're using leftovers)

This is a quick and simple way to get in a large amount of your methylation donor and adaptogen foods for the day and is my go-to breakfast and lunch combo. You can absolutely customize this to accommodate what you have in your fridge—I've included a base template before the actual recipe so that you can see the method behind the madness and make sure your version hits your basic targets.

Methyl donors: kale, spinach, red bell pepper, carrots, cabbage, sunflower seeds, thyme, parsley, rosemary, sage, dill, oregano, salmon, chicken, pork, tofu, garlic

DNA methylation adaptogens: kale, spinach, red bell pepper, carrots, cabbage, sunflower seeds, pumpkin seeds, berries, extra-virgin olive oil, thyme, parsley, rosemary, sage, dill, oregano, salmon, chicken, pork, tofu, tempeh, coconut oil, garlic, lemon

BASIC TEMPLATE:

TOTAL OF 5 CUPS VEGETABLES:

      1–2 cups dark leafy greens

      1–2 cups cruciferous vegetables

      1–3 cups colorful vegetables

½ cup seeds

½ cup berries

2 cloves garlic, minced

1–2 teaspoons dried herbs or 1–2 tablespoons fresh herbs (e.g., sage, thyme, oregano, rosemary, dill)

3–6 ounces protein of choice (e.g., salmon, chicken,
pork, or if you're vegetarian or vegan, organic
tempeh, organic tofu, or your cooked bean of choice)

2 tablespoons extra-virgin olive oil and squeeze of
lemon

FOR THE SALAD:

1 cup kale, chopped

1 cup spinach, chopped

1 cup red bell pepper, chopped

1 cup carrot, chopped

1 cup purple cabbage, chopped

¼ cup sunflower seeds

¼ cup pumpkin seeds

½ cup berries, such as blueberries, raspberries, or
strawberries

2 tablespoons Herbal Epigenetic Dressing (see page 310)

FOR THE SALMON:

1 tablespoon coconut or avocado oil

3–6 ounces salmon

1–2 cloves garlic, minced

1 slice lemon

Salt and freshly ground black pepper, to taste

1. Mix vegetables in a large glass container. Top with seeds and berries.
2. For the salmon, heat coconut oil on medium heat in a sauté pan. Add garlic and cook for 2 minutes.
3. Add salmon and cook on one side for 3 to 5 minutes until lightly brown, then flip and cook another 3 to 5 minutes until thoroughly done.
4. Squeeze lemon on top and serve alongside salad.
5. Mix salad with Herbal Epigenetic Dressing (or pack the dressing in a side container and take your salad with you).

NUTRIENTS

(analysis used ½ cup blueberries and 6 ounces salmon)

Fat: 66.4%	Calories: 626.9 kcal	Fiber: 7.9 g
Carb: 15.1%	Fat: 47.7 g	Sugar: 11.2 g
Protein: 18.4%	Carbohydrates: 25.2 g	Protein: 29.7 g

HERBAL EPIGENETIC DRESSING

YYI | K, P, VGT, V

8 servings
(1 serving = about 2 tablespoons)

Prep time: 10 minutes,
plus at least 30 minutes resoak
time for sunflower seeds

The fresh adaptogenic herbs in this dressing make a delicious and nutritious addition to a salad, stir-fry, or even cooked protein. (And it makes good use of any fresh herbs you have on hand.)

Methyl donors: sunflower seeds, garlic, apple cider vinegar, thyme, parsley, rosemary, sage

DNA methylation adaptogens: sunflower seeds, extra-virgin olive oil, coconut oil (MCT), garlic, lemon, apple cider vinegar, thyme, parsley, rosemary, sage

½ cup sunflower seeds
¼ cup extra-virgin olive oil
¼ cup MCT oil
4 cloves garlic
¼ cup lemon juice and zest of 1 lemon or
    ¼ cup apple cider vinegar
¼ cup water, or more for consistency
1 tablespoon fresh thyme (or 1 teaspoon dried)
1 tablespoon fresh parsley (or 1 teaspoon dried)
1 tablespoon fresh rosemary (or 1 teaspoon dried)
1 tablespoon fresh sage (or 1 teaspoon dried)
Salt and freshly ground black pepper, to taste

1. Soak sunflower seeds in water for at least 30 minutes; drain water.
2. Place all the ingredients in a high-powered blender and blend until smooth. Add additional water if needed to achieve desired consistency.

TIPS/VARIATIONS

Start your own mini herb garden to have these fresh herbs available anytime.

Use immediately or store on the countertop for up to one week.

NUTRIENTS

Fat: 90.8%	Calories: 158.6 kcal	Fiber: 1 g
Carbs: 6.2%	Fat: 16.9 g	Sugar: 0.4 g
Protein: 3%	Carbohydrates: 2.8 g	Protein: 1.4 g

TANGY CITRUS DILL DRESSING

YYI | K, P, VGT, V

4 servings
(1 serving = about 3 tablespoons)   *Prep time: 10 minutes*

This dressing is particularly refreshing in the early spring when citrus is in season, but it can perk up a salad, stir-fry, or protein any time. If you don't have dill, you can substitute an equal amount of whatever herb you do have on hand, such as rosemary, oregano, basil, or parsley.

Methyl donors: garlic, dill

DNA methylation adaptogens: extra-virgin olive oil, garlic, dill, lime, orange

½ cup extra-virgin olive oil
2 cloves garlic, minced
2 tablespoons fresh dill (or 2 teaspoons dried)
Juice and zest of 1 lime
Juice and zest of 1 orange
Optional: 1 teaspoon honey (omit for a vegan diet)
Salt and freshly ground black pepper, to taste

1. Place all the ingredients in a clean glass jar, shake well. Or blend in a high-powered blender for creamier dressing.

TIPS/VARIATIONS

Use immediately or store on the countertop for up to one week.

You can double or triple batch and store in the refrigerator for a week.

NUTRIENTS

Fat: 93.9%	Calories: 254.9 kcal	Fiber: 0.3 g
Carb: 5.7%	Fat: 7.1 g	Sugar: 2.2 g
Protein: 0%	Carbohydrates: 4.1 g	Protein: 0.3 g

TURMERIC-PICKLED DAIKON

YYI | P, V, VGT

72 servings   *Prep time: 5 minutes*   *Cook time: 20 minutes*
(1 serving = 1 tablespoon)   *Fermenting time: 4–5 days*

Daikon radish is a good source of nutrients such as folate, choline, and vitamin C and minerals such as potassium, magnesium, and calcium, many of which directly support methylation cycles and DNA programming. Turmeric has broad methylation adaptogenic properties. Pickling both together creates a potent probiotic (and prebiotic!) that supports a healthy microbiome, and a top-notch microbiome provides additional folate.

Pickling vegetables is a great way to not only meet your veggie requirements (and work some perhaps less common methylation-friendly vegetables into your daily diet, such as daikon radish) but also boost your intake of probiotics and optimize your gut health. Plus the briny, tangy-but-mellow taste is a delicious complement to your meals. And fermenting is much less labor intensive than you might think—really the only hard part, beyond grating the daikon, is waiting until it's ready.

While technically sugar isn't allowed on either the Younger You Intensive or Everyday, it's needed here to aid the fermentation process—the microbes convert the sugar to lactic acid, so it doesn't "count" as added sugar.

Aim to eat 1 to 3 tablespoons of this a day. It's a great accompaniment to the Not Your Mama's Burger or scrambled eggs and makes a great addition to salads, or really any savory meal. Or, eat it as a small side dish on its own.

You'll need a large glass Mason jar—the 32-ounce size is perfect.

Methyl donors: turmeric, apple cider vinegar, daikon radishes
DNA methylation adaptogens: turmeric, apple cider vinegar, daikon radishes

> 2 cups water
> ¼ cup sea salt
> ¼ cup unrefined organic sugar
> 1 teaspoon turmeric
> 3 medium daikon radishes, about 2 pounds
> ¼ cup apple cider vinegar or rice vinegar

1. Bring 1 cup of water to a simmer and add the salt, sugar, and turmeric. Stir to dissolve the salt and sugar.
2. Meanwhile, grate the radishes and pack into a glass food jar, leaving about 2 to 3 inches of space at the top.
3. Add the remaining cup of water and the vinegar to the brine and let cool. Pour gently over the radishes, making sure they are completely covered. If needed, place a small glass container or cleaned cabbage leaf inside the top of the jar to keep the radishes completely submerged.
4. Seal and keep in a dark, room-temperature place for 4 to 5 days. Every couple of days, open the jar to release pressurized air and to mix the daikon to distribute the turmeric color evenly.

   Note: Store the jar in the refrigerator, where it will last up to 1 month.

NUTRIENTS
(per tablespoon serving)

Fat: 2%	Calories: 15.4 kcal	Fiber: 0.6 g
Carb: 93.9%	Fat 0 g	Sugar: 3.2 g
Protein: 4.1%	Carbohydrates: 3.8 g	Protein: 0.2 g

LACTOFERMENTED VITAMIN D MUSHROOMS

YYI | P, V, VGT

6 servings   *Prep time: 10 minutes, plus time to sit in the sun*   *Fermenting time: 3–5 days, depending on the temperature in your kitchen*

Across cultures, mushrooms have long been viewed as a powerful superfood. They have immune-boosting properties and even some antimicrobial effects. In my practice, we love mushrooms because they contain both methyl donor and DNA methylation adaptogen nutrients, and they're full of phytonutrient compounds like polysaccharide-glucans, sterols, and lectins, as well as fiber, protein, and nutrients like selenium, potassium, magnesium, calcium, riboflavin, folate, and niacin. And . . . drum roll . . . also vitamin D—refer back to page 218 for more information on how exposing your mushrooms to the sun increases their vitamin D content.

Take those benefits one step further by fermenting those sun-exposed mushrooms. In addition to being great for you—and providing about 400 IU of vitamin D_2 per serving, they make a delicious addition to eggs and salad and are even great on their own as a simple snack.[1]

> *Tip:* You can find culture starter—a mix of microrganisms that can get the fermentation process started—online and in health food stores.

Methyl donors: mushrooms, garlic

DNA methylation adaptogens: mushrooms (vitamin D), thyme, rosemary, garlic

> 1 pound mushrooms (you can use a variety or a single favorite kind), wiped clean with a damp paper towel and sliced into uniform pieces
>
> ¼ teaspoon juice from traditionally fermented sauerkraut, or culture starter
>
> A few sprigs of fresh thyme, to taste
>
> A few sprigs of fresh rosemary, to taste
>
> 2–3 cloves garlic, smashed
>
> Saltwater brine: 1 tablespoon of salt dissolved in 1 quart of filtered water

1. Lay your mushrooms out on a flat cookie sheet and leave out in the sun for at least 15 minutes but up to 6 hours for maximum vitamin D production.
2. Place all the ingredients (except saltwater brine) in a 32-ounce, wide-mouthed Mason jar, squeezing in as much as possible.
3. Add enough brine to cover, but be sure to leave about 1 inch of space at the top.
4. Mushrooms like to float, so weigh them down. You can use a smaller jar or a cup inside your Mason jar.
5. Allow to sit on your counter for 5 days. After 5 days, your mushrooms are ready to eat. Any leftovers should be stored in the fridge.

NUTRIENTS

Fat: 11.8%	Calories: 164.7 kcal	Fiber: 11.7 g
Carb: 71.1%	Fat: 2.3 g	Sugar: 10.9 g
Protein: 17.1%	Carbohydrates: 33.1 g	Protein: 10.6 g

RED CABBAGE, BEET, AND POMEGRANATE SLAW

YYI | K, P, VGT, V

4 *servings*   *Prep time: 15 minutes*

If you have any resistance to cabbage and/or beets, try this rich, ruby-colored slaw. It has a knockout flavor, thanks to the cinnamon and pomegranate seeds, that will surprise you. It also keeps well in the fridge for up to three days; the leftovers make it easy to meet your daily beet, colorful vegetable, and cruciferous vegetable requirement without any additional chopping. If you're on the Everyday version, you can add ½ cup of crumbled goat or feta cheese for an another flavor element. (This recipe was inspired by and adapted from *Edible Rhody* to make it Younger You–friendly.)

Methyl donors: cayenne pepper, shallot, cabbage, beet, parsley, walnut, pecan, pine nut

DNA methylation adaptogens: red wine vinegar, extra-virgin olive oil, cinnamon, shallot, cabbage, beet, pomegranate, parsley, walnut, pecan

FOR THE VINAIGRETTE:
- 1 teaspoon Dijon mustard
- ¼ cup red wine vinegar
- ½ cup extra-virgin olive oil
- 1 teaspoon cinnamon
- 1 teaspoon cayenne pepper (optional for desired spice level)
- Salt and freshly ground black pepper, to taste

FOR THE SLAW:
- 1 medium shallot, thinly sliced
- 1 tablespoon red wine vinegar
- ½ head red cabbage, thinly sliced
- 1 medium beet, shredded
- Salt and freshly ground black pepper, to taste
- ½ cup pomegranate seeds
- ½ cup parsley, chopped for garnish
- Nuts, toasted and chopped, for garnish (e.g., walnuts, pecans, pine nuts)

1. Mix all the vinaigrette ingredients in a small bowl and set aside.
2. Soak the sliced shallots in a small bowl with the vinegar and a pinch of salt. Set aside.
3. Combine cabbage and beets in a large bowl and season with salt and pepper. Add pomegranate seeds and half the vinaigrette. Toss to coat the vegetables and let sit for 5 minutes.
4. Drain the shallots and add to cabbage mixture and toss again.
5. To serve, sprinkle with garnishes and additional vinaigrette as desired.

NUTRIENTS

Fat: 79.9%	Calories: 353.1 kcal	Fiber: 5 g
Carb: 17.4%	Fat: 31.8 g	Sugar: 9.1 g
Protein: 3%	Carbohydrates: 16.8 g	Protein: 3.6 g

WARM SALMON AND ROASTED CAULIFLOWER SALAD

YYI | K, P

2 servings   Prep time: 5 minutes   Cook time: 20–25 minutes

You've gotta love a one-pan meal. You'll also love how the tomatoes, parsley, capers, and chives brighten up this easy weeknight dinner.

> *Tip:* I'm a modest green thumb at best, but I can attest that chives are a super-easy-to-grow perennial herb (that my daughter endlessly picks and eats). It comes back every year and has cute, puffy, purple flowers in the spring to boot.

Methyl donors: salmon, red onion, cauliflower, tomatoes, parsley, chives

DNA methylation adaptogens: extra-virgin olive oil, salmon, red onion, cauliflower, tomatoes, parsley, capers, chives

2 tablespoons extra-virgin olive oil
2 salmon fillet portions, about 3–4 ounces each
1 small red onion, quartered and sliced
2 cups cauliflower florets, about 1 inch diameter
2 cups cherry tomatoes, halved
2 tablespoons chopped fresh parsley
2 tablespoons capers

¼ cup fresh chives, finely chopped
Salt and freshly ground black pepper, to taste

1. Preheat the oven to 375°F.
2. Drizzle a medium baking dish, or sheet pan, with olive oil.
3. Place the two salmon fillets on one side of the baking dish and drizzle with more oil. On the other side of the baking dish, toss the onion and cauliflower with a little more olive oil. Sprinkle the salmon, onion, and cauliflower with salt.
4. Bake the salmon in the oven for 15 to 20 minutes until cooked through, and the veggies a little longer, 20 to 25 minutes until softened and toasted (they may still be a little crunchy—that's OK).
5. Once out of the oven, put the salmon in a medium mixing bowl and flake it with a fork into bite-size pieces.
6. When the veggies are done, add the tomatoes, parsley, and capers to them (I like to do this in the pan they baked in, for convenience), then add them to the salmon and gently fold the ingredients together.
7. Spoon the warm mixture into two large serving dishes, such as pasta bowls. Top with the chives and season to taste with salt and pepper.

NUTRIENTS

Fat: 58.3%	Calories: 437.1 kcal	Fiber: 5.9 g
Carb: 13.9%	Fat: 28.5 g	Sugar: 8.9 g
Protein: 27.8%	Carbohydrates: 17.5 g	Protein: 30.3 g

COLORFUL QUINOA LENTIL SALAD

YYE | VGT

2 main dish–sized servings or 4 side dish–sized servings   *Prep time: 20 minutes, plus overnight for soaking lentils and quinoa*   *Cook time: 35 minutes*

This salad is a great way to cover a ton of DNA methylation–supportive bases in one bowl. And taste-wise, it's a home run. If you're vegan, just omit the eggs; the lentils and quinoa lend lots of protein even without them.

Tip: Soak the lentils and quinoa together overnight before cooking (see page 402 for soaking instructions).

Methyl donors: lentils, quinoa, garlic, cumin, ginger, red onion, carrots, egg, parsley, arugula

DNA methylation adaptogens: lentils, extra-virgin olive oil, lemon, garlic, cumin, ginger, red bell pepper, red onion, carrot, egg, parsley, arugula

1 cup lentils

½ cup quinoa

1 cup water

1 cup vegetable broth

1 tablespoon extra-virgin olive oil, plus extra for drizzling

Juice of 1 lemon

1 or 2 cloves garlic, pressed

¼ teaspoon cumin

¼ teaspoon dried ginger

Salt and freshly ground black pepper, to taste

1 red bell pepper, diced

¼ red onion, diced

2 medium carrots, grated

3 eggs, hard boiled, roughly chopped

¾ cup roughly chopped parsley

3 cups arugula

1. In a pot, bring the water and broth to boil. Add the soaked quinoa and lentils and reduce heat to simmer. Allow to cook for about 12 to 15 minutes until both are soft. Stir occasionally. When done, cover and set aside to cool.

2. Prepare the dressing: In a large mixing bowl, stir together the olive oil, lemon juice, garlic, cumin, ginger, salt, and pepper. Add the red bell pepper, onion, carrots, eggs, and parsley and toss with the dressing.

3. When the quinoa and lentils have cooled, add to the veggies and mix thoroughly. Divide the arugula between two plates and top with the quinoa lentil salad. Drizzle with olive oil and serve.

NUTRIENTS

(main dish serving size)

Fat: 37.9%	Calories: 577.4 kcal	Fiber: 13.8 g
Carb: 45%	Fat: 24.5 g	Sugar: 12.7 g
Protein: 17.1%	Carbohydrates: 66.5 g	Protein: 26.8 g

QUINOA TABBOULEH

YYE | V, VGT

2 servings   Prep time: 15 minutes,   Cook time: 30 minutes
                    plus presoak and resting
                    time for the quinoa

Traditional tabbouleh uses bulgur, a gluten-containing grain that can trigger an inflammatory response in those who have a gluten sensitivity. Replacing the bulgur with quinoa makes this refreshing, crunchy, methyl donor and DNA methylation adaptogen–rich dish a great part of your Younger You Everyday plan.

If you have the quinoa already cooked and waiting to be eaten in the fridge (a great time-saving hack to make weekday meals fast and easy), this salad comes together in 15 minutes.

Methyl donors: quinoa, cucumber, tomatoes, red onion, parsley, garlic
DNA methylation adaptogens: cucumber, tomatoes, red onion, parsley, mint, garlic, lemon, extra-virgin olive oil

    ⅔ cup quinoa, soaked for at least 20 minutes or up
        to 2 hours, then well rinsed
    1⅓ cups water, for cooking the quinoa
    ½ cucumber, diced
    3 medium tomatoes, diced
    1 medium red onion, diced
    1 cup parsley, finely chopped
    ⅓ cup mint, finely chopped
    2 cloves garlic, finely chopped
    Zest and juice of 1 lemon
    ¼ cup extra-virgin olive oil
    Salt and freshly ground black pepper, to taste

1. Place the presoaked quinoa in a saucepan with the water and bring to a simmer. Simmer on low, with the lid on, for about 15 minutes, until all the water has absorbed. Take off the heat and let sit, covered, for another 15 minutes, then fluff with a fork.
2. While the quinoa is cooking, place all the other ingredients in a medium mixing bowl. Once the quinoa is ready, add it to the mixing bowl and gently stir to combine all the ingredients thoroughly.

3. Although tabbouleh is traditionally eaten cold, you may serve this warm immediately or allow to cool before eating.

> *Note:* It's best eaten the same day it's made, though it can be refrigerated for up to 3 days.

NUTRIENTS

Fat: 51.5%	Calories: 537.8 kcal	Fiber: 9.4 g
Carb: 40.6%	Fat: 31.3 g	Sugar: 13.1 g
Protein: 7.9%	Carbohydrates: 56.8 g	Protein: 12.1 g

SPICED BUTTERNUT SQUASH AND RED LENTIL SOUP

YYE | V (if you use vegetable stock)**, VGT** (if you use vegetable stock)

4 servings　　*Prep time: 15 minutes*　　*Cook time: 25 minutes plus 30 minutes to preroast the butternut squash*

This recipe, like many listed here, is a epigenetic all-star: every ingredient except salt is a DNA methylation adaptogen! Butternut squash is high in fiber, nutrients, and antioxidants. In fact, 1 cup of diced butternut squash has more potassium than a banana and provides 50 percent of the recommended daily intake of vitamin C! Lentils are tasty, versatile, and cost-effective. They are high in dietary fiber, potassium, prebiotic carbohydrates, and beneficial phytonutrients that help to maintain health. And yet, this soup is so tasty that you won't at all feel like you're being forced to eat something uber-healthy. (It's also easy to make and satisfies even the pickiest eaters . . . promise!)

> *Tip:* To make this soup in a slow cooker, put all ingredients (except the lemon juice, salt, and spices) in and set to the low setting for 4 to 6 hours.

Methyl donors: red lentils, onion, garlic, chicken stock, cumin, turmeric, butternut squash

DNA methylation adaptogens: red lentils, onion, garlic, chicken stock, cumin, turmeric, cinnamon, butternut squash, lemon

- 1 cup red lentils
- 1 medium onion, diced
- 1–2 cloves garlic, minced
- 1 (15-ounce) can coconut milk

4 cups chicken or vegetable stock (homemade if
possible)

1 medium butternut squash, seeded, peeled, cubed, and
roasted until tender (about 30 minutes)

Juice of ½ lemon

½ teaspoon salt

1 tablespoon cumin

1 teaspoon turmeric

½ teaspoon cinnamon

1. Place all ingredients except the lemon juice, salt, and spices in a
   large, deep saucepan.
2. Bring to a boil and simmer until everything is tender, about 20
   minutes. The squash should start to melt into the soup.
3. Add the lemon juice, salt, and spices and stir to combine.

NUTRIENTS

Fat: 38%	Calories: 512.9 kcal	Fiber: 11.1 g
Carb: 47.5%	Fat: 23 g	Sugar: 11.7 g
Protein: 14.6%	Carbohydrates: 62.1 g	Protein: 20.9 g

"EVERYTHING" SEED CRACKERS

YYI | K, P, VGT, [V]

4 servings   *Prep time: 15 minutes*   *Cook time: 15 minutes*
(1 serving = about 7 crackers)

Crackers just make life better. And since these have no grains and no gluten
and are chock-full of methyl donor and DNA methylation adaptogens,
they also help make your DNA methylation better. I recommend using Bob's
Red Mill coconut flour here because it has a mild flavor; some other brands
have a stronger coconut taste.

> *Tip:* You can make these crackers vegan by replacing the two eggs with
> 2 tablespoons of ground flax seeds soaked in 6 tablespoons of water for
> 15 minutes. You can also replace the sesame seeds, poppy seeds, dried onion,
> dried garlic, and salt with a scant 2 tablespoons of an "everything" spice blend.

Methyl donors: coconut flour, flax seeds, sesame seeds, poppy seeds,
garlic, onion, eggs, almond butter

DNA methylation adaptogens: coconut flour, garlic, onion, almond butter,
coconut oil

¼ cup plus 1 tablespoon coconut flour
¼ cup coarsely ground flax seeds
1 tablespoon white sesame seeds
1 teaspoon black sesame seeds
1 teaspoon poppy seeds
½ teaspoon dried garlic
½ teaspoon dried onion
¼ teaspoon salt
2 eggs
⅓ cup almond butter
2 tablespoons coconut oil, melted

1. Preheat the oven to 350°F and prepare a baking tray lined with greased parchment paper or a silicone liner.
2. Combine the dry ingredients in a medium bowl and mix until evenly distributed.
3. In a separate bowl, whisk together the eggs, almond butter, and coconut oil.
4. Add the wet mixture to the dry and mix until a thick ball of dough forms. Press the ball of dough onto a piece of parchment paper and flatten as much as possible with your hands.
5. Place another piece of parchment paper over the top of the dough to avoid sticking and roll it out with a rolling pin until it is about ⅛ inch thick. Remove the top layer of parchment and transfer dough to prepared baking tray.
6. With a sharp knife or pizza cutter, deeply score the dough with vertical and horizontal lines to create individual crackers that are around 1½ inches square.
7. Bake in the oven for about 15 minutes, watching closely so that they don't brown. You're looking for a golden color.
8. Remove the crackers from the oven and let them cool on the tray for about 5 minutes, until you can handle them easily. Break the crackers along the scored lines and let them finish cooling on a wire rack.

   Note: Once completely cooled, the crackers can be stored in an airtight container for up to 3 days.

NUTRIENTS

Fat: 71.5%	Calories: 321.1 kcal	Fiber: 7.8 g
Carb: 16.2%	Fat: 26.6 g	Sugar: 2 g
Protein: 12.2%	Carbohydrates: 12.6 g	Protein: 10.4 g

ROSEMARY AND SEA SALT CRACKERS

YYI | K, P, VGT, [V]

4 servings   *Prep time: 20 minutes*   *Cook time: 20 minutes*
(1 serving = about 7 crackers)

These are similar to the "Everything" Seed Crackers (page 321), but since crackers are so handy for snacks or light meals, and travel well, I think you'll enjoy having an additional cracker recipe with a different flavor profile in your repertoire.

> *Tip:* You can make these crackers vegan by replacing the egg with 1 tablespoon of ground flax seeds soaked in 3 tablespoons of water for 15 minutes.

Methyl donors: almond flour, garlic, egg, rosemary

DNA methylation adaptogens: almond flour, garlic, egg, extra-virgin olive oil, rosemary

1¼ cups almond flour or almond meal
¼ teaspoon baking soda
1 egg
2 cloves garlic, finely minced
1 tablespoon extra-virgin olive oil
2 teaspoons dried rosemary (or 2 tablespoons fresh)
1 teaspoon coarse sea salt

1. Preheat the oven to 350°F and prepare a baking tray lined with greased parchment paper or a silicone liner.
2. In a medium bowl, combine the almond flour and baking soda until the baking soda is evenly distributed.
3. In a separate bowl, beat the egg, stir in the garlic, and then add to the dry mixture.
4. Work the egg through the flour mixture with your hands and form into a ball of dough.
5. Press the ball of dough onto a piece of parchment paper and flatten as much as possible with your hands.
6. Place another piece of parchment paper over the top of the dough to avoid sticking and roll it out with a rolling pin until it is about ⅛ inch thick. Remove the top layer of parchment and transfer dough to the prepared baking tray.
7. Using a pastry brush, brush the olive oil evenly over the top of the dough. Sprinkle the rosemary and sea salt evenly over the top and lightly press with your hands.

8. With a sharp knife or pizza cutter, deeply score the dough with vertical and horizontal lines to create individual crackers that are about 1½ inches square.
9. Bake in the oven for 15 to 20 minutes until golden, watching closely so that they don't get too brown.
10. Remove the crackers from the oven and let them cool on the tray for about 5 minutes, until you can handle them easily. Break the crackers along the scored lines and let them finish cooling on a wire rack.

> *Note:* Once completely cooled, the crackers can be stored in an airtight container for up to 3 days.

NUTRIENTS

Fat: 75.1%	Calories: 501.7 kcal	Fiber: 7.9 g
Carb: 12.3%	Fat: 44.4 g	Sugar: 3.4 g
Protein: 12.6%	Carbohydrates: 15.3 g	Protein: 17.6 g

NUT AND SEED "EVERYTHING" BREAD

YYI | K, V, VGT

10 servings
(1 serving = 1 slice)

Prep time: 10 minutes,
plus 2–12 hours resting time

Cook time: 1 hour

This is a versatile, nutrient-dense bread, which was adapted from a recipe by Sarah Britton of the blog My New Roots, that will help you stay energized and satiated throughout the day. Top it with our Broccoli Pesto with Pasta (page 360, hold the pasta), Herbed Beet Yogurt Dip (page 328), or eat it just by itself and savor the varied flavors and textures!

Methyl donors: hazelnut, walnuts, sunflower seeds, almonds, almond flour, shredded coconut, flax seeds, chia seeds, maple syrup, garlic powder

DNA methylation adaptogens: hazelnuts, walnuts, sunflower seeds, almonds, almond flour, shredded coconut, chia seeds, coconut oil, garlic powder

½ cup hazelnuts, walnuts, or almonds, chopped

1 cup sunflower seeds

1 cup almond flour

½ cup dried shredded coconut, unsweetened

½ cup ground flax seeds

2 tablespoons chia seeds

4 tablespoons psyllium seed husks

1 teaspoon salt

2–4 drops liquid stevia (optional, or 1 teaspoon maple syrup if you're on the Everyday)

3 tablespoons coconut oil, melted

1½ cups water

Optional: 1 teaspoon garlic powder or other seasonings of your choice

1. Line an 8 x 4-inch loaf pan with parchment paper.
2. In a medium bowl, combine all dry ingredients, stirring well.
3. Whisk stevia, coconut oil, and water together in a separate small bowl.
4. Add the wet mix to the dry ingredients and stir until dough becomes very thick (if the dough is too thick to stir, add 1 or 2 teaspoons of water until the dough is manageable).
5. Add the dough to the lined loaf pan and let it sit out on the counter at least 2 hours, or a maximum of 12 (cover with a clean kitchen towel). This is simply to allow the nuts and seeds time to soak up the liquid—it doesn't take long for the dough to be ready, but if you want to prep it at night and bake the next morning, it won't negatively affect the flavor or texture.
6. Preheat the oven to 350°F.
7. Place the loaf pan in the oven on the middle rack and bake for 20 minutes.
8. Remove bread from the loaf pan, place it upside down directly on the rack, and bake for another 30 to 40 minutes. Cool completely before slicing.

> **Note:** Store any leftovers in the refrigerator for up to 5 days or in the freezer for up to 3 months.

NUTRIENTS

Fat: 76.4%	Calories: 294.1 kcal	Fiber: 7.2g
Carb: 14.2%	Fat: 26.6g	Sugar: 1.6g
Protein: 9.3%	Carb: 10.8g	Protein: 8g

LUSCIOUS LIVER PÂTÉ

YYI | K, P

6 servings   Prep time: 15 minutes, plus   Cook time: 35 minutes
                    presoaking time for cashews

If you don't think you're a liver person, this makes a great gateway dish. Inspired by a luxurious pâté that our chief nutritionist, Romilly Hodges, had at a restaurant in the South of Spain, this version delivers a sumptuous richness *and* a heaping helping of methylation-supportive nutrients. Serve it with either "Everything" Seed Crackers or Rosemary and Sea Salt Crackers, or with crudités.

> *Tip:* Don't skip the step of presoaking the cashews—it helps make this spread so creamy. (See page 402 for more information on soaking.)

Methyl donors: onion, pork, chicken liver, cashews, rosemary, thyme

DNA methylation adaptogens: extra-virgin olive oil, onion, pork, chicken liver, cashews, rosemary, thyme

3 tablespoons extra-virgin olive oil

1 onion, diced

3 slices Irish back bacon or Canadian bacon

¼ cup cashews, presoaked in water for at least 2 and up to 12 hours

1 pound organic chicken livers, trimmed

1 teaspoon salt

2 teaspoons dried rosemary (or 2 tablespoons fresh)

2 teaspoons dried thyme (or 2 tablespoons fresh)

Freshly ground black pepper, to taste

1. In a medium saucepan on low heat, add the olive oil and onion and sauté for 5 to 7 minutes, until the onion has softened.
2. Add the bacon, cashews, and chicken livers to the pan. Continue to sauté for 12 to 15 minutes, until the livers and bacon are cooked through.
3. Add the seasonings and stir for another minute or so. Take off the heat and let cool 5 to 10 minutes.
4. Transfer the mixture to a food processor and process until completely smooth. You may need to stop intermittently to scrape down the sides and/or add a little water to achieve a spreadable consistency.
5. Once cool, store in the refrigerator until ready to use.

Note: Will store in the refrigerator for up to 3 days. It freezes well, too, if you don't want to use it all at once. (Thaw in the fridge overnight before serving.)

NUTRIENTS

Fat: 53%	Calories: 240.1 kcal	Fiber: 0.6 g
Carb: 7.3%	Fat: 14.4 g	Sugar: 1.2 g
Protein: 39.6%	Carbohydrates: 4.5 g	Protein: 22.7 g

BAKED SPINACH AND ARTICHOKE DIP

YYI | KL, P, VGT, V

6 servings
(1 serving =
about ¾ cup)

Prep time: 10 minutes, plus presoak time for the cashews

Cook time: 20 minutes

This yummy, creamy (thanks to the soaked cashews) dip means you can bring a methylation-friendly appetizer to a party—or keep it just for yourself. The artichokes make this a high-fiber feast that feels like a splurge.

Methyl donors: cashews, garlic, spinach, artichokes

DNA methylation adaptogens: cashews, garlic, lemon, spinach, artichokes, extra-virgin olive oil

1 cup raw cashews, presoaked for 2 hours in ⅔ cup water, soaking liquid reserved

4 large cloves garlic

Juice of 1 lemon

4 cups packed fresh spinach

2 (14-ounce) cans artichoke hearts, packed in water, drained and rinsed

¼ cup extra-virgin olive oil

Salt and freshly ground black pepper, to taste

1. Preheat the oven to 400°F.
2. Using a high-powered blender or food processor, blend the cashews with half of their soaking liquid until you have a completely smooth cashew cream.
3. Add the remaining ingredients and pulse until desired dip consistency. You may need to scrape the sides down intermittently and add more of the soaking liquid to keep the dip creamy.

4. Transfer to an oven-safe dish and bake until hot and bubbly, 15 to 20 minutes.
5. Serve with the "Everything" Seed Crackers (page 321), Rosemary and Sea Salt Crackers (page 323), or vegetable crudités.

NUTRIENTS

(for the dip only, not including the crackers)

Fat: 58.9%
Carb: 32.2%
Protein: 8.9%

Calories: 334.2 kcal
Fat: 22.9 g
Carbohydrates: 29.1 g

Fiber: 10.5 g
Sugar: 3.5 g
Protein: 10.2 g

HERBED BEET YOGURT DIP

YYI | V, VGT

8 servings
(1 serving = about ⅓ cup)

Prep time: 20 minutes   Cook time: 25–30 minutes

This dip will delight your taste buds *and* your eyes. It's great paired with sliced vegetables, served on top of a salad, or eaten with our "Everything" Seed Crackers (page 321). This recipe was inspired by a recipe by Melissa Clark in the *New York Times*—we adapted it to make it Younger You–compliant and even more DNA methylation–friendly.

Tip: If you hate peeling beets, boil them whole and unpeeled. They will take 45 to 60 minutes to cook through, depending on size, but the peels will slip right off.

Methyl donors: beets, walnuts, garlic, almonds, rosemary, thyme, dill
DNA methylation adaptogens: beets, walnuts, garlic, almonds, lemon, rosemary, thyme, dill

2 medium beets, peeled and cubed
½ cup walnuts
2 large cloves garlic
1 cup unsweetened nondairy yogurt, such as almond, coconut, or cashew (or regular plain yogurt if you're on the Everyday)
2 tablespoons lemon juice, or more, to taste
2 tablespoons fresh dill (or ¾ teaspoon dried)
2 teaspoons fresh rosemary (or ¾ teaspoon dried)
2 teaspoons fresh thyme (or ¾ teaspoon dried)

1 teaspoon salt

Freshly ground black pepper, to taste

1. Place beets in a pot and cover with water and a lid. Place the walnuts in a small bowl and cover with water; set aside to soak while the beets cook.
2. Bring beets to a boil, then reduce heat to a simmer. Cook the beets for 15 to 20 minutes, until tender.
3. Remove the beets from the water and let them cool. Meanwhile, drain and rinse walnuts.
4. Place all of the ingredients in a food processor and puree.

Note: Will keep in the refrigerator for up to 5 days.

VARIATIONS:

Substitute sunflower seeds for the walnuts.

Add a dash of cayenne pepper if you want a little kick.

NUTRIENTS

Fat: 49.3%	Calories: 81 kcal	Fiber: 1.8 g
Carb: 43.9%	Fat: 4.7 g	Sugar: 4.4 g
Protein: 6.8%	Carbohydrates: 9.6 g	Protein: 1.6 g

GARLIC AND ROSEMARY SUNFLOWER SEED BUTTER

YYI | K, P, VGT, V

20 servings
(1 serving = 2 tablespoons)   *Prep time: 11 minutes*

Sunflower seed butter is a great way to meet your daily ¼-cup sunflower seed requirement. This extra-savory version is great spread on crackers (especially our cracker recipes!) or on apple slices, but a little goes a long way as it is nutrient and calorie dense.

Tip: Because flaxseed oil can easily go rancid, look for a refrigerated version in an opaque bottle and use it before the "best before" date.

Methyl donors: sunflower seeds, pumpkin seeds, garlic, rosemary, flaxseed oil

DNA methylation adaptogens: sunflower seeds, garlic, rosemary, pumpkin seeds

2½ cups sunflower seeds, raw or roasted

½ cup pumpkin seeds

4 cloves garlic

¼ cup fresh rosemary (or 1 tablespoon dried)

½ cup flaxseed oil

Salt and freshly ground black pepper, to taste

1. Place all the ingredients in a food processor or high-speed blender and process until smooth and creamy. Scrape the sides down intermittently to ensure you catch all those ingredients.

Note: You can store the seed butter in a jar in the refrigerator for up to 1 week.

NUTRIENTS

Fat: 80.5%	Calories: 168.7 kcal	Fiber: 1.8 g
Carb: 10.1%	Fat: 15.9 g	Sugar: 0.5 g
Protein: 9.4%	Carbohydrates: 4.2 g	Protein: 4.6 g

ROASTED MUSHROOM TAPENADE

YYI | K, P, V, VGT

6 servings   *Prep time: 5 minutes*   *Cook time: 20 minutes*
(1 serving = about ⅓ cup)

This tapenade, paired with "Everything" Seed Crackers (page 321) or Rosemary and Sea Salt Crackers (page 323), makes a great appetizer, snack, or light meal. It also pairs well with scrambled eggs, sautéed greens, or Luscious Liver Pâté (page 326). And since a food processor does most of the work, there's little chopping to do.

Methyl donors: shiitake mushrooms, crimini mushrooms, sunflower seeds, pumpkin seeds, garlic, chives

DNA methylation adaptogens: extra-virgin olive oil, sunflower seeds, pumpkin seeds, olives, garlic, lemon, capers, chives

1 cup shiitake mushrooms, tough stalks removed

1 cup crimini mushrooms, halved

3 tablespoons plus ¼ cup extra-virgin olive oil

¼ cup sunflower seeds

¼ cup pumpkin seeds

¾ cup kalamata olives, without pits

2 medium cloves garlic

Juice and zest of 1 lemon

1 tablespoon balsamic vinegar

2 tablespoons capers

2 tablespoons chopped chives, plus more for garnish

Salt and freshly ground black pepper, to taste

1. Preheat the oven to 400°F.
2. In a large baking dish or sheet pan, toss the mushrooms with the olive oil and distribute evenly across the pan. Bake for 15 to 20 minutes, or until cooked through.
3. Place the sunflower and pumpkin seeds into a food processor and pulse until coarsely chopped.
4. Add the remaining ingredients as well as the mushrooms and continue to pulse until the tapenade is formed.
5. Transfer to a serving dish and season with the remaining chives.

NUTRIENTS

Fat: 88.3%	Calories: 281.3 kcal	Fiber: 3.3 g
Carb: 6.4%	Fat: 28.9 g	Sugar: 1.4 g
Protein: 5.3%	Carbohydrates: 5.8 g	Protein: 4.4 g

CABBAGE STEAKS WITH POMEGRANATE AND CREAMY DRIZZLE

YYI | P, V, VGT

2 servings   Prep time: 10 minutes   Cook time: 40 minutes

Cabbage truly is one of the most versatile vegetables—shredded raw it makes a great slaw, sautéed with a little bacon it makes an easy side dish. But I'm guessing you probably haven't eaten a thick slice of it that's been baked. Prepare to be blown away. Baking it makes it so mellow that it's almost sweet; dousing it with lemon juice before baking keeps the flavor bright. Drizzled with this creamy sauce and sprinkled with pomegranate seeds, you've got an easy dinner that tastes restaurant worthy.

Tip: Look for a dense head of green cabbage for this recipe—it will help the steaks stay together better. And if you can find black sesame seeds, they make the dish especially pretty.

Methyl donors: cabbage, tahini, sesame seeds

DNA methylation adaptogens: extra-virgin olive oil, cabbage, lemon, pomegranate, Mexican oregano

> **1 tablespoon extra-virgin olive oil, plus more for sprinkling**
>
> **1 small head of cabbage**
>
> **Juice of 1 lemon**
>
> **¾ teaspoon salt**
>
> **⅓ cup cold water**
>
> **2 tablespoons tahini**
>
> **⅓ cup pomegranate seeds**
>
> **2 tablespoons chopped fresh Mexican oregano (or 2 teaspoons dried)**
>
> **1 tablespoon black or white sesame seeds**
>
> **Freshly ground black pepper, to taste**

1. Preheat the oven to 375°F.
2. Lightly brush a large baking pan or sheet pan with olive oil.
3. Prepare the cabbage by trimming any dried stem and then slicing the whole head vertically into large rounds, each about ½ inch thick. A large head should yield four or five "steaks."
4. Carefully, so they don't fall apart, lay the cabbage rounds in your baking pan. It's OK if they overlap a little bit, but you want each one to make contact with the pan, as that will help it brown instead of steam.
5. Sprinkle with a little olive oil, the lemon juice, and ½ teaspoon of the salt. Bake in the oven for 35 to 40 minutes, until just tender and browned at the edges.
6. Meanwhile, prepare the creamy drizzle: In a small bowl, slowly add the cold water to the tahini, stirring continuously. It will first start to get thick, and then loosen again as you add more water. It will also get a little lighter in color. Add ¼ teaspoon salt to the drizzle.
7. Spoon the drizzle over the cabbage steaks and top with the pomegranate seeds, Mexican oregano, black sesame seeds, and pepper.

NUTRIENTS

Fat: 53.2%	Calories: 297.2 kcal	Fiber: 12.4 g
Carb: 38.2%	Fat: 18.6 g	Sugar: 16.4 g
Protein: 8.5%	Carbohydrates: 32.8 g	Protein: 8.9 g

FRAGRANT SPICED RICE

YYE | V, VGT

3–4 side dish–sized servings	Prep time: 10 minutes plus 45 minutes for precooking the brown rice	Cook time: 20 minutes

Tantalize your taste buds and give your cells a boost with this fragrant spiced rice. I like Lundberg rice as a base for this, since it is grown organically and tested for heavy metal contamination (rice can easily pick up heavy metals such as arsenic from the environment, so a good quality source is important). It goes perfectly as a side dish with chicken, lamb, whitefish, or legumes.

Methyl donors: cardamom, turmeric, cumin, curry, chili powder, onion, garlic, brown rice, cilantro

DNA methylation adaptogens: coconut oil, cinnamon, turmeric, cumin, curry, onion, garlic, cilantro

  2 tablespoons coconut oil
  1 bay leaf
  6 cardamom pods
  1 cinnamon stick
  1 teaspoon turmeric
  1 tablespoon cumin seeds
  curry or chili powder, optional, to taste (depending on
       how hot you like it)
  1 large onion, minced
  2 cloves garlic, minced
  2–5 cups cooked brown rice
  ⅓ cup cilantro leaves
  Salt and freshly ground black pepper, to taste

1. In a large sauté pan, heat the oil over medium heat. Add the bay leaf, cardamom pods, cinnamon stick, turmeric, cumin seeds, and curry, if using. Warm the spices gently until they become fragrant.
2. Add the onion and sauté for 7 to 10 minutes until translucent. Add the garlic and cook another few minutes before adding the rice.
3. Stir frequently until the rice is fully heated through and completely coated in the spices.
4. Take off the heat, remove the bay leaf, and add salt and pepper to taste. Transfer to a serving dish and top with the cilantro leaves.

NUTRIENTS

Fat: 25.8%
Carb: 67.8%
Protein: 6.4%

Calories: 308 kcal
Fat: 9 g
Carbohydrates: 51.4 g

Fiber: 4.4 g
Sugar: 2.1 g
Protein: 5.9 g

BAKED GOLDEN TEMPEH

YYI (for vegans and vegetarians only) | YYE | V, VGT

2 servings   *Prep time: 5 minutes*   *Cook time: 25 minutes*

Made from fermented soy beans, tempeh is a great vegetarian or vegan protein source—although it's good for meat eaters, too (so long as you're on the Younger You Everyday, as soy is only allowed on the Intensive for non–meat eaters.) Like tofu, tempeh tastes best when cooked with some seasoning, and this recipe adds plenty of flavor. Use it when you want to make any of the main courses that contain meat vegetarian- or vegan-friendly.

Methyl donors: garlic
DNA methylation adaptogens: tempeh, garlic, extra-virgin olive oil

8-ounce package of tempeh
1 teaspoon extra-virgin olive oil
1 tablespoon coconut aminos
½ teaspoon garlic powder (or seasonings of choice)
1 tablespoon fresh (or 1 teaspoon dried herb) of choice (e.g., rosemary, sage, dill, cilantro, oregano, thyme)
Salt and freshly ground black pepper, to taste

1. Preheat the oven to 400°F and line a baking sheet with parchment paper.
2. Cut tempeh into ½-inch cubes and place in a small bowl. Add oil, coconut aminos, seasonings, and herbs to tempeh cubes and mix thoroughly.
3. Place tempeh on baking sheet and bake for 25 minutes or until golden brown.
4. Serve warm or cold.

> *Note:* Can be stored up to 5 days in the refrigerator.

NUTRIENTS

Fat: 48%	Calories: 255.3 kcal	Fiber: 4.2 g
Carb: 20.6%	Fat: 14.5 g	Sugar: 6.1 g
Protein: 31.4%	Carbs: 12.3 g	Protein: 23.1 g

MAIN COURSES • • • • •

MIX-AND-MATCH STIR-FRY

YYI | K, P, [V], [VGT]

1–2 main dish–sized servings or 2–4 side dish–sized servings   *Prep time: 20 minutes*   *Cook time: 20 minutes*

This is an adaptive recipe where you can use most of the ingredients from the Mix-and-Match Rainbow Salad (page 308) and easily turn them into a warm stir-fry—a nice change for when the weather is cold. It is easily adaptable to vegetarian and vegan diets, too. Together, these two recipes (really, more like templates) can cover the majority of your meals if you, like me, like to keep your meal prep as simple as possible.

Methyl donors: kale, spinach, carrots, cabbage, pumpkin seeds, sunflower seeds, thyme, parsley, oregano, rosemary, sage, salmon, chicken, pork, tofu

DNA methylation adaptogens: kale, spinach, cruciferous vegetables, red bell pepper, carrots, cabbage, sunflower seeds, berries, extra-virgin olive oil, thyme, parsley, oregano, rosemary, sage, salmon, chicken, pork, tempeh, tofu, coconut oil, lemon

BASE TEMPLATE:

TOTAL OF 5 CUPS VEGETABLES:

> 1–2 cups dark leafy greens
>
> 1–2 cups cruciferous vegetables
>
> 1–3 cups colorful vegetables

½ cup seeds

2 cloves garlic, minced

2 teaspoons fresh or dried herbs (e.g., sage, thyme, oregano, rosemary, dill)

3–6 ounces protein of choice (e.g., salmon, chicken, pork, scallops, or, if you're vegetarian or vegan, organic tempeh, organic tofu, or your favorite cooked bean)

FOR THE STIR-FRY:

1 tablespoon coconut oil

1–2 cloves garlic, minced

1 cup sliced carrot

1 cup diced purple cabbage

1 cup diced red bell pepper

1 cup chopped kale

1 cup chopped spinach

¼ cup sunflower seeds

¼ cup pumpkin seeds

FOR THE SALMON:

1 tablespoon coconut or avocado oil

3 ounces salmon

1–2 cloves garlic, minced

1 slice lemon

Salt and freshly ground black pepper, to taste

1. Heat oil in a large sauté pan over medium heat. Add garlic and cook for 2 minutes, stirring frequently.
2. Add carrot, purple cabbage, and red bell pepper and cook for 3 to 5 minutes. Add kale and spinach (and plant-based protein, if using) and cook for an additional 3 to 5 minutes. Remove from heat.
3. For the salmon, heat coconut oil on medium heat in a medium sauté pan. Cook the salmon on one side for 3 to 5 minutes until lightly brown, then flip and cook another 3 to 5 minutes, until thoroughly done.
4. Squeeze lemon on top, season with salt and pepper, and serve alongside vegetables, garnished with seeds.

VARIATIONS:

Switch up your veggies, including a variety of dark leafy greens and cruciferous and colorful vegetables.

Top with various herbs and spices, such as chives, oregano, dill, rosemary, sage, thyme, and cilantro, or with the Herbal Epigenetic Dressing (page 310).

Add coconut aminos for additional flavor.

NUTRIENTS
(main dish serving size)

Fat: 66.4%	Calories: 626.9 kcal	Fiber: 7.9 g
Carb: 15.1%	Fat: 47.7 g	Sugar: 11.2 g
Protein: 18.4%	Carbohydrates: 25.2 g	Protein: 29.7 g

SPICED SALMON CAKES WITH VEGETABLE FRIES

YYI | P

2 servings
(1 serving = 3 patties)

Prep time: 30 minutes

Cook time: 50 minutes

Yes, salmon is great cooked simply, with just a little extra-virgin olive oil, salt, and pepper. But when you want a full taste sensation, try these flavorful salmon cakes.

Tip: Kohlrabi can be hard to find. Peeled broccoli stems make a great substitute, as they have a similar texture and taste. Plus, using them reduces food waste.

Methyl donors: kohlrabi, broccoli, beets, salmon, garlic, eggs, arrowroot powder, turmeric, sesame seeds, chives, avocado, onion powder

DNA methylation adaptogens: extra-virgin olive oil, kohlrabi, broccoli, summer squash, beets, salmon, red bell pepper, scallions, garlic, eggs, turmeric, chives, avocado, flaxseed oil, lemon, onion powder, red pepper flakes

FOR THE VEGETABLE FRIES:

1 kohlrabi (or 1 large or 2 small broccoli stems)

1 medium summer squash

2 medium beets

1 tablespoon extra-virgin olive oil

Salt, to taste

FOR THE SALMON CAKES:

2 tablespoons extra-virgin olive oil, plus more, for drizzling

2 salmon fillets, about 3–4 ounces each

1 red bell pepper, finely diced

2 scallions, finely diced

3 cloves garlic, minced

2 large eggs

1 tablespoon Dijon mustard

2 tablespoons arrowroot powder

2 teaspoons turmeric

1 teaspoon red pepper flakes (optional)

2 teaspoons sesame seeds

½ teaspoon salt

¼ cup chives, finely chopped

Freshly ground black pepper, to taste

FOR THE AVOCADO MAYONNAISE:

1 ripe avocado, quartered

1 tablespoon flaxseed oil

1 tablespoon fresh lemon juice

¼ teaspoon garlic powder

½ teaspoon onion powder

½ teaspoon salt (or more, to taste)

Water

1. Preheat the oven to 425°F.
2. Place salmon fillets on a medium baking tray and drizzle with a little oil. Bake for 12 to 15 minutes, or until cooked through. Remove from the oven and let cool.
3. Meanwhile, prepare the kohlrabi (or broccoli stems), squash, and beets for the fries by peeling and cutting them into ½-inch batons. Toss with 1 tablespoon olive oil and spread them out on a large baking sheet. Make sure they're not overlapping, otherwise they will steam instead of crisp. Sprinkle with salt. Cook in the oven for 20 to 30 minutes, until just tender and slightly browned.
4. Meanwhile, in a large skillet, add 1 tablespoon of the olive oil and sauté the red bell pepper over medium heat for 5 to 6 minutes. Add the scallions and garlic and cook another 1 to 2 minutes. Remove them from the heat for a few minutes, until cool enough to handle.
5. In a medium mixing bowl, whisk the eggs together with the mustard, arrowroot powder, turmeric, red pepper flakes (if using), sesame seeds, and salt.
6. Flake the salmon into the egg mixture. Add the red bell pepper mixture, along with the chives. Mix everything together well.
7. Form the mixture into six patties. Wipe down the skillet you used for the vegetables and add an extra tablespoon of olive oil.
8. Over medium heat, cook the salmon cakes for 3 to 4 minutes each side or until cooked through. Adding a lid over the pan when cooking the second side helps the middles cook well. Remove the salmon cakes to a paper towel–lined plate.
9. Lastly, combine all the avocado mayonnaise ingredients except water in a blender and process on low until smooth and creamy. Add water in very small amounts until you have a creamy but not too thin consistency.
10. Serve three patties per person with the vegetable fries on the side and a dollop of avocado mayo on top.

NUTRIENTS

Fat: 60.3%	Calories: 780.8 kcal	Fiber: 14.7 g
Carb: 19.5%	Fat: 53.4 g	Sugar: 15 g
Protein: 20.2%	Carbohydrates: 40.7 g	Protein: 39.5 g

ROSEMARY CHICKEN WITH TOMATO, AVOCADO, AND BACON

YYI | K, P

2 servings　　　　*Prep time: 10 minutes*　　　　*Cook time: 30 minutes*

There's nothing fancy about this dish—it's really just baked chicken thighs with simple accompaniments that, except for the bacon, don't need to be cooked. But the luscious combination of the fat from the avocado, the salty crunch of the bacon (which should be nitrite-free and, ideally, organic), and the brightness of the tomato makes this weeknight meal an embodiment of comfort food.

Methyl donors: chicken, rosemary, pork, avocado, tomato, garlic

DNA methylation adaptogens: chicken, pork, rosemary, tomato, avocado, garlic, olive oil

> **4 boneless chicken thighs**
> **1 tablespoon extra-virgin olive oil, plus a dash more for drizzling at the end**
> **2 tablespoons fresh rosemary**
> **2 pieces of Irish back bacon or Canadian bacon, fat trimmed**
> **4 medium tomatoes**
> **1 ripe avocado**
> **2 cloves garlic**
> **Salt and freshly ground pepper, to taste**

1. Preheat the oven to 375°F and place the chicken thighs in an oven-proof baking dish.
2. Rub the chicken with 1 tablespoon of olive oil plus the rosemary, then season with salt. Bake the chicken for 25 to 30 minutes, or until thoroughly cooked through.
3. In the meantime, cook the two pieces of bacon in a skillet over medium heat until starting to crisp. When cool enough to handle, finely dice.
4. Prepare the tomato and avocado by cutting them into bite-size pieces. Finely mince the garlic and mix in with the tomato.
5. Build your plates in layers—tomato first, then avocado, then a sprinkle of salt. Then top each mound of veggies with two chicken thighs and a sprinkle of bacon. Finish with an extra drizzle of olive oil and freshly ground black pepper.

NUTRIENTS

Fat: 54.6%	Calories: 637.4 kcal	Fiber: 7.9 g
Carb: 9.7%	Fat: 39.5 g	Sugar: 7 g
Protein: 35.6%	Carbohydrates: 17.2 g	Protein: 54.8 g

CREAMY GARLICKY CHICKEN WITH CAULIFLOWER RICE

YYI | KL, P

2 servings   Prep time: 20 minutes   Cook time: 45 minutes

This is a great, family-friendly weeknight meal. (The sauce melds with the cauliflower rice in a way that even picky eaters shouldn't care that it's not actual rice.) Or, if you're cooking for one, it's tasty enough that you'll happily eat it a second time for leftovers later in the week.

Tip: To save prep time, buy your chicken at the meat counter (not prepackaged) and ask the butcher to cut it into cubes for you.

Methyl donors: onions, chicken breast, garlic, tomatoes, cauliflower, chives

DNA methylation adaptogens: coconut oil, onions, garlic, tomatoes, cauliflower, chives

2 tablespoons coconut oil
2 medium onions, halved and thinly sliced
2 boneless chicken breasts, cut into 1½-inch cubes
4 cloves garlic, minced
6 sun-dried tomatoes, oil-packed, diced
½ cup full-fat coconut milk
⅓ cup low-sodium chicken broth (I like Kettle and Fire)
½ large head of cauliflower (about 3 cups florets), or
   1 12-ounce bag of frozen riced cauliflower
Fresh chives, finely chopped, for garnish
Salt and freshly ground pepper, to taste

1. In a medium skillet, heat 1 tablespoon of the coconut oil and add the onions. Sauté for 10 to 12 minutes over medium-low heat, until soft and translucent. Add the chicken and sauté 3 to 4 minutes more. Add the remaining ingredients, including salt and

pepper to taste, except for the cauliflower and chives, and cook for another 5 to 10 minutes, until the chicken is cooked through.

2. Meanwhile, prepare the cauliflower. If you are using fresh cauliflower, cut it into florets and then pulse in a food processor until the texture resembles rice.

3. In a separate medium skillet, heat the other tablespoon of coconut oil and sauté the cauliflower until it is just tender, about 10 minutes, adding salt and pepper as needed.

4. Serve the creamy chicken over a bed of cooked cauliflower rice topped with the fresh chives.

NUTRIENTS

Fat: 56.1%	Calories: 440.4 kcal	Fiber: 6 g
Carb: 21.2%	Fat: 28.3 g	Sugar: 11.3 g
Protein: 22.7%	Carbohydrates: 25.1 g	Protein: 25.4 g

CREAMY COCONUT CURRY WITH CHICKEN AND VEGETABLES

YYI | P, [V], [VGT]

4 servings   Prep time: 20 minutes   Cook time: 30 minutes

This flavorful meal warms the body on a cold day and can easily be made vegetarian by substituting legumes or organic tempeh for animal protein, or simply omitting the chicken, and vegan by also omitting the optional honey. You can also mix and match any vegetables you have on hand, such as cauliflower, kale, carrots, and cabbage, making it a great way to use up your produce before it goes bad. It's one of my favorite Younger You Intensive meals (and Izzy's, too!).

Methyl donors: bok choy, broccoli, carrot, arrowroot powder, cashew, cauliflower, chicken, cilantro, cumin, curry, garlic, ginger, onion, pumpkin seeds, turmeric

DNA methylation adaptogens: bok choy, broccoli, carrot, cashew, cauliflower, cilantro, coconut oil, cumin, curry, garlic, ginger, lime, onion, turmeric, zucchini, red pepper flakes, pumpkin seeds

**1 large head cauliflower (about 6 cups florets), or
2 10–12 ounce bags of frozen cauliflower rice**

3 tablespoons coconut oil

1 medium onion, diced

1 1-pound chicken breast, sliced thin

2 cloves garlic, diced

2 teaspoons ground ginger

1½ tablespoons curry powder

2 teaspoons cumin

¼ teaspoon turmeric

Optional: 1 makrut lime leaf, thinly sliced, and 1 2-inch piece of fresh lemongrass stalk

1 (13.5 ounce) can full-fat coconut milk

2 heads bok choy, chopped

1 cup diced broccoli

1 medium zucchini, sliced

1 large carrot, sliced

1 tablespoon arrowroot powder

Juice and zest of 1 lime

¼ teaspoon red pepper flakes, or to taste

Salt and freshly ground black pepper, to taste

Optional: 1 tablespoon coconut aminos and/or honey

¼ cup pumpkin seeds or cashews

½ cup cilantro, finely chopped

1. Prepare the cauliflower: If using a head of cauliflower, cut into florets and then pulse in a food processor until the texture resembles rice. If using frozen cauliflower rice, proceed to next step.
2. Heat 1 tablespoon of the coconut oil in a large skillet and sauté the cauliflower until it is just tender, about 10 minutes.
3. Meanwhile, in a separate skillet, heat the remaining 2 tablespoons coconut oil over medium heat. Add the onion and stir frequently until lightly brown, about 5 minutes.
4. Add the chicken or vegetarian protein and cook for 5 to 10 minutes, or until thoroughly cooked, stirring often.
5. Add the garlic, ginger, curry, cumin, and turmeric and cook for 2 to 3 minutes, continuing to stir. (If you want to amp the flavor, add the makrut lime leaf and lemongrass at this step.)
6. Stir in the coconut milk and bring to a boil and then reduce to medium heat.
7. Add bok choy, broccoli, zucchini, and carrot and cook until desired consistency—5 to 10 minutes.

8. Meanwhile, mix 1 tablespoon arrowroot powder with 2 tablespoons cold water and stir until dissolved. Once vegetables are cooked, add arrowroot mixture and stir until the sauce thickens.
9. Remove from heat and add lime juice and zest. Season with red pepper flakes, salt, and pepper. Add coconut aminos and honey, if using, to taste.
10. Serve on top of cauliflower rice and garnish with pumpkin seeds and cilantro.

NUTRIENTS

(calculated using pumpkin seeds)

Fat: 49%	Calories: 651.2 kcal	Fiber: 13.3 g
Carb: 21.3%	Fat: 36.9 g	Sugar: 16.4 g
Protein: 29.7%	Carbohydrates: 38 g	Protein: 51.3 g

RED LENTIL AND TEMPEH CURRY

YYE | V, VGT

4 servings | Prep time: 10 minutes *(does not include time for optional presoaking of lentils)* | Cook time: 1 hour

Doing the study and researching DNA methylation adaptogens has given me such a deep appreciation for the DNA-regulating power of spice! Curries are a fabulous way to get lots of methylation-supportive spices in one tasty bowl. And curries also make for great leftovers—in fact, I often think that they taste better the next day, after the flavors have had a chance to meld. The result is a super-healthy dish that's friendly for your taste buds and your schedule.

Red lentils are quick-cooking and don't generally require soaking, but soaking does have its benefits (see more info on page 402) . . . if you have time, presoak, but if you don't, that's OK too.

Methyl donors: cumin, turmeric, nutmeg, clove, ginger, onion, garlic, red lentils, tahini, apple cider vinegar, brown rice, bok choy

DNA methylation adaptogens: coriander, coconut oil, cumin, turmeric, cinnamon, nutmeg, clove, ginger, onion, garlic, tempeh, red lentils, apple cider vinegar, bok choy

2 tablespoons coconut oil
1 tablespoon cumin

1 teaspoon turmeric

½ teaspoon cinnamon

½ teaspoon coriander

¼ teaspoon nutmeg

⅛ teaspoon ground clove

1 onion, minced

1-inch piece of fresh ginger, peeled and grated

2 cloves garlic, minced

1 8-ounce packet of tempeh, crumbled

1 cup red lentils, soaked if you have time, otherwise debris removed and rinsed

2 cups vegetable stock

6 ounces (half a can) full-fat coconut milk

1 tablespoon tahini

2 teaspoons apple cider vinegar

1 teaspoon salt

Freshly ground black pepper, to taste

FOR SERVING:

2 cups cooked brown rice (or swap out for cauliflower or broccoli rice for a YYI-friendly option)

4 cups steamed and chopped bok choy, from 1 medium-sized head of bok choy (approximately 1½ pounds)

1. In a large saucepan, heat the oil over medium-high heat and sauté the spices for 2 to 3 minutes, until fragrant. Add the onions and cook, stirring, for 5 minutes, until translucent. Add the ginger, garlic, and tempeh and cook for another 5 to 10 minutes.
2. Add the remaining ingredients and simmer for 30 to 45 minutes, checking occasionally to see if you need more liquid—add water, a ½ cup at a time, if so. Conversely, you can transfer everything to a slow cooker and cook on low for 6 hours.
3. After everything is cooked and soft, check the seasonings and adjust to your liking. Serve with a ½ cup cooked brown rice and 1 cup steamed bok choy per person.

NUTRIENTS

Fat: 35.7%	Calories: 600.2 kcal	Fiber: 11.4 g
Carb: 47.8%	Fat: 25.1 g	Sugar: 6.2 g
Protein: 16.6%	Carbohydrates: 70.9 g	Protein: 29.1 g

EPIGENETIC CHILI

YYE | YYI (V or VGT) | [V], [VGT]

8 servings *Prep time: 20 minutes,* *Cook time: 1 hour*
plus presoak time for the beans

This filling but still brightly flavored (i.e., not heavy-tasting) chili makes a large portion that is perfect for feeding the entire family, or for having leftovers for later in the week. It tastes great eaten warm, of course, but it's also great served cold on a hot summer day. And it's easy to make vegetarian or vegan by swapping the turkey for steamed and crumbled tempeh and opting for vegetable broth or water instead of bone broth.

Methyl donors: tomatoes, garlic, red onion, turkey, cumin, chili powder, thyme, sage, black beans, kidney beans, maple syrup

DNA methylation adaptogens: tomatoes, coconut oil, bell peppers, garlic, red onion, cumin, chili powder, thyme, sage, black beans, kidney beans, green onion

5 large fresh tomatoes, 2 diced, 3 pureed, or
1 (14.5-ounce) can diced

2 tablespoons coconut oil

1 red bell pepper, chopped

1 yellow bell pepper, chopped

4 cloves garlic, minced

1 red onion, chopped

1 pound ground turkey

2 tablespoons cumin

2 tablespoons chili powder

2 tablespoons fresh thyme

2 tablespoons fresh sage

1 (7-ounce) jar tomato paste

¾ cup black beans, soaked overnight and drained, or
1 (15-ounce) can, rinsed

¾ cup kidney beans, soaked overnight and drained, or
1 (15-ounce) can, rinsed

16 ounces water (or bone or vegetable broth)

Salt and freshly ground black pepper, to taste

Dash of maple syrup, optional

Green onions, diced, for garnish

1 spoonful of dairy-free yogurt, such as almond, coconut, or cashew, per serving, for garnish

1. Prep tomato sauce by pureeing three of the large tomatoes in a blender until they reach a liquid consistency.
2. Heat coconut oil in large pot over medium heat. Add bell peppers, garlic, and onion and sauté for 3 to 5 minutes. Add turkey and stir frequently until thoroughly cooked, about 7 to 10 minutes. Add cumin, chili, thyme, and sage and cook for 2 to 3 minutes. Add diced tomatoes, tomato paste, and tomato puree.
3. Turn down to a simmer and cook for 10 minutes, allowing sauce to reduce slightly and deepen in color.
4. Add beans and water. Simmer 30 to 40 minutes.
5. Season with salt and pepper and, if using, maple syrup. Serve topped with yogurt and green onions.

NUTRIENTS

Fat: 42.9%	Calories: 309.5 kcal	Fiber: 7.8 g
Carb: 31.9%	Fat: 14.8 g	Sugar: 10.3 g
Protein: 25.2%	Carbohydrates: 26.5 g	Protein: 21.1 g

MEDITERRANEAN STUFFED PORK TENDERLOIN WITH GREEN BEANS

YYI | KL, P

4 servings   *Prep time: 10 minutes*   *Cook time: 45 minutes plus 10 minutes resting time*

If you've ever felt pork tenderloin was too bland, or too dry, this recipe will change your mind. Stuffed with flavor-rich DNA methylation adaptogens, including sun-dried tomatoes, sunflower seeds, and capers, this dish tastes like it takes a lot more time to prepare than it does. Although it's easy enough for a weeknight dinner, it's tasty enough for entertaining—and your guests will never suspect you're serving them a health-focused dinner.

Tip: If you don't have butcher's twine, you can use toothpicks to keep the tenderloin together—just leave enough of them sticking out that they are easy to remove before slicing and eating.

Methyl donors: pork, sunflower seeds, tomatoes, garlic, rosemary, flax seeds

DNA methylation adaptogens: pork, sunflower seeds, tomatoes, garlic, capers, Mexican oregano, rosemary, red chili pepper, extra-virgin olive oil, lemon, green beans

    1 pound pork tenderloin

FOR THE STUFFING:
    ¼ cup sunflower seeds
    5 sun-dried tomatoes, oil-packed
    3 cloves garlic
    ¼ cup capers
    2 tablespoons fresh Mexican oregano (or 1 teaspoon dried)
    1 tablespoon fresh rosemary (or ½ teaspoon dried)
    Pinch of red pepper flakes
    ½ teaspoon salt
    Fresh ground pepper

FOR THE GLAZE:
    2 tablespoons extra-virgin olive oil
    1 tablespoon balsamic vinegar
    Juice and zest of 1 lemon
    2 teaspoons Dijon mustard
    ½ teaspoon salt

FOR THE GREEN BEANS:
    1 pound green beans, trimmed
    1 tablespoon flaxseed oil
    2 cloves garlic, minced
    ½ teaspoon salt

1. Preheat the oven to 425°F.
2. Coarsely grind the sunflower seeds in a food processor. Add the remaining stuffing ingredients to the processor and pulse until everything comes together into a paste.
3. Slice the pork tenderloin in half lengthways, but don't cut it all the way through. Spread it out flat and place the stuffing lengthways in the center. Roll it back up and tie with butcher's string. Transfer to a baking dish.

4. Mix the glaze ingredients together in a small bowl and then brush over the tied tenderloin.
5. Bake in the oven for 15 minutes, then reduce the heat to 375°F and cook for another 20 to 30 minutes, until fully cooked through (internal temperature of 160°F or above). Allow to rest for 10 minutes, then cut into eight slices.
6. Meanwhile, steam the green beans until tender. Combine the flaxseed oil, garlic, and salt and stir through the cooked green beans.
7. Distribute the pork tenderloin slices onto four plates along with a serving of green beans. Serve immediately.

NUTRIENTS

Fat: 49%	Calories 393.9 kcal	Fiber: 5.2 g
Carb: 12.9%	Fat: 22.1 g	Sugar: 5.5 g
Protein: 38.1%	Carbohydrates: 14.6 g	Protein: 36.8 g

NOT YOUR MAMA'S BURGER WITH KOHLRABI MASH

YYI | K, P

4 servings   *Prep time: 25 minutes plus 1 hour for chilling patties*   *Cook time: 15 minutes*

A burger isn't generally considered to be health food, but if you make the beef grass-fed and combine it with the methylation superstars beets and rosemary, it's a valuable (and delicious!) (and purple!) addition to your epigenetic eating plan. The marinade here not only infuses extra flavor, it also reduces the formation of oxidative compounds formed during high-heat cooking that otherwise deplete methyl donor reserves and impair DNA methylation.

> *Tip:* Because the beets make the burger a bright purple color, it can be hard to gauge doneness. Use a meat thermometer to ensure burgers reach an internal temperature of 160°F. Also, if you can't find kohlrabi, try mashed turnips. Also delish!

Methyl donors: beef, beets, rosemary, apple cider vinegar, garlic, kohlrabi, turnip

DNA methylation adaptogens: beets, rosemary, coconut oil, extra-virgin olive oil, apple cider vinegar, garlic, grapefruit, lemon, kohlrabi, turnip

FOR THE MARINADE:
>   2 tablespoons extra-virgin olive oil
>   2 tablespoons apple cider vinegar
>   1 tablespoon grapefruit or lemon juice
>   1 teaspoon Dijon mustard
>   2 cloves garlic, crushed
>   1–2 tablespoons coconut aminos (optional)

FOR THE PATTIES:
>   1 pound organic grass-fed ground beef
>   2 medium beets, raw and grated
>   ½ teaspoon fresh or dried rosemary, finely chopped
>   (about ½ sprig fresh)
>   3 tablespoons coconut oil
>   Sea salt and freshly ground black pepper, to taste

FOR THE KOHLRABI MASH:
>   2 kohlrabi (or 2 turnips), peeled and diced
>   2 tablespoons extra-virgin olive oil
>   Salt, to taste

1. Stir together all the marinade ingredients and set aside.
2. Mix the beef with the beets and rosemary. Season with salt and pepper and form into four patties.
3. Place the burger patties in a shallow baking dish. Pour the marinade over the patties, cover and place in the refrigerator for 1 hour.
4. Meanwhile, steam or boil the kohlrabi until tender, around 15 minutes.
5. Mash the cooked kohlrabi well and mix in the olive oil and salt. Keep the mash warm in a covered pan until the burgers are done.
6. When the patties have chilled, place a large sauté pan over medium heat and wait 1 to 3 minutes until it builds up temperature. Add the coconut oil to the pan and tip the pan carefully to distribute.
7. Add the patties to the pan. Do this in batches if you need to, being careful not to crowd the pan.
8. Cook for 4 minutes on the first side, and 3 minutes on the second, using a meat thermometer to determine when they've hit 160°F. Serve patties alongside the warm kohlrabi mash.

NUTRIENTS

Fat: 71.3%	Calories: 487.1 kcal	Fiber: 4 g
Carb: 8.9%	Fat: 38.3 g	Sugar: 6.5 g
Protein: 19.8%	Carbohydrates: 11.1 g	Protein: 24.1 g

SIMPLE PAN-FRIED STEAK WITH "CREAMED" GREENS

YYI | KL, P

2 servings   Prep time: 5 minutes   Cook time: 30 minutes
plus 3 minutes resting
time for the steaks

Like a good pair of black pants, this dish is versatile—it works as a quick (if decadent) weeknight dinner, and just as well as a celebratory meal. Using frozen greens makes it that much easier to prepare—no washing or chopping required. It also reduces the amount of greens you need to process; if you prefer using fresh greens, you'll need a whopping 11 cups spinach and 8 cups kale! But I've included those options in the ingredients list, in case you have a lot of spinach or kale on hand that you need to use up.

Tip: If you'd like your "creamed" greens a little creamier, add 2 tablespoons of canned coconut milk at the end of the greens cooking process.

Methyl donors: beef, onion, spinach, kale, garlic, pine nuts

DNA methylation adaptogens: extra-virgin olive oil, onion, spinach, kale, garlic, Mexican oregano, red pepper flakes

¼ cup pine nuts, for garnish

1 tablespoon extra-virgin olive oil

1 medium onion, diced

5 ounces frozen chopped spinach (or 11 cups fresh, cleaned and chopped)

5 ounces frozen chopped kale (or 8 cups fresh, cleaned, de-stemmed, and chopped)

4 cloves garlic, minced

1 tablespoon arrowroot powder

¼ cup low-sodium chicken broth (such as Kettle and
Fire brand)

Salt and freshly ground black pepper, to taste

2–3 tablespoons full-fat coconut milk (optional)

2 small strip steaks, about 3–4 ounces each, grass-fed
if possible

1 tablespoon refined (clear) avocado oil

2 tablespoons fresh Mexican oregano, finely chopped,
for garnish

Red pepper flakes (optional), for garnish

1. Preheat the oven to 350°F. In a small oven-proof dish, toast the
   pine nuts until just golden brown and beginning to release a nutty
   odor, about 6 to 8 minutes (be careful to watch them—they can
   burn quickly).

2. Meanwhile, in a large saucepan over medium heat, warm the olive oil and sauté the onion until tender, about 10 to 12 minutes.
   Add the spinach, kale, and garlic and cook for another 5 to 7
   minutes, stirring, until all the greens have defrosted and cooked
   (if using fresh, cook until wilted, about 3 minutes).

3. Sprinkle the arrowroot powder over the greens and stir through
   evenly. Once you can no longer see any arrowroot clumps, add
   the chicken broth and continue to stir through for 2 to 3 minutes.
   Season to taste with salt and pepper, add coconut milk if using,
   then cover and set aside while you cook the steaks.

4. Preheat a skillet over medium heat. Season the steaks with salt
   and pepper. Add the avocado oil to the skillet and sear the steaks
   2 to 3 minutes each side. Continue cooking until the steaks reach
   your preferred level of doneness.

5. Let the steaks rest for 2 to 3 minutes, then cut across the grain at
   a slight diagonal into slices about ½-inch thick.

6. Place a large spoonful of creamed greens on each plate and fan
   the steak slices out against them. Top with the pine nuts, Mexican
   oregano, and red pepper flakes (if using).

NUTRIENTS

(calculated without the optional coconut milk)

Fat: 47.2%	Calories: 564.1 kcal	Fiber: 7.6 g
Carb: 13.9%	Fat: 30.7 g	Sugar: 4.9 g
Protein: 38.9%	Carbohydrates: 21.6 g	Protein: 57.2 g

PAN-FRIED CAULIFLOWER STEAK WITH CREAMY LEMON GARLIC GREENS

YYI | P, V, VGT

4 servings   Prep time: 10–12 minutes   Cook time: 45–50 minutes
(does not include soaking cashews)

I s there anything cauliflower can't do? It's great as crudités, amazing roasted, and mimics rice and even pizza dough. It's also a fabulous stand-in for steak, whether you're vegan, vegetarian, or just looking for a cost-effective and easy-to-prepare entrée option. This lemon garlic cashew cream sauce is luscious and also goes great with a variety of dishes, including salads, cooked greens or vegetables, poultry, and seafood.

As with the previous recipe, using frozen greens makes for much easier prep and reduces the volume of greens you need to wash, de-stem (in the case of kale), and chop. Again, I'm including amounts for fresh greens if you prefer, but don't let them scare you off—they will cook down considerably.

> *Tip:* Any extra bits of cauliflower will keep in the refrigerator for 5 days, or in the freezer for 3 to 4 weeks. You can use these pieces for making cauliflower rice, or steam them and mash them with a little extra-virgin olive oil, salt, and pepper for a tasty alternative to mashed potatoes, or even throw them into a smoothie or on top of a salad for extra methylation support.

Methyl donors: cauliflower, onion, spinach, kale, garlic, pine nuts, cashews
DNA methylation adaptogens: cauliflower, extra-virgin olive oil, onion, spinach, kale, garlic, Mexican oregano, lemon, cashews

FOR THE GREENS:
- ¼ cup pine nuts (optional)
- 1 tablespoon extra-virgin olive oil
- 1 medium onion, diced
- 5 ounces frozen chopped spinach (or 11 cups fresh, cleaned and chopped)
- 5 ounces frozen chopped kale (or 8 cups fresh, cleaned, de-stemmed, and chopped)
- 2 cloves garlic, minced
- ¼ cup low-sodium vegetable broth
- 2 tablespoons fresh Mexican oregano, finely chopped
- Salt and freshly ground black pepper, to taste

FOR THE CAULIFLOWER STEAKS:

    2 large heads cauliflower

    1 tablespoon extra-virgin olive oil

    2 tablespoons refined (clear) avocado oil

FOR THE CREAMY LEMON GARLIC SAUCE:

    1 cup raw cashews, soaked overnight

    2 tablespoons fresh lemon juice

    1 or 2 cloves of garlic, minced, to taste

    ½ teaspoon sea salt

    3–4 tablespoons water, to taste

1. If using pine nuts, preheat the oven to 350°F. In a small oven-proof dish, toast the pine nuts until just golden brown and beginning to release a nutty odor, 6 to 8 minutes.

2. In a large saucepan over medium heat, sauté the onions in the olive oil until tender, about 10 minutes. Add the spinach, kale, and garlic and cook for another 5 to 7 minutes, stirring until all the greens have defrosted and cooked (if using fresh, cook until wilted, 2 to 3 minutes).

3. Add the vegetable broth and stir into the greens for 2 to 3 minutes. Season with the Mexican oregano and a few pinches of salt and pepper, cover, and set aside while you cook the cauliflower steaks.

4. Cut leaves off the cauliflower heads, place the heads stem side down and cut 1-inch-thick slices vertically (top to bottom). Make sure each slice is flat on the top and bottom and a similar thickness so that they'll cook evenly. Each large head should yield two or three "steaks." You need a total of four, but you can always cook more if you have them. Brush the steaks with the olive oil, then dust with sea salt and pepper.

5. To make the sauce, place all of the sauce ingredients in a high-speed blender or food processor. Blend until the mixture is creamy and smooth, adding additional water 1 teaspoon at a time until it reaches your desired consistency. Add more salt and pepper to taste.

6. Preheat a skillet over medium-high heat, then add the avocado oil. Once hot, add two steaks to the skillet and cook each side for about 4 minutes, until they are slightly browned. Transfer to a serving plate and repeat with the other two steaks.

7. Plate the warmed greens, place a cauliflower steak on top, then drizzle the lemon garlic sauce over the steak and greens. Top with toasted pine nuts (if using).

NUTRIENTS

Fat: 59.7%
Carb: 30.1%
Protein: 10.2%

Calories: 502 kcal
Fat: 35 g
Carb: 40.6 g

Fiber: 13.1 g
Sugars: 12.8 g
Protein: 18 g

DNA METHYLATION MINESTRONE

YYI | P

6 servings

Prep time: 30 minutes plus 60 minutes cooling time for the meatballs

Cook time: 1 hour

This soup is nothing short of a DNA methylation extravaganza! Yes, it has beef liver, but it's mixed with turkey inside a delicious meatball, so it's not noticeable. There is a lot of chopping involved, but once that's done, your labor is basically over and you've got five additional servings left over (or four, if you're cooking for two).

Methyl donors: turkey, beef liver, egg, parsley, garlic, onion, carrots, tomatoes, shiitake mushrooms, butternut squash, asparagus, oregano, rosemary, spinach

DNA methylation adaptogens: turkey, beef liver, egg, parsley, olive oil, coconut oil, garlic, onion, carrots, celery, tomatoes, zucchini, butternut squash, asparagus, oregano, rosemary, spinach

FOR THE MEATBALLS:

1 pound ground turkey

3 ounces beef liver, trimmed (remove the white membrane) and chopped

1 egg

2 tablespoons parsley, minced, plus additional minced parsley, for garnish

Salt and freshly ground black pepper, to taste

2 tablespoons extra-virgin olive oil, avocado oil, or coconut oil

FOR THE MINESTRONE SOUP:

> 2 tablespoons extra-virgin olive oil, avocado oil, or coconut oil
>
> 4 cloves garlic, chopped
>
> 1 cup diced onion
>
> 1 cup chopped carrots
>
> 1 cup chopped celery
>
> 2 cups sliced shiitake mushrooms
>
> 1 (14-ounce) can diced tomatoes
>
> 3 cups water
>
> 1 small zucchini, chopped
>
> ½ large or 1 small butternut squash, peeled, seeded, and chopped into ½-inch pieces
>
> 1 pound asparagus, trimmed and chopped into ½-inch pieces
>
> 1 bay leaf
>
> 1 teaspoon oregano
>
> 2 teaspoons rosemary (or 1 fresh rosemary sprig)
>
> 2 cups spinach, de-stemmed and julienned
>
> Salt and freshly ground black pepper, to taste

1. In a food processor, blend the turkey and liver. Place the ground meat into a bowl and mix in the egg, parsley, salt, and pepper by hand. Allow mixture to set, covered, in the refrigerator for at least 1 hour.
2. Once the meat has set, form small meatballs, about 1 inch in diameter.
3. In a large stockpot or Dutch oven, heat 2 tablespoons olive oil over medium-low heat. Cook the meatballs until golden all over, 6 to 8 minutes. Set aside.
4. In the same stockpot, heat the remaining 2 tablespoons of oil. Add the garlic, onions, carrots, celery, and mushrooms. Sauté, stirring occasionally, for 3 to 5 minutes.
5. Add the tomatoes, water, zucchini, butternut squash, asparagus, bay leaf, oregano, and rosemary and bring to a low simmer.
6. Carefully place the turkey meatballs in the soup, covering them with as much broth as possible.
7. Simmer for 15 minutes. Test one meatball to make sure the meat has cooked through.

8. Once meatballs are done, turn off the heat and remove the rosemary sprig if you used one (the leaves should have fallen off) and the bay leaf. Add the spinach and stir the soup until the spinach wilts. Season with salt and pepper to taste.
9. Garnish with parsley and serve.

NUTRIENTS

Fat: 53.1%	Calories: 411.4 kcal	Fiber: 7.9 g
Carb: 20.3%	Fat: 24.5 g	Sugar: 8.5 g
Protein: 26.6%	Carbohydrates: 23 g	Protein: 28.8 g

WILD MUSHROOM RAGOUT

YYI | P, VGT, V

2 servings   *Prep time: 30 minutes*   *Cook time: 40 minutes*

The more I learn about mushrooms, with their high quantities of methyl donors and DNA methylation adaptogens, the deeper I fall in love with them. This dish puts them front and center. It also proves how hearty a plant-based meal can be. Try serving it over garlicky sautéed greens with some Rosemary and Sea Salt Crackers. (And if you're not vegan, a fried or poached egg is great with it, too.) If you can't find kohlrabi, try peeled broccoli stems—they have a similar taste and texture and are also DNA-methylation friendly.

Methyl donors: onions, carrots, kohlrabi, broccoli, shiitake mushrooms, tomatoes, garlic, arrowroot powder, parsley

DNA methylation adaptogens: extra-virgin olive oil, onions, carrots, broccoli, kohlrabi, tomatoes, garlic, parsley

- 2 tablespoons extra-virgin olive oil
- 2 medium onions, diced
- 2 medium carrots, peeled and finely diced
- 1 kohlrabi, peeled and diced (or 1 large or 2 small broccoli stalks, peeled and diced)
- 8 ounces shiitake mushrooms, sliced
- 8 ounces crimini mushrooms, sliced

4 sun-dried tomatoes, oil-packed, minced

4 cloves garlic, minced

3 tablespoons arrowroot powder

1 cup low-sodium vegetable broth

Salt and freshly ground black pepper, to taste

¼ cup finely chopped parsley, for garnish

1. In a large saucepan with a lid, gently heat the oil over medium heat and add the onions, carrots, kohlrabi, and mushrooms.
2. Cover and cook, stirring intermittently, until everything is soft, about 30 minutes.
3. Add the tomatoes, garlic, and arrowroot powder. Stir well and cook 1 to 2 minutes more.
4. Add the vegetable broth and season to taste. Bring to a boil, then turn the heat down low and cook for another 10 minutes, until the flavors have mellowed and blended together.
5. Serve in two bowls topped with the parsley.

NUTRIENTS

Fat: 39.5%	Calories: 345 kcal	Fiber: 10.7 g
Carb: 53.1%	Fat: 15.5 g	Sugar: 15.7 g
Protein: 7.4%	Carbohydrates: 48.8 g	Protein: 9.6 g

LEMON GARLIC BROCCOLI RABE AND WHITE BEAN STEW

YYE | YYI (VGT and V) | V, VGT

4 main dish–sized servings or 6 side dish–sized servings   *Prep time: 15 minutes*   *Cook time: 20 minutes*

Ever since I dated an Italian man when I was in my twenties, broccoli rabe has been my favorite green veggie. I eat an absurd amount of it every week (in season, probably around three pounds!). As a cruciferous vegetable, it has a robust complement of methyl donors (including a ton of folate) and methylation adaptogens. Personally, I like my broccoli rabe prepared very simply, with salt, pepper, lots of garlic, and a healthy glug of flavorful extra-virgin olive oil. I add the rosemary and MCT oil as little extra YY kicks.

Broccoli rabe is not for the timid: it's very bitter. The longer you cook it, the mellower it becomes; that's why I advise steaming it before sautéing it. The lemon in this dish brightens it up and the beans make it hearty enough for a meal. You can top with crushed red pepper flakes for additional heat or toasted pine nuts for crunch and texture.

Note that because of the beans, it's really not appropriate for the Younger You Intensive *unless* you are a vegan, in which case a moderate amount of beans is important for you to meet your protein requirements on the eating plan. Also note that if you are a meat eater, you can make this Intensive-approved by replacing the beans with a serving of animal protein of your choice—this version is one of my go-to meals (I usually top mine with an organic chicken sausage or some salmon).

> *Tip:* If you prefer broccoli rabe on the crunchier side, remove before adding the beans and put back once the beans are almost done. You can also remove the lemon slices at the end of the cooking process and puree everything to make a flavorful soup.

Methyl donors: lemon, garlic, great northern beans, rosemary

DNA methylation adaptogens: extra-virgin olive oil, coconut oil, lemon, broccoli rabe, garlic, rosemary, red pepper flakes

- 14–16 ounces fresh broccoli rabe, cleaned, trimmed
- 4 large cloves garlic, sliced thin
- 2 tablespoons MCT oil
- ¼ cup extra-virgin olive oil
- 1 small lemon, sliced thin with seeds removed
- ¼ teaspoon freshly ground black pepper
- 2 (15-ounce) cans of great northern or cannellini beans, rinsed
- ½ cup water
- ½ teaspoon kosher salt, or more, to taste
- ¼ teaspoon ground rosemary

1. Steam the broccoli rabe in a large covered pot until stalks are fork soft (5 to 7 minutes), adding the sliced garlic with 2 to 3 minutes remaining.

2. Transfer the broccoli rabe and garlic to a large skillet over medium heat. Add the MCT oil, ⅛ cup of the olive oil, lemon, salt, and pepper, making sure to fully coat the broccoli rabe. Cook and occasionally stir for about 3 minutes until lemon is soft and slightly brown. Broccoli rabe should be a vibrant green and slightly crisp.

3. Add the beans and water and heat until everything begins to boil. Reduce to a low heat and simmer; continue to cook and carefully stir occasionally (for about 3 to 4 minutes) until the flavors combine and the liquid is reduced by half (the remaining liquid acts as a light sauce).

4. Transfer everything to a serving plate or bowl, sprinkle the remaining olive oil and rosemary over the top, and serve.

NUTRIENTS
(main dish serving size)

Fat: 44%	Calories: 425.8 kcal	Fiber: 13.2 g
Carb: 41.5%	Fat: 21.7 g	Sugars: 1.2 g
Protein: 14.6 %	Carbs: 44.2 g	Protein: 19 g

BROCCOLI PESTO WITH PASTA

YYE | V, VGT

4 servings   Prep time: 15 minutes   Cook time: 15 minutes
plus presoak time for
walnuts and sunflower seeds

This pesto, inspired by a recipe in the *New York Times*, gets additional depth from broccoli florets (which, as a cruciferous vegetable, are both a methyl donor and a DNA methylation adaptogen) and from some of our favorite DNA methylation adaptogenic herbs. It makes a great dip on its own, or serve it over chickpea, lentil, mung bean, or kelp pasta. Top it with Rosemary, Garlic, and Lemon Olives (page 370) for even more flavor.

Methyl donors: broccoli, garlic, basil, oregano, thyme, walnuts, sunflower seeds, chickpeas, lentils, mung beans, kelp

DNA methylation adaptogens: broccoli, garlic, basil, oregano, thyme, walnuts, sunflower seeds, lemon, extra-virgin olive oil, chickpeas, lentils, kelp, red pepper flakes

8 cups water

4 cups broccoli florets

1 (8-ounce) package gluten-free chickpea, lentil, mung bean, or kelp pasta

2 cloves garlic

2 cups fresh basil leaves

2 tablespoons oregano

2 tablespoons thyme

½ cup walnuts or sunflower seeds, soaked in water for at least 1 hour

1 lemon, zested and juiced

½ cup extra-virgin olive oil, plus more for serving

Salt and freshly ground black pepper, to taste

Red pepper flakes (optional)

1. Add the water to a large pot and bring to a boil.
2. Add the broccoli and cook, stirring occasionally, until bright green, about 3 to 5 minutes.
3. Keeping the water boiling, remove the broccoli with a slotted spoon and transfer to a food processor.
4. Add the pasta into the boiling water and cook according to the package's directions. Reserve ½ cup of pasta cooking water.
5. Meanwhile, add garlic, basil, oregano, thyme, walnuts, and lemon juice and zest to the food processor and pulse until smooth. Next, add the olive oil and mix briefly.
6. Drain the pasta and transfer to a large bowl. Stir in the pesto and toss until the pasta is evenly coated. Add in the reserved pasta water to desired consistency, 1 tablespoon at a time.
7. Add salt and pepper (and red pepper flakes, if using) to taste. Serve warm.

Note: Store the pesto in the refrigerator for up to 3 days.

NUTRIENTS

(includes 2 ounces of dry chickpea pasta per serving)

Fat: 74.8%	Calories: 429.1 kcal	Fiber: 5.6 g
Carb: 17.9%	Fat: 36.8 g	Sugar: 3.5 g
Protein: 7.3%	Carbohydrates: 20.2 g	Protein: 8.9 g

TURKEY MEATBALLS

YYI | K, P

2 servings   *Prep time: 15 minutes*   *Cook time: 25 minutes*

These super-tasty meatballs are a great way to get in a lot of methylation-supportive foods in a way that your kids won't even notice. They also refrigerate and freeze well and are great for snacking or adding to meals, so consider doubling the recipe.

Methyl donors: turkey, almond flour, flax seed, spinach, Swiss chard, arugula, parsley, onion powder, garlic powder

DNA methylation adaptogens: turkey, almond flour, spinach, Swiss chard, parsley, onion powder, garlic powder

½ pound ground turkey
½ cup almond flour
3 tablespoons ground flax seed
1 cup greens (such as spinach, Swiss chard, arugula)
2 tablespoons dried parsley (or 6 tablespoons fresh; about one medium bunch), finely chopped
1 teaspoon onion powder
½ teaspoon garlic powder
¾ teaspoon salt
¼ teaspoon black pepper

1. Preheat the oven to 375°F. Using a food processor, combine all ingredients until you have a near-smooth mixture. If you don't have a food processor, you can finely chop the greens, then mix all the ingredients in a large mixing bowl until well combined.

2. Form the mixture into about 12 to 16 meatballs and place on a baking sheet lined with parchment paper. Bake for 15 to 25 minutes or until cooked through.

NUTRIENTS

Fat: 63.9%
Carb: 8.7%
Protein: 27.3%

Calories 524.6 kcal
Fat: 38.5 g
Carbohydrates: 11.5 g

Fiber: 7 g
Sugar: 1.7 g
Protein: 37.4 g

VEGGIE BALLS IN MARINARA SAUCE

YYE | YYI (VGT and V) | VGT, V

4 servings   *Prep time: 20 minutes*   *Cook time: 45 minutes*
                    plus 15 minutes
                    to cook the quinoa

These veggie balls are little nuggets of deliciousness. Try serving them over zucchini noodles for a full pasta-like experience. If you can't find Mexican oregano, regular oregano is a good substitute; it's not as high in luteolin (a powerful DNA methylation adaptogen) as Mexican oregano, but it does have some adaptogenic compounds in it.

Methyl donors: tomatoes, onion, garlic, shiitake mushrooms, broccoli, beets, quinoa, almond, eggs

DNA methylation adaptogens: tomatoes, onion, garlic, red pepper flakes, Mexican oregano, extra-virgin olive oil, broccoli, beet, almond, eggs, broccoli sprouts

FOR THE MARINARA SAUCE:

> 2 (14-ounce) cans (or 1 28-ounce can) whole peeled tomatoes, BPA-free
> 1 medium onion, minced
> 2 cloves garlic, minced
> Pinch of red pepper flakes (optional)
> 2 tablespoons fresh Mexican oregano (or 2 teaspoons dried)
> Salt and freshly ground black pepper, to taste

FOR THE VEGGIE BALLS:

> 1 onion, quartered
> 5 ounces shiitake mushrooms
> 1 cup broccoli florets
> 1 medium beet, peeled and quartered
> 3 cloves garlic
> 2 tablespoons extra-virgin olive oil
> 1 cup cooked quinoa
> 1/3 cup ground almond meal

1 egg (or replace with one "flax egg"—see ingredient
  note on page 305)
1 tablespoon arrowroot powder
½ teaspoon salt
Freshly ground black pepper

TO GARNISH:
  Broccoli sprouts

1. Start with the marinara sauce. In a medium saucepan, combine all
   the ingredients and simmer gently for about 45 minutes, stirring
   intermittently. After about 15 minutes or so, you will be able to
   start breaking up the tomatoes against the side of the pan with
   the back of a wooden spoon.
2. Meanwhile, make the veggie balls. Place the onion, mushrooms,
   broccoli, beets, and garlic in a food processor and pulse until you
   have a very finely minced mixture.
3. In a medium skillet, heat the olive oil and cook the vegetable mixture over medium heat, until tender, about 8 to 10 minutes. Cool
   slightly, then transfer back to the food processor.
4. Preheat the oven to 375°F. To the processor, add the remaining
   veggie ball ingredients. Pulse until the mixture comes together
   and is well combined. It doesn't have to be completely smooth.
5. Form the mixture into bite-size balls and lay out on a parchment-
   lined baking sheet. Bake in the oven for 20 minutes until just starting to brown.
6. Transfer the veggie balls into the marinara sauce and fold them
   in until evenly coated. Do this carefully so as not to break up the
   veggie balls.
7. Plate the veggie balls in marinara sauce and garnish with broccoli
   sprouts.

NUTRIENTS

Fat: 43.3%	Calories 287.2 kcal	Fiber: 10.1 g
Carb: 44.6%	Fat: 14.4 g	Sugar: 11 g
Protein: 12.1%	Carbohydrates: 34 g	Protein: 10.2 g

CRISPY GARLICKY TEMPEH WITH CAULIFLOWER RICE

YYE | YYI (VGT and V) | K, V, VGT

2 servings   *Prep time: 20 minutes*   *Cook time: 30–40 minutes*

Organic tempeh, made from fermented soybeans, makes a great substitution for poultry in stir-fries, cutlet-based dishes, slow cooker stews, and chili. Like tofu, it absorbs the taste of the spices and flavors of the food it's cooked with. In this dish, pan-searing the tempeh first minimizes its earthy, nutty taste and helps it mimic chicken more effectively. That means even your meat-eater family will like it.

Methyl donors: onions, garlic, tomatoes, cauliflower, chives

DNA methylation adaptogens: coconut oil, onions, tempeh, garlic, tomatoes, cauliflower, chives

- 2 tablespoons coconut oil
- 2 medium onions, halved and thinly sliced
- 8 ounces (1 package) organic, plain tempeh, cut into 1- to 2-inch cubes
- 4 cloves garlic, minced
- 6 sun-dried tomatoes, oil-packed, diced
- ½ cup full-fat coconut milk
- ⅓ cup vegetable broth
- Salt and freshly ground black pepper, to taste
- ½ head of cauliflower, or 2 12-ounce bags of frozen riced cauliflower
- Fresh chives, finely chopped, for garnish

1. In a medium skillet, heat 1 tablespoon of the coconut oil and add the sliced onions. Sauté for 10 minutes over medium-low heat, until soft and translucent.
2. Add the tempeh and sauté 5 to 6 minutes more, until it is browned with a slight "crust."
3. Add the remaining ingredients, except for the cauliflower and chives, and cook for another 6 to 8 minutes, until the tempeh is saturated with sauce and flavors.

4. Meanwhile, prepare the cauliflower: if you are using fresh cauliflower, cut it into florets and pulse in a food processor until the texture resembles rice.
5. In a separate skillet, heat the remaining tablespoon of coconut oil and sauté the cauliflower rice until it is just tender, about 10 minutes, adding salt and pepper as needed.
6. Serve the crispy garlicky tempeh over a bed of cooked cauliflower rice and top with the fresh chives.

NUTRIENTS

Fat: 59.3%
Carb: 23.4%
Protein: 17.3 %

Calories: 552.5 kcal
Fat: 38.1 g
Carbs: 33.6 g

Fiber: 9.9 g
Sugars: 14.4 g
Protein: 28.9 g

CAULIFLOWER-CRUST PIZZA

YYI | KL, P, VGT

2 servings   *Prep time: 40 minutes*   *Cook time: 30 minutes*

This yummy pizza has only a mild cauliflower flavor that supports the tangy tomato and red onion sauce. And the dough holds together well. You could make it even more DNA methylation–friendly by adding some mushrooms and colorful bell peppers as toppings.

Methyl donors: cauliflower, eggs, garlic, red onion, tomatoes, basil

DNA methylation adaptogens: cauliflower, eggs, garlic, red onion, tomatoes, basil

2 small bags of frozen riced cauliflower (or 1 head of fresh cauliflower)

2 eggs

2 tablespoons arrowroot powder

2 cloves garlic, minced

½ teaspoon salt

Salt and freshly ground black pepper, to taste

¼ cup marinara sauce (read the label to make sure there's no added sugar)

3 tablespoons tomato paste
2 medium red onions, finely sliced
¼ cup basil leaves, for garnish

1. Set the oven to 400°F and line a baking sheet with parchment paper. If you have a pizza stone, place it in the oven.
2. If you are using fresh cauliflower, chop it into 2-inch pieces and then pulse in a food processor until you have a texture that resembles rice.
3. Steam the cauliflower for fifteen minutes until tender. Allow to cool so that you can handle it, then transfer to a clean kitchen cloth, wrap it up and squeeze it well to remove as much water as possible.
4. In a medium mixing bowl, beat the eggs with the arrowroot powder, then add the garlic and salt. Stir to combine.
5. Add the riced cauliflower to the egg mixture, season with salt and pepper, and keep stirring until everything is well distributed.
6. Press the mixture onto your prepared baking sheet, forming a circular pizza shape. Aim for about ½-inch thickness. Bake the crust for about twenty minutes.
7. Meanwhile, stir the marinara sauce and tomato paste together until evenly combined.
8. Remove the crust from the oven and spread the tomato sauce carefully over it. Top with the red onions and bake for another 10 to 12 minutes or until the edges are a touch browned and the onions slightly toasted.
9. Garnish with basil and serve immediately.

NUTRIENTS

Fat: 22.1%
Carb: 60.1%
Protein: 17.8%

Calories 260.1 kcal
Fat: 6.4 g
Carbohydrates: 41.8 g

Fiber: 9.5 g
Sugar: 16.3 g
Protein: 14.3 g

SNACKS AND SWEETS   • • • • • •

SPICY BUFFALO CAULIFLOWER "POPCORN"

YYI | K, P, V, VGT

4 servings   *Prep time: 15 minutes*   *Cook time: 45 minutes*

Roasted cauliflower on its own is delicious. Cauliflower that's been tossed in this spicy and savory blend of methylation-friendly ingredients is off the charts. In fact, it's so good raw that I dare you not to keep eating pieces right off the pan before it goes in the oven.

> *Tip:* If you want your cauliflower to be extra crispy, use a food dehydrator set to 115°F for 16 hours.

Methyl donors: cauliflower, tahini, tomato, apple cider vinegar, cayenne pepper, garlic powder, onion powder, turmeric

DNA methylation adaptogens: cauliflower, extra-virgin olive oil, tomato, apple cider vinegar, garlic powder, onion powder, turmeric

- 1 head cauliflower
- 1 tablespoon tahini
- 1 tablespoon extra-virgin olive oil
- 1 tablespoon tomato paste
- 1 tablespoon apple cider vinegar
- 1 teaspoon cayenne pepper (omit if you don't want it spicy)
- 1 teaspoon garlic powder
- 1 teaspoon onion powder

1 teaspoon turmeric
1 teaspoon salt
Freshly ground black pepper, to taste
¼ cup water

1. Preheat the oven to 350°F and lightly oil a large baking sheet.
2. Chop the cauliflower into bite-size pieces. (It makes it easier to slice off any leaves first, then start separating the florets from underneath.)
3. In a large mixing bowl, stir all the remaining ingredients into a smooth paste.
4. Add the cauliflower pieces to the mixing bowl and use your hands to mix them with the paste until it is evenly distributed.
5. Spread the coated cauliflower onto the baking sheet and bake in the oven for 40 to 45 minutes, until slightly crunchy on the outside and soft on the inside.
6. Serve immediately, while still warm.

NUTRIENTS

Fat: 51%	Calories: 101.6 kcal	Fiber: 3.9 g
Carb: 38.6%	Fat: 5.9 g	Sugar: 3.5 g
Protein: 10.4%	Carbohydrates: 10.7 g	Protein: 4 g

OVEN-BAKED BEET CHIPS

YYI | K, P, V, VGT

4 servings   *Prep time: 5 minutes*   *Cook time: 45–60 minutes*

Earthy. Salty. Crunchy. These beet chips satisfy the urge for a processed snack without the high sodium and low-quality oils most chips are cooked in.

Methyl donors: beets
DNA methylation adaptogens: beets, extra-virgin olive oil

2 medium beets, peeled or very well scrubbed
2 teaspoons sea salt
2 tablespoons extra-virgin olive oil

1. Preheat the oven to 300°F. Lightly oil two large baking sheets.
2. Cut the ends off and slice the beets very thin. I highly recommend a mandolin or the slicer disc of your food processor for this, but a sharp chef's knife will do in a pinch.
3. Place the beets in a medium bowl and sprinkle with the salt. Work the salt into the beet slices so that they are all well salted. Let sit for 30 minutes.
4. Drain any water that comes off the beets and pat them dry with a paper towel. Drizzle the olive oil over the beets and toss with your hands to evenly coat them. (Beware—this will turn your hands purple temporarily!)
5. Lay the beet slices onto the baking sheets and bake for 30 minutes. Then check them every 5 minutes, removing the beets that have curled and crisped up each time you check. (It could take up to another 30 minutes for all the chips to finish cooking.)

Note: Any leftover chips can be stored in a glass container on the counter for up to a week, but they're so yummy I doubt they'll last that long!

NUTRIENTS

Fat: 78.1%	Calories: 77.3 kcal	Fiber: 1.1 g
Carb: 19.5%	Fat: 6.8 g	Sugar: 2.8 g
Protein: 2.4%	Carbohydrates: 3.9 g	Protein: 0.7 g

ROSEMARY, GARLIC, AND LEMON OLIVES

YYI | K, P, V, VGT

6 servings   Prep time: 5 minutes   Cook time: 5 minutes
plus 5–10 minutes for cooling

Take the flavor of your favorite olives up several notches with garlic, rosemary, and lemon zest—a great-tasting combination that's also superfood for your genes. These olives are yummy as a snack, or pair with roasted chicken and a green salad for a satisfying meal.

Tip: You can use olives that have been pitted or that still have their pits.

Methyl donors: rosemary, garlic

DNA methylation adaptogens: extra-virgin olive oil, lemon, rosemary, garlic, olives

3 tablespoons extra-virgin olive oil

Zest from 1 lemon

1 tablespoon fresh rosemary (or 1 teaspoon dried)

2 cloves garlic, minced

2 cups mixed olives such as kalamata, cerignola, niçoise, picholine, or gaeta

1. To a medium saucepan over medium heat, add the olive oil, zest, rosemary, and garlic and cook, stirring, until the garlic just starts to brown, about 5 minutes. Be careful not to let the garlic burn.
2. Remove from the heat and let cool.
3. Stir the olives into the seasoning mixture.

> Note: The olives will keep in the refrigerator for up to 5 days. Best served at room temperature or slightly warmed.

NUTRIENTS

Fat: 95.4%	Calories: 201.7 kcal	Fiber: 4.1 g
Carb: 0%	Fat: 22.8 g	Sugar: 0 g
Protein: 3.8%	Carbohydrates: 2.4 g	Protein: 2.1 g

CINNAMON NUT CRUNCH

YYI | K, P, V, VGT

6 servings   Prep time: 10 minutes   Cook time: 20 minutes
(1 serving = about ½ cup)

Nuts and seeds are great to eat completely unadorned. But when you add a little cinnamon, a touch of sweetener, and *just a bit* of salt, they become a taste sensation. You honestly won't feel like you're following any kind of healthy eating plan with these.

Methyl donors: pecans, pumpkin seeds, sunflower seeds, sesame seeds

DNA methylation adaptogens: pecans, sunflower seeds, pumpkin seeds, shredded coconut, cinnamon, extra-virgin olive oil

2 cups pecans, roughly chopped

1 cup pumpkin seeds

1 cup sunflower seeds

½ cup sesame seeds

1 teaspoon cinnamon

¼ teaspoon stevia or monk fruit powder

1½ tablespoons extra-virgin olive oil

Pinch of salt

1. Preheat the oven to 325°F and lightly grease a large baking sheet.
2. In a large mixing bowl, combine the pecans and all the seeds and mix together.
3. In a separate small bowl, stir together the cinnamon, stevia, and olive oil. Add this to the nuts and seeds and use your hands to coat them all with the cinnamon mixture.
4. Spread the nuts and seeds on the baking sheet and cook in the oven for 15 to 20 minutes until lightly browned.

> **Note:** Once cooled, the nut crunch can be stored in an airtight container for 2 to 3 weeks.

NUTRIENTS

Fat: 81%	Calories: 610.2 kcal	Fiber: 8.5 g
Carb: 9.6%	Fat: 58.8 g	Sugar: 2.4 g
Protein: 9.4%	Carbohydrates: 14.5 g	Protein: 16.6 g

NO-BAKE GOLDEN ENERGY BALLS

YYI | P, V, VGT

4 servings
(1 serving = 3 balls)

Prep time: 30 minutes
plus 2 hours to set

These energy balls are a seed extravaganza! They're also super handy to have on hand for snacking or being on the go. They last a full two weeks in the fridge (and also freeze well), so make a double batch to ensure that you always have something methylation friendly on hand for those times when you need something *now*.

Methyl donors: sunflower seeds, pumpkin seeds, shredded coconut, flax seeds, turmeric

DNA methylation adaptogens: sunflower seeds, pumpkin seeds, shredded coconut, dates, turmeric, coconut oil, lemon

1 cup sunflower seeds

¼ cup pumpkin seeds

¼ cup dried shredded coconut, unsweetened,
plus extra for coating

¼ cup sunflower seed butter

4 Medjool dates, pits removed

2 tablespoons ground flax seeds

1 tablespoon turmeric

1 tablespoon coconut oil, melted

2 tablespoons water

Zest of 2 lemons

1 teaspoon real vanilla extract

Pinch of salt

1. Combine all ingredients in a food processor and blend until you have a medium-coarse mixture with a consistency resembling dough. You may need to stop and scrape the sides down intermittently.
2. Form the mixture into twelve balls and roll them in the extra shredded coconut.

Note: Store in an airtight container in the refrigerator for up to 2 weeks or in the freezer for up to 3 months.

NUTRIENTS

Fat: 64.5%	Calories: 168.4 kcal	Fiber: 2.8 g
Carb: 25.5%	Fat: 12.9 g	Sugar: 6.4 g
Protein: 9.5%	Carbohydrates: 11.3 g	Protein: 4.6 g

BLUEBERRY GUMMY SQUARES

YYI | P, [VGT, V] (if you use agar-agar in lieu of gelatin)

12 servings
(1 serving = 1 square)

Cook time: 15 minutes
plus 2 hours to set

These gummies have a rich purple color and a tart flavor with a hint of coconut. You can cut them into squares, or use small cookie cutters to cut them into kid-friendly shapes. Agar-agar is a plant-based alternative to gelatin derived from algae. It's available online and at health food stores.

And coconut butter is a cream spread made of pureed dried coconut meat that's rich in protein, carbs, fiber, and healthy fats.

Methyl donors: coconut butter, agar-agar

DNA methylation adaptogens: blueberries, lemon, coconut butter

1 cup blueberries

½ cup lemon juice

½ cup coconut butter

½ teaspoon stevia or monk fruit powder
(or 3 tablespoons maple syrup if you're on the YYE)

4 tablespoons gelatin or powdered agar-agar

1. Line an 8 x 8-inch glass dish with parchment paper and set aside.
2. In a small saucepan over low heat, bring the first four ingredients to a gentle boil. Take off the heat and stir until the coconut is melted and well combined.
3. Put the warm blueberry mixture into a blender and add the gelatin or agar-agar powder. Process until completely smooth (it will be fairly thick).
4. Pour the mixture into the lined glass dish and refrigerate for 2 hours.
5. When set, gently tease out the contents onto a cutting board and cut into twelve squares, each approximately 1½ inches square.

Note: Store in a sealer container in the refrigerator for up to 5 days.

NUTRIENTS

Fat: 67%	Calories: 83.9 kcal	Fiber: 1.7 g
Carb: 19.9%	Fat: 6.1 g	Sugar: 2.3 g
Protein: 13.1%	Carbohydrates: 4.5 g	Protein: 2.8 g

MATCHA GUMMIES

YYI | K, P, [VGT, V] (if you use agar-agar in lieu of gelatin)

12 servings
(1 serving = 1 square)

Cook time: 10 minutes
plus 3 hours to set

f you don't love drinking green tea (as I admit, I don't), these matcha gummies are a great way to get a concentrated dose of EGCG from green tea in just a bite. The coconut milk makes them luscious. If you don't like or don't have coconut milk, you can use an unsweetened nut milk if you prefer. The gummies will be less creamy, but still tasty. And if you're vegan, substitute agar-agar for gelatin.

Tip: You can use molds or an 8 x 8-inch pan.

Methyl donors: agar-agar

DNA methylation adaptogens: matcha powder

> 1 can full-fat coconut milk (13.5 fluid ounces)
> ½ cup water
> 1 tablespoon matcha powder
> ½ teaspoon stevia or monk fruit powder (or 2 tablespoons honey if you are following the YYE)
> Pinch of salt
> 3 tablespoons gelatin or powdered agar-agar

1. Heat the coconut milk and water over medium heat until just simmering.
2. Add the remaining ingredients except the gelatin and stir. Sprinkle the gelatin (or agar-agar) over the top and stir until it has completely dissolved. Continue stirring over the heat for another 3 to 5 minutes.
3. Distribute the mixture into lightly oiled molds or pour into an 8 x 8-inch baking pan that you've lined with parchment paper.
4. Chill in the refrigerator for at least 3 hours, until solidified.
5. Lift the parchment paper out of the pan and cut gummies into 12 squares, approximately 1½ inches square each.

Note: Store in a sealed container in the refrigerator for up to 4 days.

NUTRIENTS

Fat: 68.3%	Calories: 68.8 kcal	Fiber: 0.6 g
Carb: 19.2%	Fat: 5.6 g	Sugar: 2.6 g
Protein: 12.5%	Carbohydrates: 3.5 g	Protein: 2.3 g

RASPBERRY CACAO TRUFFLES

YYI | V, VGT

6 servings　　　　　*Prep time: 20 minutes*
(1 serving = 2 truffles)　*plus 1–2 hours to set*

These luscious, chocolaty treats come together quickly and will kick any feelings of deprivation straight to the curb. The freeze-dried raspberries add a little crunch as well as a pop of brightness.

Methyl donors: cocoa, sunflower seed butter, coconut flour

DNA methylation adaptogens: cocoa, raspberries, coconut flour, sunflower seed butter

FOR THE TRUFFLES:

> 3 ounces of dairy-free dark chocolate (70 percent cacao or higher), broken into small pieces
>
> ¾ cup unsweetened sunflower seed butter
>
> 1 tablespoon coconut flour
>
> ¼ cup freeze-dried raspberries
>
> ½ teaspoon real vanilla extract
>
> ¼ teaspoon stevia or monk fruit powder (or 1 tablespoon maple syrup if you're on the YYE), to taste
>
> Pinch of salt

FOR DUSTING:

> 3 tablespoons unsweetened cocoa powder

1. In a medium heat-proof bowl set over a saucepan with 2 inches of gently boiling water, place the chocolate pieces/chips and stir until they melt.
2. Meanwhile place the remaining ingredients in a food processor.
3. Carefully remove the bowl from the saucepan and add the melted chocolate to the food processor. Blend until you have a smooth dough-like mixture. You may need to scrape the sides down intermittently so that everything gets incorporated evenly. Place the mixture in the refrigerator for 1 hour to reach a soft but solid state.
4. Form into twelve bite-size balls and refrigerate for 1 more hour to harden.
5. Sift the additional 3 tablespoons cocoa powder into a bowl and gently roll each ball in the powder to coat.

> *Note:* Store in the refrigerator for up to 1 week or in the freezer for up to 3 months.

NUTRIENTS

(using stevia)

Fat: 66%
Carb: 25.5%
Protein: 8.3%

Calories: 315 kcal
Fat: 24.3 g
Carbohydrates: 38.5 g

Fiber: 5.9 g
Sugar: 11.1 g
Protein: 7.5 g

NO-BAKE SUNBUTTER CHOCOLATE SQUARES

YYI | K, P, V, VGT

24 servings
(1 serving = 1 square)

Prep time: 20 minutes
plus 45 minutes to chill

These squares are easy to make and deliciously filling (and calorically dense, which is why the serving size is small). They're also a tasty way to meet your seed requirements for the day.

Methyl donors: sunflower seeds, pumpkin seeds, ground almonds, cocoa
DNA methylation adaptogens: sunflower seeds, pumpkin seeds, ground almonds, coconut oil, cocoa

FOR THE BASE LAYER:

⅔ cup sunflower seeds

⅔ cup pumpkin seeds

⅓ cup ground almonds or almond flour

¼ cup unsweetened sunflower seed butter

½ teaspoon stevia or monk fruit powder (or 2 tablespoons maple syrup if you're on the YYE)

¼ teaspoon salt

FOR THE MIDDLE LAYER:

2 tablespoons coconut oil

1 cup unsweetened sunflower seed butter

¾ teaspoon stevia or monk fruit powder (or 3 tablespoons maple syrup if you're on the YYE)

2 tablespoons unsweetened nondairy milk

4 tablespoons coconut flour

½ teaspoon real vanilla extract

Scant ½ teaspoon salt

FOR THE TOP LAYER:

> 1¼ cups dairy-free stevia-sweetened dark chocolate (either chocolate chips or broken-up chocolate bars)
>
> 2 tablespoons unsweetened sunflower seed butter

1. Lightly grease an 8 x 8-inch baking pan and line it with parchment paper.
2. To make the base layer, combine the sunflower and pumpkin seeds in a food processor and pulse until finely chopped. Add the remaining base layer ingredients to the food processor and continue pulsing until everything is just combined.
3. Press the mixture into the bottom of the prepared baking pan so that you have an even, tightly packed layer. Place in the refrigerator while you prepare the middle layer.
4. For the middle layer, gently melt the coconut oil in a medium-size saucepan. Add the sunflower seed butter, stevia, and nondairy milk. Stir to combine and warm through.
5. Take off the heat and add the coconut flour, vanilla, and salt to the mixture. Stir well.
6. Take the base layer out of the refrigerator and pour the middle layer mixture on top of it, smoothing it out evenly and making sure it reaches all the corners. Return the baking pan to the refrigerator.
7. For the top layer, place a saucepan on the stove and add 1 or 2 inches of water. Bring to a boil. Place the chocolate in a heat-safe mixing bowl nested inside the saucepan without touching the water. Stir gently until the chocolate is melted. Add the sunflower seed butter and stir to combine. Remove from the heat.
8. Remove the baking pan from the refrigerator once more and drizzle the melted chocolate mixture over the top. Return it to the refrigerator for a further 45 minutes.
9. Gently release from the baking pan and cut into 24 (four rows of six) bite-size squares.

Note: Store in an airtight container in the refrigerator for up to 1 week.

NUTRIENTS

Fat: 71.5%	Calories: 213.4 kcal	Fiber: 3 g
Carb: 19.1%	Fat: 17.8 g	Sugar: 4.1 g
Protein: 9.3%	Carbohydrates: 10.1 g	Protein: 5.6 g

NO-BAKE CHOCOLATE ALMOND CUPS

YYE | K, P, V, VGT

24 servings   Prep time: 5 minutes   Cook time: 30–40 minutes
(1 serving = 2 cups)

These Chocolate Almond Cups are *really* good *and* super healthy. Use them for entertaining or gift giving, or just keep them in the refrigerator for when you need a little treat! I admit that there are a lot of steps to take, but that work yields forty-eight mini cups—enough to keep you going for a while.

Thanks to Angela Liddon of the blog Oh She Glows, whose 3-Layer Dream Cups were the inspiration for this recipe.

Methyl donors: coconut butter, almond flour, almond butter, maple syrup, cocoa, coconut shavings

DNA methylation adaptogens: coconut butter, almond flour, almond butter, coconut oil, cocoa

FOR THE CRUST:
   ½ cup coconut butter
   1 cup almond flour
   1 dropperful liquid stevia
   ¼ teaspoon salt

FOR THE MIDDLE LAYER:
   1 cup almond butter
   1 tablespoon coconut oil
   ½ teaspoon real vanilla extract
   1 tablespoon maple syrup
   1 dropperful liquid stevia

FOR THE TOP LAYER:
   1½ cups dairy-free stevia-sweetened dark chocolate chips
   ½ cup coconut shavings, unsweetened (optional)

1. Prepare a mini-cupcake tray with liners, set aside.
2. First make the crust layer: Warm the coconut butter in a small saucepan on the stove. When soft, mix in the almond meal, stevia, and salt, combining thoroughly. By the teaspoonful, press the mixture into the bottom of the cupcake liners so that it forms a compact and flattened base layer.

3. Next make the creamy middle layer: Warm all the ingredients in that same saucepan. It should be slightly creamy, but not runny. Again, by the teaspoonful, add the mixture as the next layer to your cupcake liners, pressing down and out to the edges with a wet finger if necessary.

4. Finally, melt the chocolate: The best way to do this is over a double boiler to prevent the chocolate from burning. If you have an electric stove, you can place the chocolate in a cleaned small saucepan and set it on the now turned-off burner you were just using; it will be warm enough to melt the chocolate with the occasional stir to help. Add teaspoons of melted chocolate to the cupcake liners to make the last layer.

5. If you'd like to get the top layer very flat, place the tray in the oven on the lowest setting for 10 minutes. Then you can just gently tap the tray to help the chocolate settle into a flat layer.

6. Top with the coconut shavings, then place the tray (cooled) in the freezer or refrigerator to get very hard. Serve either in the cupcake liners or out.

> *Note:* Keep any cups you don't eat in the refrigerator until you're ready to use to prevent them from melting.

NUTRIENTS

Fat: 73.1%	Calories: 107 kcal	Fiber: 1.9 g
Carb: 19.1%	Fat: 9 g	Sugar: 2.2 g
Protein: 7.7%	Carbohydrates: 5.1 g	Protein: 2.3 g

INDIVIDUAL COCONUT CACAO CHIA PUDDINGS

YYE | V, VGT

6 servings
(1 serving = ½ cup)

Prep time: 2 minutes

Cook time: 10 minutes
plus at least 3 hours
of chilling time

Sometimes you just need something creamy and chocolaty. This chia pudding satisfies that important need while also doing your body a *lot* of good, as every ingredient delivers multiple health benefits, including optimizing DNA methylation—even the maple syrup contains important phytonutrients! I do recommend using as little as possible to get a sweetness that appeals; although the recipe calls for a quarter cup, you might be able to use less without sacrificing taste.

Methyl donors: maple syrup, cacao, chia seeds

DNA methylation adaptogens: raspberries, blueberries, cacao, chia seeds

> ¾ cup raspberries
> ¾ cup blueberries or blackberries
> 1 can unsweetened, full-fat organic coconut milk
> ¼ cup pure maple syrup
> 2 teaspoons real vanilla extract
> 1 tablespoon cacao powder (unsweetened)
> ⅓ cup chia seeds
> 1 bar dairy-free dark chocolate (at least 70 percent cacao) for grating on top (optional)
> Extra berries for top (optional)

1. Divide the raspberries and blueberries between six small bowls or ramekins.
2. In a medium-size bowl, mix the coconut milk, maple syrup, vanilla, and cacao powder until very smooth.
3. Add the chia seeds and mix well. Pour approximately ⅓ cup of liquid over the berries in each container.
4. Refrigerate at least 3 hours, or overnight, until firm.
5. For optional garnish, top each serving with berries and finish with a small grating of the chocolate bar.

NUTRIENTS

Fat: 55.2%	Calories: 248.5 kcal	Fiber: 6.9 g
Carb: 39.8%	Fat: 16.3 g	Sugar: 15.6 g
Protein: 5%	Carbohydrates: 25.7 g	Protein: 3.5 g

ROSEMARY LEMON TART

YYI | P, [VGT, V] (if you use agar-agar in lieu of gelatin)

6 servings   *Prep time: 30 minutes plus*
                              4 hours to set

Like a kid with a favorite cake, I make this lemon tart for every birthday and holiday—it is definitely celebration worthy. (It's also one of the most commented-upon recipes on my website.) I warn you: the flavor is on the tart side. But the sweetness of the dates (which are legal on the Intensive, so long as your fruit consumption for the day stays less than 1 cup total) in the crust tempers the sourness of the lemon filling and makes a great (and pleasing) combination. To make this recipe vegan, use agar-agar instead of gelatin.

Methyl donors: sunflower seeds, pumpkin seeds, shredded coconut, cashews, rosemary

DNA methylation adaptogens: sunflower seeds, pumpkin seeds, shredded coconut, dates, coconut oil, cashews, lemons, rosemary, raspberries

FOR THE CRUST:
>   1 cup mixed sunflower/pumpkin seeds
>   ¾ cup dried shredded coconut, unsweetened
>   6 Medjool dates, pitted
>   2 tablespoons coconut oil
>   ¼ teaspoon salt

FOR THE FILLING:
>   Juice and zest of 6–10 lemons, enough to make 1 cup of juice
>   1 tablespoon gelatin or powdered agar-agar
>   1 can (13.5 ounces) full-fat coconut milk
>   ¼–⅓ cup Lakanto monk fruit syrup, to taste (or use 3–6 tablespoons maple syrup, to taste, if on the YYE)
>   1 cup cashews
>   1 teaspoon chopped fresh rosemary (or ¼ teaspoon dried)
>   ¼ teaspoon salt

FOR THE GARNISH:
>   1 cup fresh raspberries

1. Line an 8-inch springform pan or an 8- or 9-inch pie dish with waxed paper.
2. In a food processor, combine all the crust ingredients and process until the seeds are very small and it starts to stick together. You may need to scrape down the sides of the food processor intermittently. Empty the crust mixture into your prepared pan/dish and press down to coat the bottom evenly with no gaps.
3. For the filling, heat the lemon juice in a small pan on the stove until it just begins to simmer. Then pour it into a high-speed blender, add the gelatin, and blend until frothy.
4. Add the remaining filling ingredients and blend until everything is completely smooth. This may take a few minutes, but you want there to be no remaining traces of cashew pieces.
5. Pour the filling on top of the crust and place in the refrigerator for about 4 hours to firm completely.
6. Serve garnished with raspberries.

NUTRIENTS

Fat: 63.7%	Calories: 480.5 kcal	Fiber: 6.2 g
Carb: 28.4%	Fat: 36.2 g	Sugar: 22 g
Protein: 7.9%	Carbohydrates: 37.1 g	Protein: 11 g

SUNBERRY SORBET

YYE | P, V, VGT

2 servings   *Prep time: 20 minutes*

Think of this as the methylation-friendly version of frozen yogurt, with a smooth frozen base and plenty of toppings for extra flair. It's also vegan friendly. Although it has a lot of natural sugar from the fruit, it also has plenty of fiber to keep the impact on your blood sugar manageable. If you know that you have insulin sensitivity, save this dessert for after a strenuous workout.

Methyl donors: beets, banana, flax seeds, sunflower seeds

DNA methylation adaptogens: raspberries, blueberries, beets, banana, lemon, kiwi, sunflower seeds, mint

FOR THE SORBET:

    1 cup raspberries, frozen

    ½ cup cooked beets, frozen

    ½ banana, frozen

    1 tablespoon ground flax seeds

    Juice of 1 lemon

    ¼ teaspoon stevia or monk fruit powder (optional)

FOR THE TOPPINGS:

    ¼ cup raspberries

    ¼ cup blueberries

    1 kiwi, peeled and diced

    2 tablespoons sunflower seeds, finely chopped

    Sprig of mint

1. Blend all the sorbet ingredients in a high-speed blender until completely smooth.
2. Divide the blended ingredients into two serving bowls. Arrange the toppings on top and serve.

NUTRIENTS

Fat: 26.4%	Calories: 241.8 kcal	Fiber: 12.4 g
Carb: 65.2%	Fat: 7.6 g	Sugar: 23.1 g
Protein: 8.4%	Carbohydrates: 43.3 g	Protein: 6.2 g

BEVERAGES · · · · · · · · · ·

ENERGY BOOST GREEN SMOOTHIE

YYI | KL, P, V, VGT

1 serving   *Prep time: 5 minutes*

This anytime smoothie has it all: matcha gives a little bit of caffeine for energy; nutrient-dense avocado and sunflower seeds give you energy when you need it; and the tanginess of the lemon and turmeric balance the richness of the avocado—it all makes for a delicious pick-me-up.

Methyl donors: avocado, sunflower seed butter, turmeric

DNA methylation adaptogens: avocado, matcha powder, sunflower seed butter, lemon, turmeric

½ ripe avocado
1 teaspoon matcha powder
1 tablespoon sunflower butter
Juice and zest of 1 lemon
1 teaspoon turmeric
1 cup almond or coconut milk, unsweetened
Pinch of salt

1. Place all ingredients into a high-speed blender and blend until completely smooth.
2. Serve immediately.

NUTRIENTS

(almond milk used for calculations)

Fat: 68.3%	Calories: 325.2 kcal	Fiber: 8.3 g
Carb: 23.4%	Fat: 26.4 g	Sugar: 5.5 g
Protein: 8.4%	Carbohydrates: 20.9 g	Protein: 7.8 g

VEGAN MEGABOOST SHOT

YYI | P, V, VGT

2 servings   *Cook time: 5 minutes*

It can be challenging for vegans to get the full suite of amino acids. This recipe helps you cover those bases with its addition of hemp seeds. It also contains iron (from the spinach), vitamin C (which helps with iron absorption, from the mango), and zinc (from the pumpkin seeds)—other nutrients that are often at risk with vegan diets. If you're on the Intensive, omit the banana and know that this recipe will fill your daily allowance of fruit for the day.

Methyl donors: hemp, spinach, banana, pumpkin seeds

DNA methylation adaptogens: pumpkin seeds, banana, mango, spinach

- 1 cup cold water
- 3 tablespoons hemp seeds
- 2 tablespoons pumpkin seed butter, unsweetened (or use 3 tablespoons pumpkin seeds)
- ½ banana
- Pinch of salt
- 1 cup spinach leaves, packed
- ½ cup frozen mango

1. Place all ingredients into a high-speed blender and blend until completely smooth. Serve immediately.

NUTRIENTS

(pumpkin seeds used in calculation)

Fat: 53.1%	Calories: 229.6 kcal	Fiber 3.7 g
Carb: 31.1%	Fat: 13.1 g	Sugar: 11.9 g
Protein: 15.8%	Carbohydrates: 19.2 g	Protein: 9.3 g

GOLDEN TURMERIC MILK

YYI | K, P, V, VGT

1 serving   *Prep time: 2 minutes*   *Cook time: 5 minutes*

It's a drink. It's a snack. It's a time-honored Ayurvedic self-care ritual called "Haldi Ka Doodh." And now we know that it's a DNA methylation powerhouse. I'm talking about golden milk (although in this case, I suggest a non-dairy milk, such as coconut or almond milk). This tasty beverage gets its color from turmeric—the "clean-up crew" for life's inevitable biochemical messes. Mix yourself up a cup whenever you need a pick-me-up.

> *Tip:* You can triple or even quadruple the amounts of spices and store the blend in a glass jar for future cups—just add a rounded 1½ teaspoons to your nondairy milk and sweetener of choice.

Methyl donors: turmeric, ginger

DNA methylation adaptogens: turmeric, ginger, cinnamon

1½ cups coconut or almond milk, unsweetened
1 teaspoon turmeric
¼ teaspoon ginger
¼ teaspoon cinnamon
⅛ teaspoon black pepper
A few drops of liquid stevia, to taste (or 1 teaspoon honey or maple syrup if you are on YYE)

1. Combine all ingredients in a saucepan and bring to a simmer.
2. Turn off the heat and let sit for 5 minutes for the spices to mellow and blend together. Enjoy while still warm.

NUTRIENTS

Fat: 46.6%	Calories: 67.6 kcal	Fiber: 1.9 g
Carb: 43.6%	Fat: 3.6 g	Sugar: 3 g
Protein: 9.8%	Carbohydrates: 7.8 g	Protein: 1.8 g

MATCHA LATTE

YYI | K, P, V, VGT

1 serving   *Cook time: 5 minutes*

You don't have to patronize a fancy coffee shop to enjoy a delicious matcha latte. This DIY version makes getting your daily green tea a tasty treat.

DNA methylation adaptogens: matcha powder

1½ teaspoons matcha powder
1 cup hot almond or coconut milk, unsweetened
¼ teaspoon stevia or monk fruit powder (optional)

1. Pour your matcha powder into a mug.
2. Add 1–2 tablespoons of the hot milk first and stir into the matcha powder until smooth. While stirring, slowly add the remaining milk. Add sweetener if desired and enjoy immediately.

NUTRIENTS

Fat: 39%
Carb: 41.5%
Protein: 19.4%

Calories: 59.5 kcal
Fat: 2.7 g
Carbohydrates: 6.7 g

Fiber: 2.9 g
Sugar: 2 g
Protein: 3.3 g

BEET BUBBLY

YYI | KL, V, VGT

1 serving   Prep time: 1 minute

This drink is a great way to use up beet juice from other recipes (such as the Blueberry Beet Scones, page 305). Even better, it makes a tasty spritzer, especially with a squeeze of lemon. For DNA methylation bonus points, muddle a little fresh rosemary in the bottom of the glass before pouring in the spring water and beet juice.

Methyl donors: beet juice
DNA methylation adaptogens: beet juice, lemon

½ cup beet juice
1 cup sparkling water
Sliced lemon and ice cubes to serve (optional)

1. Place all the ingredients into a glass and enjoy!

NUTRIENTS

Fat: 3.7%
Carb: 82.4%
Protein: 13.8%

Calories: 42.7 kcal
Fat: 0.2 g
Carbohydrates: 9.2 g

Fiber: 1.9 g
Sugar: 4.3 g
Protein: 1.5 g

ICED OOLONG TEA WITH ORANGE AND ROSEMARY

YYI | K, P, V, VGT

2 servings

*Prep time: 20 minutes
plus 1–2 hours to chill*

This is a great summer refresher. Oolong tea is nearly as high in EGCG as green tea. Be sure to let it steep for ten full minutes as that process helps extract the EGCG.

Methyl donors: rosemary

DNA methylation adaptogens: oolong tea, orange, rosemary

- 4 cups water
- 3 bags oolong tea
- 1 medium orange, cut into slices
- 1 sprig fresh rosemary
- 1 cup ice cubes

1. Bring the water to a boil in a medium saucepan.
2. Add the tea bags, turn off the heat, and let steep for 10 minutes. Remove the teabags.
3. Place the orange slices and rosemary sprig in a pitcher and pour the tea over them. Let cool and then put in the fridge to chill.
4. To serve, add the ice cubes, stir gently with a long wooden spoon, and bring to the table.

NUTRIENTS

Fat: 2.6%
Carb: 90.7%
Protein: 6.7%

Calories: 31.2 kcal
Fat: 0.1 g
Carbohydrates: 7.8 g

Fiber: 1.6 g
Sugar: 6.1 g
Protein: 0.6 g

CALMING HERBAL TONIC

YYI | K, P, V, VGT

2 servings   *Prep time: 15 minutes*

Take your chamomile tea to the next level—both flavor-wise and DNA methylation–wise—by adding fresh ginger, lemon, and rosemary.

Methyl donors: ginger, rosemary

DNA methylation adaptogens: chamomile, ginger, lemon, rosemary

   4 cups water
   4 bags chamomile tea
   1-inch piece of fresh ginger, sliced
   1 small lemon, quartered
   2 sprigs rosemary

1. Bring the water to a boil in a medium saucepan. Remove from heat.
2. Add the chamomile tea bags, ginger, lemon, and rosemary and let steep for 10 minutes.
3. Remove tea bags and strain out the solids, reserving the liquid. Serve warm or cold.

   Note: This will last in the refrigerator up to 3 days.

NUTRIENTS

Fat: 11.3%	Calories: 3.7 kcal	Fiber: 0.3 g
Carb: 77.3%	Fat: 0.1 g	Sugar: 0.3 g
Protein: 11.3%	Carbohydrates: 1.1 g	Protein: 0.1 g

EXERCISE RECOVERY DRINK

YYE | P, V, VGT

1 serving   *Prep time: 5 minutes*

After exercise, food sources of antioxidants (in other words, all the ingredients in this recipe) are fabulously regenerative for the body. This recipe is chock-full of electrolytes (such as the potassium, chloride, and magnesium in cantaloupe and coconut water) and trace minerals (from the small pinch of

Himalayan pink salt) to replace what you sweated out; it also delivers protein (in the flax seeds and almonds) to aid in muscle building and repair.

> *Tip:* Keep your ground flax seed in the freezer to preserve its delicate fat and antioxidant content.

Methyl donors: flax seed, almond

DNA methylation adaptogens: blackberries, blueberries, cantaloupe, almond, coconut water

½ cup blackberries or blueberries
½ cup cantaloupe melon, seeded and peeled
1 teaspoon ground flax seeds
6–8 almonds
1 cup coconut water
Pinch of Himalayan pink salt
2–3 ice cubes, optional

1. Place all the ingredients into a high-speed blender and blend until completely smooth. Serve immediately.

NUTRIENTS

Fat: 31.3%	Calories: 167.1 kcal	Fiber: 8.9 g
Carb: 57%	Fat: 6.3 g	Sugar: 16.6 g
Protein: 11.7%	Carbohydrates: 25.1 g	Protein: 5.7 g

FIRE CIDER

YYI | [V], VGT

64 servings   *Prep time: 30 minutes*   *Curing time: 30 days*
(1 serving = 1 tablespoon)

Fire cider is an all-around tonic—the ginger and apple cider vinegar promote digestion, while the horseradish, cayenne, and garlic boost immunity. My team of nutritionists turned it into a DNA-methylation powerhouse by adding rosemary, orange, and turmeric. Just grating the horseradish will clear your sinuses!

In this version, the flavor of orange shines through immediately, followed by a mild spicy tingle and flavor of garlic at the end. You can combine it with olive oil to make a pungent salad dressing, or drink a small amount straight. Some of my patients have used a morning shot of this fire cider as a way to help dial down their coffee habit—it certainly has a pick-you-up kick! The tiny amount of honey per serving makes this still OK to consume on the Younger You Intensive. If you're vegan, either swap the honey for maple syrup or omit.

Methyl donors: ginger, horseradish, onion, garlic, orange, rosemary, turmeric, apple cider vinegar

DNA methylation adaptogens: ginger, horseradish, onion, garlic, jalapeño, orange, rosemary, turmeric, apple cider vinegar

> 1 medium ginger root, about 5 inches long, peeled and grated
>
> 1 medium horseradish root, about 5 inches long, scrubbed well and grated
>
> 1 small onion, roughly chopped
>
> 10 cloves garlic, crushed
>
> 2 jalapeño peppers, stems removed and chopped in half lengthwise
>
> Zest and juice of 1 orange
>
> 2 tablespoons fresh rosemary (or 2 teaspoons dried)
>
> 2 teaspoons turmeric
>
> 32 ounces raw apple cider vinegar, enough to cover the above ingredients
>
> ⅛ cup honey, or to taste

1. Prepare your roots, fruits, herbs, and spices and place them in a 32-ounce sterilized glass jar (or two if your jars are smaller), leaving 2 to 3 inches of room at the top.
2. Pour the apple cider vinegar into the jar until it reaches just below the top. The other ingredients should be well covered.
3. If you are using a metal lid, place a piece of natural parchment paper under the lid to keep the vinegar from touching the metal. Otherwise use a plastic lid if you have one.
4. With the lid on tightly, shake the jar well and then pack down the solid ingredients again with a spoon.
5. Store in a dark, cool place for a month and remember to shake daily.

6. After 1 month, strain out the pulp using a cheesecloth, reserving the liquid. Squeeze out as much liquid from the solids as you can. Pour the liquids into a fresh, sterilized glass jar or bottle.
7. Add the honey and stir to dissolve.
8. Consume by the tablespoon, or add it to a veggie juice, splash it over food, or incorporate it into a salad dressing.

> *Note:* Keeps for 3–4 months in the refrigerator.

NUTRIENTS

Calories: 8.4 kcal	Carbs: 1.4 g	Sugar: 0.9 g
Fat: 0 g	Fiber: 0.1 g	Protein: 0.1 g

SHOPPING LISTS

Younger You Intensive, Menu Version, Week 1

As you'll soon see, this list is made up mostly of fresh produce. To make the most of your food budget dollars, you can look for frozen fruits and vegetables, shop at your local farmers' market to buy produce that's in season, and buy your nuts and seeds in bulk (since you'll be eating plenty more over the rest of the eight-week program). Remember to look for organic where possible.

If you need to stock up on the things on the staples list because they're not already in your pantry, know that you won't have to restock them for a while; meaning, your grocery bill on the second week will be significantly less.

FOR ONE PERSON, FOR WEEK 1

- 5½ cups spinach (about 2 medium bunches)
- 4 cups kale (about 1 extra-large bunch, or 2 small bunches)
- 3 cups arugula (about 1 large bunch)
- 1½ cups Swiss chard (less than one bunch)
- ½ cup collard greens (or use leftover Swiss chard in its place)
- 1 medium head broccoli
- 1 medium head cauliflower
- 1 large or 2 medium kohlrabi
- 1 small bunch radishes
- 1–2 daikon radishes

- 1 head red cabbage, as small as possible
- 5 medium tomatoes
- ½ pound shiitake mushrooms
- 2 medium red onions
- 3 large red bell peppers
- 1 large orange bell pepper
- 1 (14-ounce) can of artichoke hearts, in water
- 1 small bunch celery
- 1 small bag of whole carrots
- 1½ cups green beans
- 1¼ cups snap peas
- 1 large leek
- 1 small bunch fresh parsley
- 1 small bunch fresh chives
- 1 pint cherry tomatoes
- 11 beets
- 6–10 lemons (enough to yield 1 cup juice)
- 6 Medjool dates
- 1 pint blueberries
- 1 medium Granny Smith apple
- 1¾ cups sunflower seeds (1 12-ounce bag)
- 1¾ cups pumpkin seeds

- 1 (8-ounce) bag cashews
- 1 (8-ounce) bag walnuts
- 1 (8-ounce) bag almonds
- 1 (16-ounce) jar organic sunflower butter
- 1 (13.5-ounce) can full-fat coconut milk
- 1 (12-ounce) jar beet juice
- 1 bag freeze-fried raspberries
- 1 pound organic chicken livers
- 1 dozen eggs (you'll use ½ dozen this week and ½ dozen next week)
- 4 bone-in chicken thighs (about 1 pound)
- 1 pound pork tenderloin
- 12 ounces wild or responsibly farmed salmon
- ¼ pound Irish back bacon or Canadian bacon (or buy ½ pound, as you'll need it next week, too)
- 1 pound grass-fed ground beef
- Small container (generally around 3 ounces) matcha green tea powder, culinary grade

PANTRY ITEMS (BUY IF YOU DON'T HAVE):

- Extra-virgin olive oil
- Avocado oil
- Coconut oil
- Flaxseed oil
- MCT oil
- Balsamic vinegar
- Apple cider vinegar
- Dijon mustard
- Almond flour
- Coconut flour
- Arrowroot powder
- Baking powder
- Vanilla extract
- Dairy-free milk (such as almond or macadamia — not soy)
- Coconut aminos
- Turmeric
- Rosemary (fresh or dried)
- Thyme (fresh or dried)
- Sage (fresh or dried)
- Mexican oregano or regular oregano (fresh or dried)
- Red pepper flakes
- Sun-dried tomatoes

- Capers
- Pine nuts (not called for until Week 2, so you can delay this purchase by a week if needed)
- Garlic
- 1 bar 70% cacao or higher dark chocolate (preferably dairy- and sugar-free, like Lily's)
- Gelatin or agar-agar

- Oolong tea
- Green tea
- Stevia (comes in both powdered and liquid form; although our recipes call for both types, they can be used interchangeably, so you only need to purchase one kind), monk fruit, or erythritol
- Sea salt

Younger You Intensive, Menu Version, Week 2

Definitely look in your fridge and pantry and assess what you have left over from Week 1; there may be items on this list that you already have. While the recipes call for a wide variety of greens, you can absolutely use them interchangeably—if you only need a ½ cup of Swiss chard for the Savory Onion and Chard Muffins recipe, but you have extra spinach or mustard greens, you can use those instead and skip buying the chard.

- 6 cups spinach (about 2 medium bunches)
- 3 cups kale (about 1 large bunch)
- ½ cup Swiss chard (or use leftover spinach or beet greens)
- 2½ cups mustard greens (1 small bunch)
- ½ cup collard greens (about 2 leaves; or use leftover spinach or beet greens)
- 1 small bunch cilantro
- ¾ cup arugula (less than 1 small bunch)
- 13 beets
- 7 cups cauliflower (2 medium or 1 extra-large head)
- 2½ cups broccoli (1 medium bunch)
- 4½ cups purple cabbage (1 large or 2 small heads)
- About 2 cups of kohlrabi (1 large or 1 small)

- 1 cup Brussels sprouts (about ½ pound before removing outer leaves and de-stemming)
- 1 bunch celery
- 3 medium onions
- 1 small bag carrots
- ½ pound cremini mushrooms
- ½ pound shiitake mushrooms
- 4 small tomatoes
- 2 medium zucchini
- 1 small butternut squash
- 3 large red bell peppers
- 1 pound asparagus
- 1 avocado
- 1 medium summer squash
- 1 (14-ounce) can diced tomatoes
- 2 lemons
- 1 bulb garlic
- 1 shallot
- 1 bunch scallions
- 1 small bunch basil
- 1 pomegranate

- 2 small bags frozen cauliflower rice
- 1 quart nondairy milk, unsweetened
- 1 quart low-sodium vegetable broth
- 1 small jar no-sugar marinara sauce
- 1 small jar tomato paste
- 1 pound ground turkey

- ¼ pound beef liver
- ¼ pound Irish back bacon or Canadian bacon
- 1 pound organic chicken livers
- 2 small strip steaks, about 3–4 ounces each, grass-fed if possible
- 2 4-ounce salmon fillets
- 12–16 ounces organic chicken thighs or breast (skinless, boneless)

THINGS YOU SHOULD STILL HAVE ON HAND FROM WEEK 1:

- Matcha
- Sunflower seeds (if you bought a large bag)
- Pumpkin seeds (if you bought a large bag)
- Sunflower butter
- Eggs (if you bought a dozen; you'll need another 6 this week)
- Turmeric
- Rosemary

- Green tea
- Oolong tea
- Beet juice
- Almond flour
- Cashews
- Pine nuts
- Stevia
- Parsley
- Chives

PANTRY ITEMS (BUY IF YOU DON'T HAVE):

- Tapioca flour
- Garlic powder
- Red pepper flakes
- Baking powder
- Baking soda
- Bay leaf
- Oregano
- Rosemary
- Sun-dried tomatoes
- Arrowroot powder
- Unsweetened shredded coconut

- Flax seeds (buy whole and grind just before using, if possible, otherwise buy preground and store in refrigerator)
- Coconut oil
- Vanilla extract
- Mexican oregano
- Ground cinnamon
- Dijon mustard
- Red wine vinegar
- Coconut flour
- Sesame seeds

Younger You Intensive, Improv Version, Shopping List

This is the list of foods we gave to our study participants; most of whom opted to follow the improv version of the Younger You Intensive rather than follow a scripted version. Keep in mind, they had weekly calls with a nutritionist to help them figure out how to meet their nutrient targets (for a refresher, refer to the Cheat Sheet on page 122).

Remember to look for organic where possible. Frozen vegetables and berries are OK.

FOR ONE PERSON, FOR ONE WEEK:

METHYL DONORS:
- 14 cups of fresh dark leafy greens, such as kale, Swiss chard, collard greens, spinach, dandelion, mustard greens (1 medium bunch is about 2½ cups, packed)
- Alternative: 7 cups of frozen dark leafy greens
- 14 cups cruciferous vegetables, choosing from broccoli, cabbage, cauliflower, Brussels sprouts, bok choy, arugula, kale, mustard greens, watercress, rutabaga, kohlrabi, radish, Swiss chard, turnip
- 21 cups of additional colorful vegetables (excludes white potato and sweet corn)
- 7–14 medium beets
- 1¾ cups pumpkin seeds (1 12-ounce bag)
- 1¾ cups sunflower seeds (1 12-ounce bag)
- 9 ounces liver (chicken or beef, organic preferred)
- 5–10 eggs (buy a half dozen if you plan on eating liver, a dozen if you don't, as you'll need to eat more eggs to make up for some of the nutrients in liver)
- 60–80 ounces of good-quality meat, poultry, fish and/or seafood (3¾ pounds–5 pounds)

DNA METHYLATION ADAPTOGENS

Choose at least one, but remember that DNA methylation adaptogens appear to be even more effective when used in combination. See Nutrient Reference for additional options.

- 3½ cups berries
- 3½ teaspoons dried rosemary, or 1 bunch fresh rosemary
- 3½ teaspoons turmeric

- 14 green tea bags
- 21 oolong tea bags
- 14 cloves garlic (about 2 bulbs)

OTHER USEFUL ITEMS TO HAVE:
- Oils—olive, coconut, flax seed, pumpkin seed, for example

- Salt and pepper
- Nondairy milk, unsweetened (such as almond milk or coconut milk)

PRODUCT TIPS (LOOKS FOR THESE IN YOUR LOCAL HEALTH FOOD STORE, WHOLE FOODS MARKET, OR ONLINE):

- Cost saver: check the freezer section for dark leafy greens (2 cups fresh is equivalent to 1 cup frozen)
- Rice alternative: check the freezer section for cauliflower rice
- Pasta alternative: look for vegetable "noodles" or kelp noodles for the Intensive, or chickpea, lentil, or mung bean pasta for the Everyday
- Bread alternative: Julian Bakery Paleo Bread, or look for unsweetened paleo breads made with nut flours
- Cracker alternative: Simple Mills almond crackers, or look for unsweetened paleo crackers
- Wrap alternative: Julian Bakery Paleo Wrap or Nuco Coconut Wrap
- Half-and-half alternative: Califia Farms Better Half (almond and coconut)
- Cream cheese alternative: Kite Hill Farms cream cheese
- Sauce-thickening alternative to flour: arrowroot powder
- Online source for liverwurst: www.grasslandbeef.com

Younger You Everyday, Menu Version, Week 1 Shopping List

- 1 bunch basil
- 1 bunch kale
- 1 bunch or small bag spinach
- 1 bunch or small bag arugula
- 1 small bunch Swiss chard
- 1 small bunch collard greens (or use leftover spinach or chard)
- 1 medium head broccoli
- 1 medium head cauliflower
- 1 small head purple cabbage
- 1 small bunch bok choy, or 2–3 baby bok choy
- 1 medium butternut squash
- 1 medium zucchini
- 5 large tomatoes or 1 (14-ounce) can diced tomatoes
- Small bag rainbow carrots
- 2 red bell peppers
- ¼ pound shiitake mushrooms
- 2 heads garlic
- 4 red onions
- 1 bunch parsley
- ½ pound snap peas
- 3 medium beets
- 4 lemons
- 1 banana
- Fresh dill (or use dried)
- Fresh rosemary (or use dried)
- Fresh thyme (or use dried)
- Fresh sage (or use dried)
- Pint of berries of your choice
- 1 apple
- 1 small bag fresh cranberries (or ¼ cup dried)
- 1 small bag dried black beans
- 1 small bag dried kidney beans

- 1 small jar applesauce (no sugar added)
- 1 quart chicken or vegetable broth
- 1 (13.5-ounce) can full-fat coconut milk
- 1 (7-ounce) can tomato paste
- 1 pint plain yogurt (nondairy preferable)
- 1 8-ounce box chickpea pasta
- 1 8-ounce bag pumpkin seeds
- 1 8-ounce bag sunflower seeds
- 1 small bag wild rice
- 1 small canister steel-cut or thick-cut rolled oats
- 1 small can chickpeas (make sure label says BPA-free)
- 1 small jar coconut butter
- 1 small jar almond butter (unsweetened)
- 1 small jar sunflower seed butter (unsweetened)
- 1 12-ounce bag dairy-free stevia-sweetened dark chocolate chips
- 1 quart nondairy milk (almond or coconut preferred, unsweetened)
- 1½ pounds ground turkey
- 1 dozen eggs
- Small package smoked salmon
- ¼ pound Irish back bacon or Canadian bacon
- 1 pound organic chicken livers
- ½ pound boneless skinless chicken thighs or breasts
- Beet juice
- Green tea
- Oolong tea
- Matcha powder

PANTRY ITEMS (BUY IF YOU DON'T ALREADY HAVE):

- Red lentils
- Walnuts
- Almonds
- Cashews
- Hazelnuts
- Almond flour
- Shredded unsweetened coconut
- Flax seeds (buy whole and grind just before using if possible, otherwise buy preground and store in refrigerator)
- Chia seeds
- Psyllium seed husks
- Garlic powder
- Onion powder
- Cumin
- Turmeric
- Ground ginger
- Chili powder
- Cinnamon
- Oregano
- Nutmeg
- Cloves
- Vanilla
- Stevia
- Gluten-free flour
- Baking soda
- Baking powder
- Organic cane sugar
- Maple syrup
- Extra-virgin olive oil
- Coconut oil
- Quinoa

SOAKING LEGUMES, GRAINS, AND NUTS FOR BETTER BIOAVAILABILITY

Soaking and sprouting techniques have been used for millennia across Eastern and Western cultures to improve the digestibility and nutritional value of whole grains, legumes, and beans. Soaking and sprouting helps improve the digestibility of beans and the bioavailability of their nutrients by breaking down and reducing saccharides and antinutrients, making for a much more health-promoting food.

If you are new to handling your legumes this way, start with the basic soaking method. It doesn't really take any more time, just a little more advanced planning. Once you feel comfortable with that, move on to sprouting: it's always exciting to see the first little shoots! (Note that you can use this method with grains as well.)

BASIC METHOD: SOAKING

- To soak legumes, first pick out any debris, then rinse thoroughly. Place in a large bowl, cover with two to three inches of warm water, and add one to two tablespoons of raw apple cider vinegar or raw coconut vinegar for every cup of legumes. The vinegar helps ferment the legumes, which improves their nutritional profile and reduces antinutrients that can hinder absorption and provoke the gut.
- Soak, uncovered, for twelve to twenty-four hours. Drain into a fine-mesh strainer and rinse. They are now ready for cooking, or you can store them in the refrigerator until you're ready to cook them. Cook these straight away, keep them in the refrigerator, or use them for sprouting. . . .

ADVANCED METHOD: SPROUTING

- Once your legumes have been soaked and rinsed, return them to the large bowl. They should be damp, but not submerged in any water. Cover with a clean dishcloth and leave for two to three days, rinsing them twice a day and then returning them to the bowl. When you start to see little "tails" appearing from your legumes (these are the sprouts that would grow into a full plant if you planted them), either store them in the fridge until you're ready to cook them, or cook them right away.

- You can use sprouted legumes just as you would regular legumes. Although the amount of liquid you need to cook them in and the time it takes for them to cook will likely be reduced, so don't go wandering off while they're on the stove!

INGREDIENT NOTES

SOME OF THE FOODS INCLUDED ON THESE SHOPPING LISTS MAY BE new to you or may be referred to more specifically than you are used to. Here are a few I wanted to introduce you to.

Agar-agar [YYI and YYE]

Agar-agar, which is made from seaweed, is a plant-based alternative to gelatin, which is derived from animal products. In addition to using it to replace gelatin, you can also use it as a thickener—it's particularly helpful in gluten-free baking. It comes in many forms, but the powder is easiest to use (it's a 1-to-1 replacement for gelatin) and to source.

Coconut aminos [YYI and YYE]

Made by fermenting the sap of unopened coconut tree flowers, coconut aminos has a similar savory taste to soy sauce without the soy and wheat that are typically found in soy sauce.

Dairy-free yogurt [YYI and YYE]

There are yogurts made from coconut milk, almond milk, and cashew milk that fit both the Younger You Intensive and Everyday programs. You want to make sure there is no added sugar, so check the ingredients list and stick to the plain version. Brands we like include Anita's Coconut Yogurt, Lavva Plant-Based Yogurt, and Forager Project Dairy-Free Cashew Yogurt.

Extra-virgin olive oil [YYI and YYE]

Extra-virgin olive oil is a component of many diets followed in areas with the highest percentage of centenarians. Making sure to buy extra virgin means you will get the highest possible levels of numerous beautiful polyphenols. Signs to look for that connote a high-quality olive oil include a cloudy appearance, a sharp and slightly bitter taste, and perhaps even a little tingle at the back of your tongue.

MCT oil

Made from coconut oil or palm oil, MCT oil is comprised of medium-chain triglycerides that are absorbed quickly by the bloodstream because they are easier to digest. I think of it as easy fuel for the body. It offers the following benefits:

- Improved energy production in cell mitochondria
- Improved satiety and prevention of excess food intake
- Supports cognitive function and overall brain health
- Encourages the production of anti-inflammatory ketones, especially when used as part of a ketogenic or keto-leaning diet

Mexican oregano

Mexican oregano is from a totally different plant family than the oregano typically used in Italian cuisine; it's got a lemony flavor and is one of the best sources of luteolin, a DNA methylation adaptogen. The same is not true of regular oregano, although it does have some different DNA methylation adaptogenic compounds in it. In the United States, you can typically only find dried Mexican oregano—often at Latin markets or gourmet markets (and of course, online), although I have seen it at Target.

Stevia

Stevia is three hundred times sweeter than sugar, so it's best to start with the smallest amount. Avoid stevia products that have added artificial sweeteners or dextrose or maltodextrin. Some brands may have a bitter aftertaste, so you may need to experiment to find one that you like. Stevia comes in both powdered and liquid forms—powdered tends to work better in baking and liquid is more easily added to drinks, but in truth you can use them interchangeably (so if you only want to buy one form to save on costs and/or storage space, that's fine). Brands we recommend include:

- NuNaturals NuStevia—Alcohol Free
- SweetLeaf Sweet Drops SteviaClear
- Organic Traditions Stevia Leaf Powder

Erythritol

A sugar alcohol found naturally in fruits, vegetables, and fermented foods, erythritol is only about 70 percent as sweet as sugar, so you may need to use more of it. For some people, erythritol may cause gas and bloating. If you tend to react to sugar alcohols in general, start with a smaller amount of erythritol to see how it impacts your gut.

- NOW Real Food Erythritol
- Swerve Granular erythritol

Monk Fruit (Lo Han)

Native to northern Thailand and China, monk fruit is similar in sweetness to stevia but has no bitter aftertaste.

- Lakanto Monkfruit Sweetener
- NuNaturals Monk Fruit Sweetener

NUTRIENT REFERENCE

FULL LIST OF DNA METHYLATION ADAPTOGEN AND METHYL DONOR FOODS

This is as complete a list of DNA methylation–supportive epi-nutrients and the foods that contain them as we could possibly make at this time—yet know that as research continues and our understanding of orthomolecular nutrition evolves, so will this list.[1]

You'll also notice that many foods appear in multiple places. For example, blueberries contain many DNA methylation adaptogenic polyphenols as well as vitamin C, which is an active demethylation nutrient, while liver is rich in multiple methyl donors as well as active demethylation nutrients. Call me nerdy, but I think it's exciting and fun to see how many DNA methylation–smart foods you can fit into your diet on a daily basis. And that's what this list can help you do. Anytime you start wondering, "What should I eat?" refer to these pages and find a new staple that likely also helps you keep your bio age low.

Note: Foods containing each nutrient are listed in descending order of how much of that nutrient they contain. Foods legal on both the Younger You Intensive and Younger You Everyday plans are included. Nut milks are likely rich sources of some DNA methylation-supportive nutrients, but it's difficult for us to know their exact polyphenol content and therefore we are excluding them from this list.

DNA Methylation Adaptogens

Below are the compounds—and the foods that contain them—that we currently know of that assist in balancing DNA methylation, helping to ensure that, when eaten in conjunction with methyl donor foods, we're methylating the genes we want off or actively inhibiting (or removing) methylation marks from genes we want on.

In general, you want to be consuming ample amounts of as broad a variety of these adaptogenic foods on a daily basis, as consuming combinations of these nutrients probably improves absorption and DNA methylation action. For example: in addition to the one-plus serving of methylation adaptogens the Younger You Intensive requires, the daily allotments for low-glycemic fruits, cruciferous veggies, and colorful veggies can all be selected from the examples listed here.

Anthocyanin	**Vegetables and fruits:** blackberry, blackcurrant, blueberry, raspberry, strawberry, cranberry, grape, açai berry, red hibiscus, red rose, black carrot, red cabbage, purple potato, red seaweed, brown seaweed **Legumes/nuts/seeds/grains:** Tartary buckwheat **Spices/herbs/sweeteners/condiments/drinks:** red wine, red wine vinegar, blue rosemary, purple mint, purple sage, purple basil, lavender, bay leaf
Apigenin	**Vegetables and fruits:** rutabaga, celery, spinach, artichoke, beet, Brussels sprouts, cabbage, celeriac, cauliflower, kale, kohlrabi, lettuce, hot pepper, sweet pepper **Spices/herbs/sweeteners/condiments/drinks:** thyme, parsley, peppermint, annual sow thistle leaves, coffee, chamomile, oregano, basil, fennel leaves, horseradish root, rosemary
Catechins	**Vegetables and fruits:** cocoa, reishi mushroom, apple, peach, coconut, nectarine, plum, grape, apricot, rhubarb, green seaweed, red seaweed, brown seaweed **Legumes/nuts/seeds/grains:** Tartary buckwheat, pecan, almond, hazelnut, chestnut, pea **Spices/herbs/sweeteners/condiments/drinks:** Green tea, oolong tea, black tea, red wine, red wine vinegar, coffee, nutmeg, ginger, rosemary
Chlorogenic acid	**Vegetables and fruits:** blackberry, blackcurrant, blueberry, raspberry, strawberry, peach, prune, potato, tomato, apple, pear, eggplant **Legumes/nuts/seeds/grains:** Tartary buckwheat, sunflower seed **Spices/herbs/sweeteners/condiments/drinks:** green tea, coffee, parsley

Curcumin	**Spices/herbs/sweeteners/condiments/drinks:** turmeric, curry
Diindolylmethane (DIM)	**Vegetables and fruits:** Brussels sprouts, garden cress, mustard greens, collard greens, turnip, kale, radish, watercress, kohlrabi, cabbage, cauliflower, bok choy, broccoli, horseradish
Ellagic acid (and its metabolite urolithin A)	**Vegetables and fruits:** blackberry, blackcurrant, blueberry, raspberry, strawberry, pomegranate, grape, brown seaweed, green seaweed **Legumes/nuts/seeds/grains:** walnut **Spices/herbs/sweeteners/condiments/drinks:** green tea, coffee
Epicatechin	**Vegetables and fruits:** cocoa, blackberry, cherry, apple, peach, strawberry, black grape, custard apple, red raspberry, cranberry, apricot, pear, nectarine, plum, persimmon, green bean, avocado, rhubarb, green grape, blackcurrant, kiwi **Legumes/nuts/seeds/grains:** fava bean, pea, cashew, pecan, pistachio, almond, hazelnut **Spices/herbs/sweeteners/condiments/drinks:** green tea, red wine, black tea, red wine vinegar, oolong tea, apple cider vinegar
Epigallocatechin gallate (EGCG)	**Vegetables and fruits:** cranberry, blackberry, raspberry, Fuji apples, Golden Delicious apple, Granny Smith apple, Red Delicious apple (skin only), plum, avocado, pear, strawberry, sweet onion **Legumes/nuts/seeds/grains:** hazelnut, pecan, pistachio **Spices/herbs/sweeteners/condiments/drinks:** green and white tea (far and away the best source, with ten times more EGCG than any other food), oolong tea, brewed black tea, carob
Equol (produced by the gut microbiome when we consume soy that contains daidzein)	**Vegetables and fruits:** kudzu root, currant, raisin, red seaweed, brown seaweed **Legumes/nuts/seeds/grains:** natto, soy protein isolate, miso, tofu, tempeh, soybean, pistachio (refer to page 137 for guidance on eating soy) **Spices/herbs/sweeteners/condiments/drinks:** Red clover
Fisetin	**Vegetables and fruits:** strawberry, apple, mango, persimmon, kiwi, grape, tomato, onion, cucumber **Spices/herbs/sweeteners/condiments/drinks:** red wine, green tea, black tea
Genistein	**Vegetables and fruits:** red seaweed, brown seaweed **Legumes/nuts/seeds/grains:** natto, miso, soybean, pistachio (refer to page 137 for guidance on eating soy) **Spices/herbs/sweeteners/condiments/drinks:** red clover
Hesperidin	**Vegetables and fruits:** orange, tangerine, lemon, lime, grapefruit, reishi mushroom, Welsh onion, green seaweed (chlorella), red seaweed, brown seaweed **Spices/herbs/sweeteners/condiments/drinks:** peppermint

Kaempferol	**Vegetables and fruits:** caper, reishi mushroom, kale, turnip greens, endive, black bean, broccoli, cabbage, red raspberry, lingonberry, cranberry, red onion, potato, leek, blueberry, currant, green grape, strawberry, tomato, broccoli sprouts, chive, apricot, apple, green bean, green seaweed (chlorella), red seaweed, brown seaweed **Legumes/nuts/seeds/grains:** Tartary buckwheat, almond, white bean **Spices/herbs/sweeteners/condiments/drinks:** oolong tea, saffron, cumin, dill, clove, basil, caraway, green tea, red wine, coffee, black tea, coconut oil, cinnamon, ginger
Luteolin	**Vegetables and fruits:** onion leaves, broccoli, globe artichoke, celery leaves, carrot, black olive, green pepper, red lettuce, lemon juice, green olive, white radish **Legumes/nuts/seeds/grains:** pistachio, lentil, pumpkin seeds **Spices/herbs/sweeteners/condiments/drinks:** peppermint, Mexican oregano, celery seed, bird's eye chili, thyme, basil, parsley, peppermint, mint, dandelion, lemon verbena, chamomile, green chili, rosemary, coffee, olive oil, red chili pepper
Lycopene	**Vegetables and fruits:** guava, tomato, watermelon, pink grapefruit, papaya, red bell pepper, persimmon, carrot, apricot, asparagus, red cabbage, mango **Spices/herbs/sweeteners/condiments/drinks:** rosehip
Myricetin	**Vegetables and fruits:** blueberry, reishi mushroom, cranberry, Welsh onion, blackcurrant **Legumes/nuts/seeds/grains:** walnut, lentil **Spices/herbs/sweeteners/condiments/drinks:** turmeric, red wine, coffee, oolong tea, dill, parlsey, coconut oil, green tea
Naringenin	**Vegetables and fruits:** grapefruit, reishi mushroom, lemon, lime, orange, tangerine, grape, tomato, seaweed **Legumes/nuts/seeds/grains:** pistachio, almond **Spices/herbs/sweeteners/condiments/drinks:** Mexican oregano, basil, peppermint, nutmeg, red wine
Proanthocyanidin	**Vegetables and fruits:** cocoa, chokeberry, blueberry, cranberry, currant, lingonberry, black plum, rhubarb, gooseberry, strawberry, bilberry, red, white, and green grape, apple, yellow plum, pear, sea buckthorn berry, peach, custard apple, apricot, red raspberry, elderberry, nectarine, blackberry, mango, cherry, date, blackcurrant, marionberry, avocado, quince, banana, carob, kiwi **Legumes/nuts/seeds/grains:** sorghum, hazelnut, kidney bean, adzuki bean, pecan, pistachio, fava bean, almond, buckwheat, black-eyed pea, walnut, red rice, black rice, pinto bean, black bean, cashew, lentil **Spices/herbs/sweeteners/condiments/drinks:** cinnamon, rosehip, hops, red wine, curry, black tea, green tea

Pterostilbene	**Vegetables and fruits:** blueberry, cranberry, bilberry, lingonberry, huckleberry, red grape **Legumes/nuts/seeds/grains:** almond
Quercetin	**Vegetables and fruits:** cranberry, black chokeberry, black olive, black elderberry, caper, cocoa, red lettuce, blueberry, lingonberry, kale, blackberry, chive, black grape, green pepper, cherry tomato, shallot, broccoli, strawberry, green lettuce, green grape, arugula, Swiss chard, Brussels sprouts, zucchini, red onion, bilberry, orange, sea buckthorn, scallion, turnip greens, green bean, peach, nectarine, garlic, red chili pepper, apple, yellow onion, plum, pomegranate, pear, green seaweed (chlorella), red seaweed, brown seaweed **Legumes/nuts/seeds/grains:** Tartary buckwheat, chia seed, almond, lentil **Spices/herbs/sweeteners/condiments/drinks:** dill, Mexican oregano, clove, basil, apple cider vinegar, garlic, green tea, black tea, oolong tea, ginger, fennel tea, cilantro, marjoram, fenugreek, coffee, turmeric, red wine, cinnamon, coconut oil
Resveratrol	**Vegetables and fruits:** lingonberry, cranberry, blueberry, red currant, bilberry, strawberry, mulberry, black grape, cocoa, green grape **Legumes/nuts/seeds/grains:** Tartary buckwheat, pistachio, lentil, almond **Spices/herbs/sweeteners/condiments/drinks:** red wine, rosé wine, white wine, apple cider vinegar
Rosmarinic acid	**Spices/herbs/sweeteners/condiments/drinks:** peppermint, rosemary, spearmint, mint, thyme, sage, oregano, basil, lemon balm, marjoram
Silibinin	**Vegetables and fruits:** artichoke **Spices/herbs/sweeteners/condiments/drinks:** milk thistle
Sulforaphane	**Vegetables and fruits:** broccoli sprouts, radish sprouts, broccoli, Brussels sprouts, kale, cauliflower, kohlrabi, collard greens, Chinese kale, daikon radish **Spices/herbs/sweeteners/condiments/drinks:** mustard seed
Ursolic acid	**Vegetables and fruits:** apple, cranberry, blueberry, prune, raisin **Spices/herbs/sweeteners/condiments/drinks:** rosemary, marjoram, lavender, thyme, oregano, holy basil, elderflower, peppermint

Active Demethylating Nutrients

The following nutrients are a subgroup of DNA methylation adaptogens that support the function of the enzymes used to remove methyl groups from hypermethylated genes (the TET enzymes I mention on page 262). One other key player essential for TET functionality is alpha ketoglutarate

(AKG). As there are no food sources of AKG (our body makes it from protein break down), it's not listed in this table, but I do cover it as a supplement on page 222.

NUTRIENT	FOODS	FUNCTIONS
Iron (eat with vitamin C–rich foods to boost absorption)	**Vegetables and fruits:** spinach, tomato, raisin **Animal protein:** oyster, beef liver, salmon, beef **Legumes/nuts/seeds/grains:** Tartary buckwheat, white bean, lentil, tofu, kidney bean, chickpea, cashew **Spices/herbs/sweeteners/condiments/drinks:** dark chocolate	Cofactor for TET enzymes (and many other proteins and enzymes) Contributes to DNA synthesis Plays a role in producing blood and transferring oxygen from lungs to tissue Both too little iron and too much are harmful—too little can lead to anemia and fatigue and poor cognition in kids; too much can damage vital organs like the heart and liver and is potently proaging Deficiency common in premenopausal women, especially if vegan Men who consume a lot of red meat are at risk of excessive intake A common genetic condition, hereditary hemochromatosis, can cause increased absorption and excessive levels of iron
Vitamin A	**Vegetables and fruits (contain carotenoids—vitamin A precursors):** sweet potato, spinach, pumpkin, carrot, cantaloupe, butternut squash, red pepper flake, collard greens, kale, turnip greens, mustard greens, dandelion greens, beet greens, turnip greens, Swiss chard, winter squash, green onion, chili pepper, garden cress, plum, sweet red pepper, broccoli rabe, brown seaweed (kelp), apricot, date, persimmon, grapefruit, orange tomato, broccoli, broccoli sprouts, green bean, purslane, vegetable broth, tangerine, scallion **Animal protein (contains preformed vitamin A):** liver, herring, egg **Fats/oils (contains preformed vitamin A):** fish oil, cod liver oil	Increases TET expression levels Works with vitamin C to increase stem cell reprogramming (mice)[2] Fat soluble Major player in the growth and specialization of all cells in the body Plays a large role in immune function, eye development, and vision Potent antiviral There are hundreds of carotenoids, including beta-carotene, 10 percent of which are capable of being synthesized into vitamin A Not everybody converts their carotenoids as readily (particularly people with hypothyroidism), so getting some preformed vitamin A is a good idea

| Vitamin C | **Vegetables and fruits:** acerola cherry, guava, red bell pepper, currant, spinach, orange, kiwi, lemon, broccoli, strawberry, Brussels sprouts, grapefruit, kohlrabi, papaya, pineapple, bitter melon, tangerine, passion fruit, lime, cantaloupe, chili pepper, mango, cabbage, cauliflower, tomato, elderberry, mulberry, bok choy, sweet potato, avocado, turnip greens, mustard greens, clementine, beet greens, rutabaga, collard greens, garden cress, raspberry, broccoli rabe, Swiss chard, butternut squash, honeydew melon, blackberry, turnip, plantain, okra, zucchini, kale, parsnip, potato, dandelion greens, plum, cranberry, pomegranate, jalapeño pepper, green bean, apricot, artichoke, kale, blueberry, goji berry, banana, collard green, watermelon, celeriac, purslane, onion, leek, peach

Legumes/nuts/seeds/grains: Tartary buckwheat, soybean, green pea, chestnut, lima bean

Spices/herbs/sweeteners/ condiments/drinks: parsley, fennel, coconut water, coriander | Key antioxidant and infection fighter

Cofactor with iron in enzymatic reactions, including TET

Works with vitamin A to increase stem cell reprogramming (mice)

Used to make collagen, heal wounds, and promote healthy skin

Helps burn fat and make neurotransmitters

Mitigates the effect of toxins and the damage of oxidative stress on different structures

Regenerates other antioxidants, like vitamin E

Plays a role in reactivating anti-inflammatory genes and tumor suppressor genes as a cofactor for TET and other epigenetic enzymes. For this reason, vitamin C is a very important player in the anti-aging space, and is associated with a lower risk of all of the main diseases of aging, including cancer, heart disease, hypertension, stroke |
| Vitamin D | **Vegetables and fruits:** mushrooms that have been exposed to sunlight

Animal protein: trout, mackerel, cod liver oil, salmon, sardine, flounder, beef liver, egg yolk, trout, pork, turkey, chicken, oyster | Needed for bone, hormonal, immune, and heart health

An important regulator of the epigenome, regulating the expression of hundreds of genes

D deficiency is associated with accelerated aging and all the diseases of aging

A 2019 study of D-deficient obese African Americans found that supplementing with 4,000 IU of vitamin D dailiy—and no other interventions—reduced their age by 1.85 years on the Horvath clock[3] |

Methyl Donors

These nutrients are also listed in alphabetical order for ease of reference, but the primary methyl donors are folate, vitamin B_{12}, betaine, and choline. All the other nutrients included in this section play a support role in the methylation cycle, either directly or indirectly.

DONOR	FOOD SOURCES	
Betaine (AKA trimethylglycine, or TMG)	**Vegetables and fruits:** spinach, beet, lambsquarters **Animal protein:** egg yolk (contains choline), liver **Legumes/nuts/seeds/grains:** quinoa, rye, sunflower seed, kamut	
Biotin (B7)	**Vegetables and fruits:** mushrooms, carrot, avocado, berries, banana, cauliflower, sweet potato, onion, Swiss chard **Animal protein:** beef liver, egg, salmon, pork, beef, tuna, turkey **Legumes/nuts/seeds/grains:** sunflower seed, almond, berries, walnut, legumes (chickpea, green pea, soybean, lentil), oat	
Choline	**Vegetables and fruits:** maitake mushroom, enoki mushroom, cauliflower, shiitake mushroom, seaweed (kelp) **Animal protein:** liver, egg yolk, whitefish, beef, salmon, trout **Legumes/nuts/seeds/grains:** lentil, flax seed, soybean	
Cobalamin (B_{12})	**Vegetables and fruits:** lesser quantities in some seaweeds, including nori, shiitake mushrooms **Animal protein:** liver (beef, turkey, duck, goose, chicken), oyster, mackerel, clam, herring, trout, snapper, crab, salmon, lamb, beef, cod, lobster, whitefish, egg, goose, pork, chicken **Spices/herbs/sweeteners/condiments/drinks:** nutritional yeast	

WHY
- Donates a methyl group to convert homocysteine back to methionine - Can be converted (through an enzymatic reaction) into folate - Helpful in regulating blood pressure, reducing homocysteine levels, and reducing fatty deposits in the liver - Choline is a precursor to betaine
- Involved in metabolizing fats, protein, and carbohydrates - Regulates blood sugar - Behind-the-scenes role in many epigenetic processes, including DNA methylation - Works with folate to turn off pro-inflammatory genes - A healthy microbiome produces biotin - Raw egg white inhibits biotin absorption
- Involved in synthesis of neurotransmitters and healthy lipid membranes - Essential for cognitive development in fetuses—so it's extra important for pregnant women to get ample amounts - Also needed for brain function later in life - Deficiency causes muscle damage and abnormal fat deposition in the liver (and nonalcoholic fatty liver disease is increasingly common in America) - A precursor to betaine - We can make choline, but the process requires methylation, and some of us have genetic differences that make our ability to produce it less efficient; for this reason, choline is considered "conditionally essential," therefore, eating plenty of choline is a good idea for most folks
- A key player in folate metabolism and synthesis of SAMe in the methylation cycle - Essential in mitochondrial energy synthesis - Essential component of the membranes that surround neurons (known as the myelin sheath) - Involved in making of neurotransmitters - Has a relatively involved absorption journey in the gut, requiring a number of different specialized proteins - Pernicious anemia is a serious, but fairly common, autoimmune disease that involves an inability to absorb B_{12} because the proteins are damaged by autoantibodies; treatment includes B_{12} injections or lozenges - Older people, those on acid-blocking medication, individuals with untreated celiac disease, or those with small intestinal bacterial overgrowth all tend to absorb B_{12} less efficiently - Because it's mostly found in animal proteins, vegans are often deficient - Low B_{12} is associated with an increased risk for cancer, as—to a lesser extent—are high levels, which can lead to abnormal epigenetic patterns associated with cancer

Cysteine	**Vegetables and fruits:** spirulina, butternut squash
	Animal protein: egg, beef, cod, pork, whitefish, fish roe, goose (skin removed), duck breast, buffalo, lamb, chicken, quail, octopus, halibut, clam
	Legumes/nuts/seeds/grains: sesame seed, tofu, soybean, black walnut, watermelon seed, oat, pumpkin seed, pistachio, flax seed
Docosahexaenoic acid (DHA)	**Vegetables and fruits:** algae contains DHA and, to a lesser extent, EPA
	Animal protein: mackerel, salmon, fish roe, anchovy, whitefish, herring, trout, bass, tilefish, sardine, halibut, oysters, squid, flatfish, mussel, shrimp, crab, perch, scallop
	Fats/oils: fish oil, cod liver oil
	Legumes/nuts/seeds/grains: DHA may be synthesized from precursor fatty acid alpha linoleic acid (ALA), which is found in chia seed, flax seed, walnut, perilla seed, hemp seed
Folate (B$_9$)	**Vegetables and fruits:** turnip greens, wakame seaweed, spinach, kelp seaweed, okra, collard greens, artichoke, asparagus, leek, enoki mushroom, daikon radish, maitake mushroom, mustard greens, shiitake mushroom
	Animal protein: liver, turkey, chicken, beef, goose, egg
	Legumes/nuts/seeds/grains: legumes (soybean, lentil, chickpea), sunflower seed, quinoa
	Spices/herbs/sweeteners/condiments/drinks: parsley, oregano, rosemary, marjoram, tarragon, thyme, bay leaf, basil, sage, cilantro, dill
Magnesium	**Vegetables and fruits:** seaweed, cocoa, leek, spinach, avocado, lambsquarters, daikon radish, horseradish
	Legumes/nuts/seeds/grains: hemp seed, Tartary buckwheat, buckwheat, pumpkin seed, amaranth, Brazil nut, sunflower seed, cashew, almond, black bean, oat, great northern bean, teff, hazelnut, mung bean, tofu, walnut, chickpea, chia seed, kidney bean, pecan, sesame seed, rye, poppy seed, quinoa, flax seed
	Spices/herbs/sweeteners/condiments/drinks: molasses, curry, nutmeg, apple cider vinegar
Methionine	**Vegetables and fruits:** spirulina
	Animal protein: anchovy, bison, buffalo, chicken, goose, pork, snapper, tilapia, duck, haddock, halibut, herring, mackerel, salmon, turkey, sardine, whitefish, beef, cod, lamb, lobster, egg
	Legumes/nuts/seeds/grains: Brazil nut, pumpkin seed, sunflower seed, sesame seed

- This sulfur amino acid is produced after methionine is broken down into SAMe and then converted to homocysteine; homocysteine can either be recycled back to methionine, or converted to cysteine, which goes on to make glutathione, sulfate, and taurine
- Ingesting sufficient cysteine in our diet indirectly helps the methylation cycle and SAMe production

---

- An omega-3 essential fatty acid that regulates multiple enzymes in the methylation cycle[4]
- Has DNA methylation adaptogenic properties
- Powerful anti-inflammatory that's essential for brain health and cognitive function
- A host of nutrients produced from DHA (and its cousin EPA) called specialized pro-resolving lipid mediators (SPMs) are potently anti-inflammatory and involved in a variety of beneficial pathways
- It's highly likely that as research on epigenetics grows we will see DHA and EPA becoming star players

---

- Although it works in concert with many nutrients, folate is the single most important nutrient involved in genetic expression, including DNA methylation
- Essential for DNA synthesis and repair
- A key methyl donor in the methylation cycle, it works with B_{12} to produce SAMe and recycle homocysteine into methionine. Because folate and B_{12} work so closely, if you're deficient in one, you're likely deficient in the other; for this reason, both are often prescribed together
- There are a number of different natural folates used in the body that are produced via the folate cycle
- A classic sign of deficiency is megaloblastic anemia, which impairs the ability to make red blood cells efficiently
- Folate deficiency can cause far-reaching problems—increasing risk of cancer, heart disease and neurological diseases; in pregnancy folate deficiency may lead to birth defects
- Folate excess has been associated with increased risk of certain cancers, especially in older individuals
- Some cancer and cholesterol-lowering drugs can inhibit synthesis and absorption of folate, and there's speculation that birth control drugs can, too
- Not to be confused with folic acid, which is synthetic (refer back to page 54 for more on the difference between the two)

- Ubiquitous and vitally important mineral involved in at least four hundred enzymatic reactions
- Essential for all ATP energy–requiring reactions
- Essential for mitochondrial function
- Helps make ATP, DNA, and proteins
- Involved in intercellular communication and intracellular transport
- Magnesium deficiency is associated with all the chronic diseases of aging, and half the US population ingests insufficient magnesium

---

- The only essential sulfur-containing amino acid, meaning your body needs it and you can't manufacture it—therefore, you must get it from your diet
- Because it is primarily found in animal protein, it can be challenging for vegans to get enough methionine (although it is in spirulina and some nuts and seeds)
- Converted to SAMe in the methylation cycle
- Also provides the sulfur for glutathione, taurine, and sulfate

Niacin B₃	**Vegetables and fruits:** enoki mushroom, maitake mushroom, shiitake mushroom, spirulina, tomato **Animal protein:** beef liver, anchovy, lamb liver, chicken, duck, chicken liver, salmon, mackerel, game meats, lamb, trout, pork, beef, cod **Legumes/nuts/seeds/grains:** sunflower seed, pecan, sesame seed **Spices/herbs/sweeteners/condiments/drinks:** cilantro, parsley, tarragon, mustard seed, chili powder
Potassium	**Vegetables and fruits:** potato, yam, dried apricot, avocado, arrowroot, tomato, spinach, portabella mushroom, Swiss chard, enoki mushroom, shiitake mushroom, lambsquarters, daikon radish, cocoa, maitake mushroom, coconut, apple **Animal protein:** salmon, cod, pork, clam **Legumes/nuts/seeds/grains:** lima bean, adzuki bean, white bean, great northern bean, pinto bean, Tartary buckwheat, lentil, kidney bean, flax seed, pistachio, mung bean, pumpkin seed, hazelnut, sunflower seed, cashew, pine nut, pecan, tahini, chia seed **Spices/herbs/sweeteners/condiments/drinks:** dried herbs, turmeric, maple syrup, cumin, oregano, apple cider vinegar, chili powder, nutmeg
Pyridoxine B₆	**Vegetables and fruits:** potato, prune, chestnut, ancho pepper, garlic, leek, shiitake mushroom, palm heart, daikon radish, dried apricot, chive **Animal protein:** turkey liver, salmon, chicken liver, octopus, goose, pork, beef, trout, cod, game meats **Legumes/nuts/seeds/grains:** rice bran, Tartary buckwheat, pistachio, sunflower seed, sesame seed, pecan, amaranth, hazelnut, black walnut, soybean, lentil, English walnut, chickpea, soybean, brown rice, pecan **Spices/herbs/sweeteners/condiments/drinks:** baker's yeast, molasses, fenugreek seed, paprika, chili powder, sage, cayenne pepper, tarragon, basil, turmeric, bay leaf, rosemary, dill, parsley, oregano, marjoram, curry powder, chervil, celery seed, ginger, cilantro, clove, thyme
Riboflavin B₂	**Vegetables and fruits:** spirulina, chive, shiitake mushroom, daikon radish **Animal protein:** lamb liver, beef liver, egg, chicken liver, duck liver, goose liver, game meats, mackerel, fish roe **Legumes/nuts/seeds/grains:** Tartary buckwheat, almond, soybean, pecan, sesame seed **Spices/herbs/sweeteners/condiments/drinks:** paprika, cilantro, spearmint, tarragon, parsley, cayenne pepper, chili powder, chervil **Dairy:** goat cheese, brie cheese

- When activated, niacin is transformed into a compound called NAD (nicotinamide), which is a cofactor in many enzymatic reactions, including those involved in the methylation cycle
- An important player in gene stability, DNA repair, mitochondrial function, and overall health
- NAD decreases with age, and thus a variety of compounds that are converted to NAD in the body—including nicotinamide riboside (NR) and nicotinamide mononucleotide (NMN)—are considered to be rising stars in the anti-aging world

---

- Key electrolyte and fundamental player in the electrochemical system, helping heart to pump, nerves to fire, muscles to contract, and cellular transport
- The vast majority of Americans aren't getting enough potassium; it is considered "a nutrient of public concern" according to the 2015–2020 Dietary Guidelines for Americans
- Insufficient potassium is associated with heart disease, hypertension, heart arrythmias
- Works with sodium in cellular transport, so important to maintain a close potassium-to-sodium ratio; which most Americans do not successfully do, as the standard American diet is a high-sodium, low-potassium diet
- Humans are the only mammals to ingest more sodium than potassium

---

- Essential for over one hundred enzymatic reactions
- Involved in the folate cycle and the synthesis of glutathione, sulfate, and taurine from homocysteine
- A number of drugs can interfere with B_6 metabolism, including nonsteroidal anti-inflammatory drugs (such as ibuprofen), birth control, and certain Parkinson's disease medications

---

- Required for many enzymatic reactions
- Along with niacin, riboflavin is essential for both the methylation and folate cycles
- Deficiency of riboflavin can lead to a secondary folate deficiency by impairing the folate cycle; this can then in turn impair the methylation cycle
- Helps synthesize ATP, our body's main energy source
- Some individuals with MTHFR variant (see page 266) may require extra riboflavin

Sulfur	**Vegetables and fruits:** alliums (chive, leek, garlic, onion, shallot), cruciferous vegetables (arugula, bok choy, broccoli, Brussels sprouts, cabbage, cauliflower, collard greens, daikon, horseradish root, kale, kohlrabi, mustard greens, radish, rutabaga, tatsoi, turnip, watercress, wasabi), garden cress, coconut, spinach
	Animal protein: egg, cod, haddock, salmon, sardine, scallop, lamb, beef, chicken, pork, duck, goose, turkey, whey and casein
	Legumes/nuts/seeds/grains: lentil, pea, butter bean, barley, oat, haricot bean, hazelnut, chickpea, Brazil nut, almond, walnut
	Spices/herbs/sweeteners/condiments/drinks: ginger
Taurine	**Animal protein:** scallop, mussel, clam, oyster, squid, egg, octopus, cod, pork, veal, beef, chicken, turkey, shrimp
	Spices/herbs/sweeteners/condiments/drinks: brewer's yeast
Zinc	**Vegetables and fruits:** shiitake mushroom, cocoa, seaweed (agar)
	Animal protein: oyster, beef, lamb, lobster, crab, bison, pork, game meats, turkey
	Legumes/nuts/seeds/grains: rice bran, dark rye, pumpkin seed, Tartary buckwheat, pine nut, poppy seed, sesame seed
	Spices/herbs/sweeteners/condiments/drinks: celery seed, chervil, cardamom, mustard seed, thyme, parsley, basil

- Along with calcium and phosphorus, sulfur is the most abundant mineral in the body
- We use methionine, an essential sulfur-containing amino acid, to make SAMe
- SAMe (after it donates its methyl group) becomes homocysteine, which is recycled back to methionine or donates its sulfur to make the important compounds glutathione, taurine, and sulfate
- Vegans and older individuals typically take in lower amounts of sulfur-containing amino acids

- Sulfur-containing amino acid that is a derivative of methionine
- Considered to be conditionally essential, as we tend not to make enough taurine, especially if methionine intake is low (typically that means older people and/or vegetarians/vegans)
- Major player in heart muscle, skeletal muscle, vision, the central nervous system, and detoxification
- Functions as antioxidant
- Can be an important intervention for cardiac arrhythmias and hypertension

- Essential for a number of enzymes, including one of the enzymes involved in the methylation cycle
- Required to stabilize DNA and many proteins in the body, giving it far-reaching importance
- Deficiency associated with impaired growth, pregnancy complications, immune dysfunction, and increased risk of infections
- Excess zinc intake may result in a copper deficiency

THE METHYLATION CYCLE

I N ORDER TO UNDERSTAND HOW METHYL DONORS LIKE B_{12} AND FOLATE actually work to support DNA methylation, it helps to have a basic understanding of how methylation—of all types, including DNA methylation—works. The image below shows you a very simplified version of the methylation cycle.

Ingredients

PRIMARY PLAYERS

Folate	Vitamin B_{12}	Betaine

SECONDARY NUTRIENTS USED DIRECTLY IN THE METHYLATION CYCLE

Methionine	Riboflavin (B_2)	Potassium
Choline	Niacin (B_3)	Zinc
Pyridoxine (B_6)	Magnesium	

NUTRIENTS THAT SUPPORT THE NUTRIENTS USED IN THE METHYLATION CYCLE

Sulfur	Cysteine	DHA
Taurine	Biotin (B_7)	

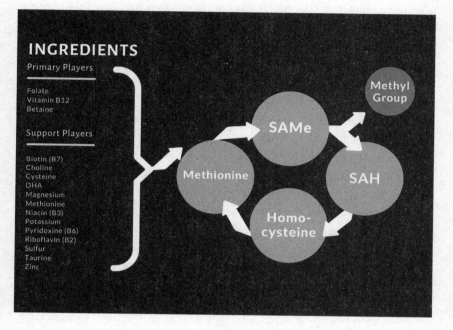

The ingredients of the methylation cycle listed above help convert methionine (an amino acid we get from animal protein) into S-adenosylmethionine (SAMe)—the universal methyl donor used in most forms of biochemical methylation, including DNA methylation. SAMe quite literally donates a methyl group to the hundreds of methylation enzymatic reactions that are happening all of the time throughout the body, including on strands of DNA.

Once SAMe delivers its methyl group, it becomes S adenosyl homocysteine (SAH). Then SAH is converted to homocysteine. With the addition of B_{12} and folate, or betaine, homocysteine is then converted back to SAMe. The methylation cycle is whirring through these steps nonstop, over and over again, all the time, throughout our lives.

DNA Methylation: Common Terms and Definitions

With few exceptions, in humans, DNA methylation happens at the fifth carbon position on the DNA nucleotide cytosine, but only when cytosine is sitting next to guanine, hence the common DNA methylation abbreviation CpG, where "p" refers to the phosphate that connects the nucleotides. Most often, DNA methylation occurs on the gene's promotor region (a regulatory region that directs whether a gene is on or off). Scientific figures denote a methylated site using a red ball on a black line stuck atop a strand of DNA (making them look like red lollipops).

- **Hypomethylation** describes a state where a gene's promoter region is only lightly methylated or not at all (and there are few to no little red lollipops present). Hypomethylation allows the gene to be turned on. You can think of it almost like a traffic light—the less red there is, the more the gene gets the signal to go. Generally speaking, hypomethylation is a negative descriptor of a gene that should be off (e.g., a proinflammatory gene) having been inappropriately methylated and, therefore, turned on.

- **Hypermethylation** is just the opposite—a gene that has an overabundance of methyl groups attached and, therefore, can't be turned on. In this case, it's more like a parking lot—those red lollipops take up all the available spaces so that there's no room for transcription factors—proteins that activate DNA—to land. Hypermethylation is generally used to describe a state in which a good gene, like a tumor-suppressor gene, is inappropriately turned off.

- **Demethylation** is an essential epigenetic process by which a hypermethylated gene can be re-expressed. Depending on circumstance, it can be beneficial or harmful. There are two types of demethylation: (1) *passive demethylation*, which is when the DNA methylation marks that are present on a DNA strand are not copied during DNA replication. This can happen for a few reasons, such as a lack of available methyl donors, toxin interference, or enzyme inhibition. While all passive demethylation isn't necessarily healthy, we think that DNA methylation adaptogens, like EGCG, support the re-expression of good genes through passive demethylation; and (2) *active demethylation*, which occurs when enzymes actively remove the attached methyl group so that it no longer has influence over the gene (more information on the enzymes that perform this function below).

Enzymes Involved in DNA Methylation

Methyl groups don't decide to plop down on, or pop off of, DNA on their own. There are specific enzymes that do the deciding of which cytosine gets the methyl group, or which methyl groups are removed. It's difficult to overstate how important these enzymes are; different members of these enzymatic families direct the development of embryos, tell pluripotent stem cells what types of cells they'll develop into, remove DNA methylation marks from parental DNA, and direct DNA methylation in response to a wide array of inputs. These enzymes, listed below, are on the front line of the interface between living your life and your genetic material and are influenced by many things—nutrients, stress, toxins, hormones, exercise, sleep, meditation . . . basically everything. So while we say we are seeking to support healthy DNA methylation, the way we do that is by supporting the healthy function of the enzymes that regulate DNA methylation.

The enzymes involved in DNA methylation include:

- **DNA methyltransferase (DNMT)** family of enzymes puts the methyl groups on DNA. Research suggests that the polyphenols we're calling DNA methylation adaptogens generally work by inhibiting DNMT.
- **Ten-eleven translocation (TET)** family of enzymes takes methyl groups off of DNA via a multistep process of oxidation. Nutrients that work with TET include vitamin C, vitamin A, iron, and alpha ketoglutarate (AKG).

RESOURCES

My Website

My website is home to:

- My blog, where I cover research related to bio age and DNA methylation and other topics in functional medicine
- My podcast, *New Frontiers in Functional Medicine*, where I interview thought leaders in the functional medicine space
- Links to bio age testing and supplements

Website: www.drkarafitzgerald.com

Younger You Digital Program

While helping our patients succeed with the Younger You Intensive and Everyday programs, we noticed that what they needed most was an easy way to track their progress. As a result, we created an app that is your digital support guide to everything Younger You. With features that enable you to track your daily food intake, sleep, relaxation, exercise, fasting window, and more, it offers insight, motivation, and accountability. It also keeps tabs on your biological age with an interactive version of the Bio Age Self-Assessment (BASA, which appears in print form on page 77 of this book) and automated evaluation of your lab results. Additionally, you can order some of the blood tests I mention on page 89, supplements, and even an epigenetic assessment of your DNA methylation so that you can see the results of your efforts to reduce your biological age for yourself—which offers the best motivation to keep going. Younger You digital program users can also individualize the Younger You plan via access to our digital nutrition coaches.

Website: YoungerYouProgram.com

Institute for Functional Medicine

Functional medicine offers a powerful new operating system and clinical model for assessment, treatment, and prevention of chronic disease to replace the outdated and often ineffective acute-care models carried forward from the twentieth century.

Functional medicine translates the latest clinical and scientific research (including omics: genome, epigenome, microbiome, etc.) into safe, whole-person medicine that recognizes the influence of environment and lifestyle factors on emergence and progression of disease.

You can find one near you by using the Institute for Functional Medicine's Find A Practitioner referral network—a comprehensive, searchable network of clinicians in various specialties and health-care professions.

The listings that feature an "IFM Certified Practitioner" badge are licensed and practicing health-care professionals who have completed the IFM Certification Program, which is the highest level of education available in functional medicine. All practitioners in the network have attended IFM's five-day foundational course, Applying Functional Medicine in Clinical Practice (AFMCP) and are also current IFM members.

Website: www.ifm.org/find-a-practitioner/

My Sandy Hook Clinic

My clinic, which is located in the Sandy Hook Village section of Newtown, Connecticut, consists of a multidisciplinary team of MDs, NDs, and nutritionists. Our core team of practitioners at the Sandy Hook Clinic are all IFM Certified.

If you can't make it to the clinic in person, we offer telehealth consultations via Zoom and other platforms as an alternative.

We have a world-renowned nutrition program, including a highly competitive nutritional training program. We offer nutritional consultations via Zoom and other platforms. In my experience, nutrition support is essential for good outcomes in functional medicine, regardless of how experienced (or trained) a patient may be. Having that additional help dialing in a therapeutic plan is vital. Every patient in our clinic receives nutrition support; we also offer nutrition consults as a stand-alone option—that is, no doctor required.

Website: www.drkarafitzgerald.com/our-clinic/

GrowBaby Health

This Grants Pass, Oregon, clinic, led by the mother-daughter team of Ob/Gyn Leslie Stone, MD, and certified nutrition consultant Emily Rydbom, CN, BCHN, CNP, uses nutrition and a focus on methylation to improve birth outcomes. They work with women and couples who are seeking to conceive in person; they also offer online group programs and educational videos for each trimester.

Website: http://growbabyhealth.com

DNA METHYLATION CLOCKS
TO ASSESS BIO AGE

THESE ARE THE BIO AGE CLOCKS THAT ARE AVAILABLE TO CONSUMers at the time of this writing. Note that some laboratories require blood to do their testing while others require saliva. Whichever lab you choose to take your baseline bio age measurement, make sure you get your follow-up test from the same lab using the same specimen type. After you've gotten your initial baseline and follow-up tests, you can change labs for your next series of tests if you like. Because different laboratories use different DNA methylation clocks, you cannot expect results from different tests to be the same. Although whether your bio age is increasing or decreasing should be consistent regardless of laboratory or test.

YY BioAge Plus

This is the suite of tests that my team and I created; it assesses multiple bio age clocks as well as the DNA methylation status of select nutrient-responsive genes.

www.drkarafitzgerald.com

epiAge

This bio age assessment is from Dr. Moshe Szyf's laboratory.
www.hkgepitherapeutics.com

TruAge Epigenetic Test Kit

Requires a clinician to order.
www.trudiagnostic.com

Elysium Index

www.elysiumhealth.com/en-us/index

Epimorphy

www.myDNAge.com

NONTOXIC CLEANING PRODUCTS

Visit the Environmental Working Group (www.ewg.org/guides/cleaners) to peruse their cleaning product recommendations. Ratings include: the presence of known hazardous materials, ingredient disclosure and transparency, other potential risks such as high acid or caustic agent content, potentially toxic packaging, and unclear ingredient verbiage ("natural cleansers," "eco-friendly," "nontoxic") without further ingredient disclosure. They also note whether each product is using animal testing methods or not.

Specific products we recommend, based on EWG's guidance:

- AspenClean Natural Bathroom Cleaner, the safest-rated bathroom cleaner.
- CLR Mold & Mildew Clear, the safest-rated shower mildew/mold remover.
- Seventh Generation Disinfecting Bathroom Cleaner, highly rated disinfecting bathroom spray.
- CloroxPro Disinfecting Bio Stain & Odor Remover, scores an A overall but has some less favorable ingredients.

ENVIRONMENTAL TESTING

Air Pollution Testing

While it is not possible to determine exact levels of heavy metals in the air through these sites, you can get some idea of the levels of air pollution in your home, which can include heavy metal particulates.

- https://www.epa.gov/indoor-air-quality-iaq/care-your-air-guide -indoor-air-quality
- www.airnow.gov
- www.lung.org/our-initiatives/healthy-air/sota

Water Testing

We recommend National Testing Laboratories for water testing.
https://watercheck.com

Soil Testing

We recommend anyone starting a vegetable garden check for soil contamination by toxins such as PCBs and lead. In the United States, many state universities and local governments offer basic soil testing for low or no cost. Do an internet search for "soil testing" and your state to see what's available near you.

SUPPLEMENTS

Beef Liver Supplements

For those of us who are a little less gung ho on buying and preparing liver (me included), you can get clean-sourced, encapsulated freeze-dried liver in supplement form. I suggest getting products that are not defatted, so the fat soluble vitamins, including preformed vitamin A (retinol), D, E, and K, are present, just as they would be if you ate liver.

ENVIROMEDICA PASTURED BEEF LIVER FOR ALLERGY CONCERNS

- Only contains liver and gelatin
- Free of dairy, wheat, yeast, gluten, corn, sugar, soy, shellfish, tree nuts, stearates, fillers, flow agents, or any other potentially irritating ingredients

WHOLESOME WELLNESS GRASS-FED DESICCATED BEEF LIVER CAPSULES

- Cows humanely pasture-raised in New Zealand without chemicals or hormones
- No fillers, no flow agents, GMO-free
- Freeze-dried to preserve all of the nutrients and cofactors

PALEOVALLEY GRASS FED ORGAN COMPLEX

- Beef liver, heart, and kidney
- Freeze-dried
- Non-GMO
- Grass-fed

ADAPT NATURALS BIO-AVAIL ORGAN

- Freeze-dried
- Grass-fed and finished organ meat
- Pesticide-, hormone-, antibiotic-free
- No artificial or synthetic ingredients

Beet Supplements

I recognize that beets can also be viewed unfavorably, yet betaine is so important to DNA methylation that you don't want to forego them altogether. If you truly can't stomach beets—or learn to love them—take them in supplement form instead, either as powder or capsules. Follow instructions on label to determine dosage.

PEAK PERFORMANCE ORGANIC BEET ROOT POWDER AND CAPSULES

- The capsules contain only cellulose and organic beets and their powder contains just organic beets
- Sugar content is 1 gram per serving
- Free of yeast, wheat, gluten, milk, eggs, fish, shellfish, and tree nuts

HUMAN N BEETELITE POWDER

- Non-GMO
- Fermented beets
- 7 grams sugar per serving

QULTURED™ FERMENTED BEETS

- Contains only organic fermented beets and less than 1 gram sugar
- Fermenting reduces the sugar content of beets and increases their nutrient content

Greens Powders

Adding a quality greens powder to a smoothie, plant-based yogurt, or even a glass of water or Beet Bubbly is a convenient and easy way to help ensure that you meet your daily greens requirement on both the Younger You Intensive and Everyday.

ORGANIC GREENS AND REDS, DOUGLAS LABORATORIES

- In addition to greens, this also includes green tea extract, beet powder, and vitamin C, covering a lot of bases

PALEOGREENS, DESIGNS FOR HEALTH

- Over 90 percent organic ingredients
- No grains, legumes, gluten, or fructose
- In addition to greens, includes apple, blueberry, cranberry, raspberry, camu camu berry, and grape skin powders

PHYTOGANIX® METAGENICS

- Non-GMO, gluten-free, and vegetarian
- Blend of seeds, vegetables, fruits, herbs, mushrooms, green tea, enzymes, and probiotics

Vegan Protein Powders

Putting some protein powder in a morning smoothie is a great way for vegans to ensure that they're getting adequate protein. These are the specific powders we recommend in our practice because their ingredients are clean and most have a full panel of amino acids.

OMEGA NUTRITION ORGANIC PUMPKIN SEED PROTEIN POWDER

- Gluten-free

INNATE RESPONSE FORMULAS VEGAN PROTEIN POWDER

- Vanilla flavored
- Pea protein
- Uses stevia and cinnamon for sweetness

JARROW FORMULAS PUMPKIN SEED PROTEIN POWDER

- Gluten-free
- Soy-free

DESIGNS FOR HEALTH PURE PEA PROTEIN

- Comes in chocolate, vanilla, and unflavored
- Uses stevia for sweetness

NUZEST CLEAN LEAN PROTEIN

- Raw
- Paleo-friendly
- 0 grams sugar

Supplement Companies Our Clinic Uses and Trusts

For other supplements I suggest in Chapter 8, these are the companies I rely on to provide the highest-quality supplements for our patients. Full disclosure: some, but not all, of these companies may sponsor our blogs, podcasts, and/or social media content.

- Metagenics
- Integrative Therapeutics
- Big Bold Health
- Designs for Health
- Ortho Molecular Products
- Klaire Labs
- Jigsaw Health
- Optimum Nutrition

- Life Extension
- Thorne
- Vital Nutrients
- NeuroProtek
- Real Mushrooms
- Tru Niagen
- T.A. Sciences
- Biotics Research
- NutriDyn
- Biocidin
- Women's International Pharmacy

ACKNOWLEDGMENTS

I T WAS AROUND 2013 WHEN I REALLY STARTED TO TUSSLE WITH THE literature on epigenetics and became entranced (and somewhat horrified) by the science regarding DNA methylation as it relates to cancer. The more I learned, the more I saw that other chronic diseases—including aging itself—share some of the same pathological DNA methylation signatures as cancer.

My next question was obvious: how might we tend to DNA methylation, through a functional medicine lens, in patient care? Unbeknownst to me at the time, answering this question would change my career. There are so many people who have helped me expand my understanding and spread the word about all I've learned.

Romilly Hodges, MS, CNS, my sister in science and the founding director of our nutrition programs at Sandy Hook Clinic, you have been deeply in the "tussle" with me, as we dialoged endlessly about the meaning of what we were reading, and how we might favorably, safely influence DNA methylation patterns. The 2016 e-book that you and I cowrote for other functional medicine professionals, *Methylation Diet and Lifestyle: Whole Being Support for Healthy Methylation and Epigenetic Expression*, laid the foundation for this book. I am deeply indebted to you for walking with me for so many years on this methylation journey. You did the heavy lifting on designing the nutrient ratios to ensure our epi-nutrient targets were achieved, and that our recipes were palatable and doable in our study and in the real world.

Jeff Bland, PhD, you have been a mentor to me—as you have for so many of us in functional medicine—for twenty-plus years, since I was a medical student and heard your brilliant lecture on the biochemistry of hops and estrogen. You have been a constant source of strength and encouragement. Having you as a bedrock of unwavering faith in me and my team's ability to execute our vision has been essential to our success.

Brent Eck, CEO, Metagenics, Inc. Thank you, thank you, thank you for having those early, open, honest, and sometimes scary conversations with me on how our interventions might be influencing epigenetic expression (favorably or not) and providing us with the unrestricted funding and support to dig in and answer our questions. I am forever indebted to you and the entire Metagenics team, including **Nikky Contractor, PhD, Kim Koch, and Kirti Salunkhe, MD**.

Executing a multivariable trial such as ours is no small feat; it takes a village of brilliant, committed scientists, nutritionists, and support staff. Thank you to my coprincipal investigator at National University of Natural Medicine's Helfgott Research Institute, **Ryan Bradley, ND, MPH**. You helmed the ship of this study with the utmost scientific rigor and integrity. Thank you also to your team at NUNM, **Doug Hanes, PhD, and Emily Stack**.

I am deeply indebted to **Moshe Szyf, PhD,** pioneer in the field of epigenetics. In 2017 I had the opportunity to podcast with you, where I introduced you to what was then just a bud of a study idea. Your guidance in all phases helped it flourish. While I know we've written the book for a broader audience, I hope we've done the science sufficient justice. Also at McGill, **David Cheishvili, PhD,** assisted us with endless questions and statistical analysis. I look forward to continued collaborations.

It's handy to become good friends with a brilliant biostatistician and gerontologist. **Josh Mitteldorf, PhD,** worked on the DNAmAge clock data analysis and continues to be willing to spend a lot of time dialoging with me on everything pertaining to longevity epigenetics. I look forward to our continued work together and the successful launch of your DataBeta study.

It's been argued that our study nutrition team (most of them graduates of our clinic internship program) were the difference between our study's success vs. failure. Of course, I am wildly appreciative to all of you for volunteering your time and I hope we continue to collaborate: **Despina Giannopoulou, CNS, Janine Henkel, CNS, Josette Herdell, CNS, Sally Logan, CNS, and Melissa Twedt, CNS**.

An extra thanks to **Josette Herdell, CNS**, for analyzing the epinutrient content on the recipes. Thank you also to our nutrition interns who helped: **Michelle Didner, MS, Miranda Kusi, MS, Jacquelyn Lombari, MS, Carrie A Newsome, BSN, RN, MSACN, CNS, Megan Pfiffner, MS, Andrew Sisisky, JD, MS, Hili Ben-David, MD, IFMCP, Gretchen DePalma, MS, CNS, CDN, Carrie J. Ettinger, MS, CNS, Tammi Hall, MS, Ann Haren, MS, Sally Logan, MS, CNS, Karin Michalk, MS, PT, CN, CNS, Amy Pabbi, MS, INHC, Dione Sordi**.

Thank you to **Melissa Parker, CNS**, who not only worked on our vegan recipe development (and is another brilliant program graduate), but shared her own personal journey of recovery from cancer in Chapter 10.

I am indebted to the **Institute for Functional Medicine**, specifically **Patrick Hanaway, MD, Laurie Hoffman, David Jones, MD, Robert Luby, MD, Dan Lukaczer, ND, Amy Mack, and Chris D'Adamo, PhD**, for your support of our work. My gratitude runs deep. Thank you to my FM peeps for your support (and challenges): **Cheryl Burdette, ND, Sara Gottfried, MD, Shalesh Khalsa, MD, PhD, Todd LaPine, MD, Helen Messier, MD, PhD, Amy Myers, MD, Cass Nelson-Dooley, MS, Joe Pizzorno, ND, Bob Rountree, MD, Tom Sult, MD, Sam Yanuck, DC**, and the early adopters at **Cleveland Clinic Center for Functional Medicine**.

Thank you to **Lucia Aronica, PhD**, nutritional epigeneticist and Stanford faculty who has cheerleaded our project since the start. I am so grateful for your support, insight, understanding, and friendship. Thank you for your scientific review of *Younger You* and the late-night responses to my urgent inquiries. I look forward to our continued collaboration.

To **Drs. Michael** and **Leslie Stone** and daughter **Emily Rydbom CNP** at Stone Medical and GrowBabyHealth: I am honored that you are incorporating ideas from Younger You into your program and research.

Thank you to the journal *Aging* for publishing our first study. We appreciate your enthusiasm and support.

Stephanie Tade, my agent: thank you, thank you, thank you for your years-long commitment to our work. I adore you and appreciate your support and belief in our project.

Mary Ann Naples, Renée Sedliar, and the team at Hachette: I knew as soon as we all met that you were the badass team to launch this project. Thank you for your extraordinary skills in making this book happen.

And to **Kate Hanley**, my cowriter supreme: could I be working with a better, more entertaining soul sister and translator of really tough science? Who hits deadlines and is uberorganized? We wrote this bad boy during COVID. How 'bout that! You have been more in the trenches with me over the last year-plus than, really, anyone else! Thank YOU.

Thank you to **Victor Chapla, Shai Rosen, and Erica Sanders at Suggestic**. You are bringing the digital platform of Younger You to life, enabling us to make the bio age testing, program, nutritionists, book, products, and future research accessible to anyone, anywhere.

To my team at **Accelerate360, Weston Gardner and Jonathon Jacobs**: Thank you for walking our work out into the world in such a beautiful way.

As some of you may know, for the last six years, I've been hosting the podcast *New Frontiers in Functional Medicine*. As I say every episode, I am interviewing the best minds in functional medicine, specifically **Dale Bredesen, MD, Randy Jirtle, PhD, Volter Longo, PhD, David Perlmutter, MD, and David Sinclair, PhD**. Their interest in this work bolstered my confidence that we might be onto something. And thank you to our producer **Kate Mayer** for making it happen each month.

Thank you to my dearest mentor: **Richard Lord, PhD**. Without your mentorship during my time at the laboratory, your endless teaching, your unending passion for nutritional biochemistry, your thinking outside of the box, and your "embracing the uncertainty," I don't know that these next phases of my career would've happened. I am indebted to you.

To our study participants: Thank you for your time, energy, attention, and commitment.

To our many patients at SHC practicing the program: Thank you!

THANK YOU to the extraordinary group of super smart, hardworking, and creative physicians and nutritionists that make our clinic a one-of-a-kind place to practice medicine. Thank you for hanging in with the insanity of our study and our book. You are my touchstones, and I practice medicine better because of all of you: **Lizzie Bird, MD, Stacey Cantor-Adkins, MD, Gretchen DePalma, CNS, Darisa Espinal, ND, Karen Herb, CNS, Jessica Kovalchik, DC, CNS, Ken Litwin, MD, Rachel Surprenant, ND, and Lara Zakaria, PharmD, MS, CNS**.

Our clinic management team, who have patiently put up with my madness and absence for the last three-plus-plus years, and who've coordinated a bear of a schedule, juggled crazy finances, and supported all of us to reach higher and dig deeper in the practice of functional medicine: THANK YOU, thank you thank you: **Sam Bucur, Karen Frank, Karen Herb, and Rhonda Timmons**.

Thank you to Brigid Krane and Samantha Bucur for the book illustrations.

And finally, to my family and my amazing care team.

Yolanda, you are my nanny as much as Isabella's. You make our lives work seamlessly. Thank you for loving my daughter and taking such good care of us. Yo te quiero.

Mom, Evan, Brigid, Dad, Jim, Rob, Chloe, Jay, and Connie: I appreciate your endless interest in this work. Mom, because "methylation is good for you," you make a delish version of our lemon tart at every holiday occasion. Iz and I can't get enough. XXOO

NOTES

INTRODUCTION

1. S. H. Woolf and H. Schoomaker, "Life Expectancy and Mortality Rates in the United States, 1959–2017," *JAMA* 322, no. 20 (2019): 1996–2016, doi: 10.1001/jama.2019.16932.

2. World Health Organization, "Top 10 Causes of Death," May 24, 2018, www.who.int/en/news-room/fact-sheets/detail/the-top-10-causes-of-death.

3. Tim Peterson, "Healthspan Is More Important Than Lifespan, So Why Don't More People Know About It?," May 30, 2017, https://publichealth.wustl.edu/heatlhspan-is-more-important-than-lifespan-so-why-dont-more-people-know-about-it/.

4. J. F. Fries, "Aging, Natural Death, and the Compression of Morbidity," *New England Journal of Medicine* 303, no. 3 (July 17, 1980): 130–135, doi: 10.1056/NEJM198007173030304.

CHAPTER 1

1. Zion Market Research, "Anti-Aging Market to Touch US $216.5 Billion by End of 2021, Globally: ZMR Report," August 30, 2018, www.globenewswire.com/news-release/2018/08/30/1563523/0/en/Anti-Aging-Market-To-Touch-US-216-52-Billion-By-the-End-of-2021-Globally-ZMR-Report.html.

2. Sarah Corapi, "Why Slowing the Aging Process Could Save the U.S. Trillions," *PBS Newshour*, October 7, 2013, www.pbs.org/newshour/health/why-delaying-aging-might-be-possible-and-very-important.

3. Rabah Kamal, Daniel McDermott, Giorlando Ramirez, and Cynthia Cox, "Health System Tracker," Peterson-KFF, December 23, 2020, www.healthsystemtracker.org/chart-collection/u-s-spending-healthcare-changed-time/#item-usspendingovertime_3.

4. A. J. Scott, M. Ellison, and D. A. Sinclair, "The Economic Value of Targeting Aging," Nature Aging 1 (2021): 616–623, doi: 10.1038/s43587-021-00080-0.

5. Hannah Ashworth, "How Long Is Your DNA?," *BBC Science Focus Magazine*, www.sciencefocus.com/the-human-body/how-long-is-your-dna/.

6. Moshe Szyf, "Episode 22," *New Frontiers in Functional Medicine* (podcast), www.drkarafitzgerald.com/2017/03/15/episode-22-gene-whispering-with-dr-moshe-szyf/.

7. S. R. Moore et al., "Epigenetic Correlates of Neonatal Contact in Humans," *Development and Psychopathology* 29, no. 5 (December 2017): 1517–1538, doi: 10.1017/S0954579417001213.

8. Dr. Kara Fitzgerald and Dr. David Sinclair, "Understanding Genetics of Aging with Harvard Professor Dr. David Sinclair, *New Frontiers in Functional Medicine* (podcast), www.drkarafitzgerald.com/2020/08/01/understanding-genetics-of-aging-with-harvard-professor-dr-david-sinclair/.

9. A. El-Osta et al., "Transient High Glucose Causes Persistent Epigenetic Changes and Altered Gene Expression During Subsequent Normoglycemia," *Journal of Experimental Medicine* 205, no.10 (2008): 2409–2417, doi: 10.1084/jem.20081188.

10. V. Vigorelli et al., "Abnormal DNA Methylation Induced by Hyperglycemia Reduces CXCR4 Gene Expression in CD34+ Stem Cells," *Journal of the American Heart Association* 8, no. 9 (2019), doi: 10.1161/JAHA.118.010012.

11. E. Barrón-Cabrera et al., "Epigenetic Modifications as Outcomes of Exercise Interventions Related to Specific Metabolic Alterations: A Systematic Review," *Lifestyle Genomics* 12, no. 1–6 (2019): 25–44, doi: 10.1159/000503289.

12. Josh Mitteldorf and Dorion Sagan, *Cracking the Aging Code* (New York: Flatiron Books, 2017).

13. A. Lu et al., "Universal DNA Methylation Age Across Mammalian Tissues," (2021), doi: 10.1101/2021.01.18.426733.

14. G. M. Fahy et al., "Reversal of Epigenetic Aging and Immunosenescent Trends in Humans," *Aging Cell* 18, no. 6 (2019): e13028, doi: 10.1111/acel.13028.

15. A. A. M. Berendsen et al., "Changes in Dietary Intake and Adherence to the NU-AGE Diet Following a One-Year Dietary Intervention Among European Older Adults—Results of the NU-AGE Randomized Trial," *Nutrients* 10, no. 12 (2018): 1905, doi: 10.3390/nu10121905.

16. N. Gensous et al., "One-Year Mediterranean Diet Promotes Epigenetic Rejuvenation with Country- and Sex-Specific Effects: A Pilot Study from the NU-AGE Project," *GeroScience* 42 (2020): 687–701, doi: 10.1007s11357-019-00149-0.

17. L. Chen et al., "Effects of Vitamin D$_3$ Supplementation on Epigenetic Aging in Overweight and Obese African Americans with Suboptimal Vitamin D Status: A Randomized Clinical Trial," *Journals of Gerontology Series A: Biological Sciences and Medical Sciences* 74, no. 1 (January 1, 2019): 91–98, doi: 10.1093/gerona/gly223.

CHAPTER 2

1. Antonio Regaldo, "More Than 26 Million People Have Taken an At-Home Ancestry Test," *MIT Technology Review*, February 11, 2019, www.technologyre

view.com/2019/02/11/103446/more-than-26-million-people-have-taken-an-at
-home-ancestry-test/.

2. National Center for Health Statistics, "Obesity and Overweight," Centers for Disease Control and Prevention, www.cdc.gov/nchs/fastats/obesity-overweight .htm.

3. L. O. Schulz and L. S. Chaudhari, "High-risk Populations: The Pimas of Arizona and Mexico," *Current Obesity Reports* 4, no. 1 (March): 92–98, doi: 10.1007 /s13679-014-0132-9.

4. C. Ling and T. Rönn, "Epigenetics in Human Obesity and Type 2 Diabetes," *Cell Metabolism* 29, no. 5 (May 7, 2019):1028–1044, doi: 10.1016/j.cmet.2019 .03.009.

5. Jordan Imhoff, "Health Inequality Actually Is a 'Black and White' Issue, Research Says," University of Michigan Health, June 3, 2020, https://healthblog .uofmhealth.org/lifestyle/health-inequality-actually-a-black-and-white-issue-research -says.

6. Francine E. Garrett-Bakelman et al., "The NASA Twins Study: A Multi-dimensional Analysis of a Year-Long Human Spaceflight," *Science* 364, no. 6436 (April 12, 2019): eaau8650, doi: 10.1126/science.aau8650.

7. Erike Hayasaki, "Identical Twins Hint at How Environments Change Gene Expression," *The Atlantic*, May 15, 2018, www.theatlantic.com/science/archive /2018/05/twin-epigenetics/560189/.

8. Breast Cancer Prevention Partners, "Organic Solvents," www.bcpp.org/re source/organic-solvents/.

9. Andrea Baccarelli et al., "Rapid DNA Methylation Changes After Exposure to Traffic Particles," *American Journal of Respiratory and Critical Care Medicine* 179, no. 7 (April 1, 2009): 572–578, doi: 10.1164/rccm.200807-1097OC.

10. R. A. Waterland and R. L. Jirtle, "Transposable Elements: Targets for Early Nutritional Effects on Epigenetic Gene Regulation," *Molecular and Cellular Biology* 23, no. 15 (August 2003): 5293–5300, doi: 10.1128/MCB.23.15.5293-5300 .2003.

11. E. W. Tobi et al., "DNA Methylation as a Mediator of the Association Between Prenatal Adversity and Risk Factors for Metabolic Disease in Adulthood," *Science Advances* 4, no. 1 (January 31, 2018): eaao4364, doi: 10.1126/sciadv .aao4364.

12. Ibid.

13. Carl Zimmer, "The Famine Ended 70 Years Ago, but Dutch Genes Still Bear Scars," *New York Times*, January 31, 2018, www.nytimes.com/2018/01/31/sci ence/dutch-famine-genes.html; Elmar W. Tobi et al.,"DNA Methylation as a Mediator of the Association Between Prenatal Adversity and Risk Factors for Metabolic Disease in Adulthood," *Science Advances* 4, no. 1 (January 31, 2018): EAAO4364, doi: 10.1126/sciadv.aao4364.

14. Marcus Pembrey et al., "Human Transgenerational Responses to Early-Life Experience: Potential Impact on Development, Health and Biomedical Research," *Journal of Medical Genetics* 51, no. 9 (September 2014): 563–572, doi: 10.1136 /jmedgenet-2014-102577.

15. Lei Cao-Lei et al., "DNA Methylation Signatures Triggered by Prenatal Maternal Stress Exposure to a Natural Disaster: Project Ice Storm," *PlosOne* (September 19, 2014), doi: 10.1371/journanl.pone.0107653; Anne-Marie Turcotte-Tremblay et al., "Prenatal Maternal Stress Predicts Childhood Asthma in Girls: Project Ice Storm" *Biomedical Research International* 2014 (2014): 201717, doi: 10.1155/2014/201717.

16. D. L. McCartney et al., "Investing the Relationship Between DNA Methylation Age Acceleration and Risk Factors for Alzheimer's Disease," *Alzheimer's & Dementia* (Amsterdam, Netherlands) 10 (2018): 429–437, doi: 10.1016/j .dadm.2018.05.006.

17. Y. Zhou et al., "FTO Genotype Associations with FTO Methylation Level Influences Body Mass and Telomere Length in an Australian Rural Population," *International Journal of Obesity* (London, England) 41, no. 9 (2017): 1427–1433, doi: 10.1038/ijo.2017.127.

18. M. Samblas, F. I. Milagro, and A. Martinez, "DNA Methylation Markers in Obesity, Metabolic Syndrome, and Weight Loss," *Epigenetics* 14, no. 5 (2019): 421–444, doi: 10.1080/15592294.2019.1595297.

19. F. H. Xiao, H. T. Wang, and Q. P. Kong, "Dynamic DNA Methylation During Aging: A 'Prophet' of Age-Related Outcomes," *Frontiers in Genetics* 10 (2019): 107, doi: 10.3389/fegene.2019.001707.

20. L. Xiaolei, J. Bin, and S. Lu, "The Epigenetics of Alzheimer's Disease: Factors and Therapeutic Implications," *Frontiers in Genetics* 9 (2018): 5790, doi: 10.3389/fgene.2018.00579; T. Pi, B. Liu, and J. Shi, "Abnormal Homocysteine Metabolism: An Insight of Alzheimer's Disease from DNA Methylation," *Behavioural Neurology* (2020): 8438602, doi: 10.1155/2020/8438602.

21. Y. Zhu et al., "Epigenetic Modification and Its Role in Alzheimer's Disease," *Integrative Medicine International* 2 (2015): 63–72, doi: 10.1159/000437329.

22. K. Toups et al., "Precision Medicine Approach to Alzheimer's Disease: Successful Proof-of-Concept Trial," medRxiv (preprint), (May 2021), doi: 10.1101/2021.05.10.21256982.

23. A. D. Smith et al., "Homocysteine and Dementia: An International Consensus Statement," *Journal of Alzheimer's Disease* 62, no. 2 (2018): 561–570, doi: 10.3233/JAD-171042.

24. L. Lind et al., "Methylation-Based Estimated Biological Age and Cardiovascular Disease," *European Journal of Clinical Investigation* 48, no. 2 (February 2018), doi: 10.1111/eci.12872.

25. C. Soler-Botija, C. Gálvez-Montón, and A. Bayés-Genís, "Epigenetic Biomarkers in Cardiovascular Diseases," *Frontiers in Genetics* 10 (October 2019): 950, doi: 10.3389/fgene.2019.00950.

26. E. M. Vidrascu et al., "Effects of Early- and Mid-Life Stress on DNA Methylation of Genes Associated with Subclinical Cardiovascular Disease and Cognitive Impairment: A Systematic Review," *BMC Medical Genetics* 20, no. 1 (March 12, 2019): 39, doi: 10.1186/s12881-019-0764-4.

27. S. G. Chrysant and G. S. Chrysant, "The Current Status of Homocysteine as a Risk Factor for Cardiovascular Disease: A Mini Review," *Expert Re-*

view of Cardiovascular Therapy 16, no. 8 (August 2018): 559–565, doi: 101.1080 /14779072.2018.1497974.

28. J. C. Earls et al., "Multi-Omic Biological Age Estimation and Its Correlation with Wellness and Disease Phenotypes: A Longitudinal Study of 3,558 Individuals," *Journals of Gerontology, Series A* 74 (November 13, 2019 [Suppl. 1]): S52–S60, doi: 10.1093/geronaglz220.

29. S. A. H. Ahmed et al., "The Role of DNA Methylation in the Pathogenesis of Type 2 Diabetes Mellitus," *Clinical Epigenetics* 12 (2020): 104, doi: 10.1186/ s13148-020-00896-4.

30. F. H. Xiao, H. T. Wang, and Q. P. Kong, "Dynamic DNA Methylation During Aging: A 'Prophet' of Age-Related Outcomes," *Frontiers in Genetics* 10 (February 18, 2019): 107, doi: 10.3389/fgene.2019.00107.

31. Y. M. Lee, D. R. Jacobs Jr., and D. H. Lee, "Persistent Organic Pollutants and Type 2 Diabetes: A Critical Review of Review Articles," *Frontiers in Endocrinology* (Lausanne, Switzerland) 9 (November 27, 2018): 712, doi: 10.3389 /fendo.2018.00712.

32. D. H. Lee et al., "A Strong Dose-Response Relation Between Serum Concentrations of Persistent Organic Pollutants and Diabetes: Results from the National Health and Examination Survey 1999–2002," *Diabetes Care* 29, no. 7 (July 2006):1638–1644, doi: 10.2337/dc06-0543.

33. M. Szyf, "The Implications of DNA Methylation for Toxicology: Toward Toxicomethlomics, the Toxicology of DNA Methylation," *Toxicological Sciences* 12, no. 2 (April 2011): 235–255, doi: 10.1093/toxsci/kfr024.

34. M. Li et al., "What Do DNA Methylation Studies Tell Us About Depression? A Systematic Review," *Translational Psychology* 9, no. 1 (February 4, 2019): 68, doi: 10.1038/s41398-019-0412-y.

35. R. L. Simons et al., "Methylation of the Oxytocin Receptor Gene Mediates the Effect of Adversity on Negative Schemas and Depression," *Development and Psychopathology* 29, no. 3 (August 2017): 725–736, doi: 10.1017/S0954579416 000420.

36. A. A. Akil et al., "Reading Between the (Genetic) Lines: How Epigenetics Is Unlocking Novel Therapies for Type 1 Diabetes." *Cells* 9, no. 11 (2020): 2403.

37. S. Vordenbäumen et al., "Methyl Donor Micronutrients, CD40-ligand Methylation and Disease Activity in Systemic Lupus Erythematosus: A Cross-sectional Association Study," *Lupus* (July 20, 2021): 9612033211034559, doi: 10 .1177/09612033211034559.

38. C. Perrier and B. Corthésy, "Gut Permeability and Food Allergies," *Environmental Health Perspectives* 107, no. 10 (November 11, 2010): doi: 10.1111/j.1365-2222.2010.03639.x.

39. G. P. Pfeifer, "Defining Driver DNA Methylation Changes in Human Cancer," *International Journal of Molecular Sciences* 19, no. 4 (April 12, 2018): 1166. doi: 10.3390/ijms19041166.

40. E. M. Michalak et al., "The Roles of DNA, RNA and Histone Methylation in Ageing and Cancer," *Nature Reviews Molecular Cellular Biology* 20, no. 10 (October 2019): 573–589, doi: 10.1038/s41580-019-0143-1.

41. Y. Hashimoto, T. J. Zumwalt, and A. Goel, "DNA Methylation Patterns as Noninvasive Biomarkers and Targets of Epigenetic Therapies in Colorectal Cancer," *Epigenomics* 8, no. 5 (May 2016): 685–703, doi: 10.2217/epi-2015-0013.

42. A. Niedzwiecki et al., "Anticancer Efficacy of Polyphenols and Their Combinations," *Nutrients* 8, no. 9 (September 9, 2016): 552, doi: 10.3390/nu8090552.

43. I. Arora, M. Sharma, and T. O. Tollefsbol, "Combinatorial Epigenetics Impact of Polyphenols and Phytochemicals in Cancer Prevention and Therapy," *International Journal of Molecular Sciences* 20, no. 10 (September 14, 2019): 4567, doi: 10.3390/iljms20184567.

CHAPTER 3

1. B. A. Ames, I. Elson-Schwab, and E. A. Silver, "High-dose Vitamin Therapy Stimulates Variant Enzymes with Decreased Coenzyme Binding Affinity (Increased Km): Relevance to Genetic Disease and Polymorphisms," *American Journal of Clinical Nutrition* 75, no. 4 (April 2002): 616–658, doi: 10.1093/ajcn/75.4.616.

2. R. A. Waterland and R. L. Jirtle, "Transposable Elements: Targets for Early Nutritional Effects on Epigenetic Gene Regulation," *Molecular and Cellular Biology* 23, no. 15 (August 2003): 5293–5300, doi: 10.1128/MCB.23.15.5293-5300.2003.

3. L. J. Williams et al. "Prevalence of Spina Bifida and Anencephaly During the Transition to Mandatory Folic Acid Fortification in the United States," *Teratology* 66, no. 1 (2002): 33–39, doi: 10.1002/tera.10060.

4. M. S. Morris et al., "Circulating Unmetabolized Folic Acid and 5-Methyltetrahydrofolate in Relation to Anemia, Macrocytosis, and Cognitive Test Performance in American Seniors" [published correction appears in *American Journal of Clinical Nutrition* 92, no. 4 (October 2010):1002], *American Journal of Clinical Nutrition* 91, no. 6 (2010): 1733–1744, doi: 10.3945/ajcn.2009.28671.

5. J. B. Mason et al., "A Temporal Association Between Folic Acid Fortification and an Increase in Colorectal Cancer Rates May Be Illuminating Important Biological Principles: A Hypothesis," *Cancer Epidemiology, Biomarkers & Prevention* 16, no. 7 (July 2007): 1325–1329, doi: 10.1158/1055-9965.EPI-07-0329.

6. Ibid.

7. K. Wallace et al., "Association Between Folate Levels and CpG Island Hypermethylation in Normal Colorectal Mucosa," *Cancer Prevention Research* (Philadelphia) 3, no. 12 (December 2010): 1552–1564, doi: 10.1158/1940-6207.CAPR-10-0047.

8. Confirmed via email exchange with Marvin Singh, MD, coeditor of *Integrative Gastroenterology*, Oxford University Press (2019).

9. Z. Sadighi, I. J. Butler, and M. K. Koenig, "Adult-Onset Cerebral Folate Deficiency," *Archives of Neurology* 69, no. 6 (2012): 778–779, doi: 10.1001/archneurol.2011.3036.

10. J. P. van Wijngaarden et al., "Effect of Daily Vitamin B-12 and Folic Acid Supplementation on Fracture Incidence in Elderly Individuals with an Elevated Plasma Homocysteine Concentration: B-Proof, a Randomized Controlled Trial," *American Journal of Clinical Nutrition* 100 (2014): 1578–1586.

11. Sadaf Oliai Araghi et al., "Folic Acid and Vitamin B$_{12}$ Supplementation and the Risk of Cancer: Long-term Follow-up of the B Vitamins for the Prevention of Osteoporotic Fractures (B-PROOF)," *Trial Cancer Epidemiology, Biomarkers and Prevention* 28, no. 2 (February 1, 2019): 275–282, doi: 10.1158/1055-9965 .EPI-17-1198.

12. Young-In Kim, "Folate and Cancer: A Tale of Dr. Jekyll and Mr. Hyde?," *American Journal of Clinical Nutrition* 107, no. 2 (February 2018): 139–142, doi: 10.1093/ajcn/nqx076.

13. Dr. Kara Fitzgerald and Dr. Valter Longo, "Episode 43: Fasting Mimicking Diet: Beyond Caloric Restrictions with Dr. Valter Longo," *New Frontiers in Functional Medicine* (podcast), www.drkarafitzgerald.com/2018/06/08/fasting-diet -beyond-caloric-dr-valter-longo/.

14. H. Zheng et al., "Life-Long Body Mass Index Trajectories and Mortality in Two Generations," *Annals of Epidemiology* 56 (2021): 18–25, doi: 10.1016/j .annepidem.2021.01.003.

15. Dr. Kara Fitzgerald and Dr. Valter Longo, "Episode 43: Fasting Mimicking Diet: Beyond Caloric Restrictions with Dr. Valter Longo," *New Frontiers in Functional Medicine* (podcast), www.drkarafitzgerald.com/2018/06/08/fasting-diet -beyond-caloric-dr-valter-longo/.

16. N. Gensous et al., "One-Year Mediterranean Diet Promotes Epigenetic Rejuvenation with Country- and Sex-Specific Effects: A Pilot Study from the NU-AGE Project," *GeroScience* 42 (2020): 687–701, doi: 10.1007s11357-019-00149-0.

17. M. Montgomery and A. Srinivasan, "Epigenetic Gene Regulation by Dietary Compounds in Cancer Prevention," *Advances in Nutrition* (Bethesda, MD) 10, no. 6 (2019): 1012–1028, doi: 10.1093/advances/nmz046.

18. K. A. Kang et al., "Luteolin Promotes Apoptotic Cell Death via Upregulation of Nrf2 Expression by DNA Demethylase and the Interaction of Nrf2 with p53 in Human Colon Cancer Cells," *Experimental & Molecular Medicine* 51, 1–14 (2019): doi: 10.1038/s12276-019-0238-y.

19. N. F. Watson et al., "Recommended Amount of Sleep for a Healthy Adult: A Joint Consensus Statement of the American Academy of Sleep Medicine and Sleep Research Society," *Sleep* 38, no. 6 (2015): 843–844, doi: 10.5665/sleep.4716.

20. J. E. Carroll et al., "Epigenetic Aging and Immune Senescence in Women with Insomnia Symptoms: Findings from the Women's Health Initiative Study," *Biological Psychiatry* 81, no. 2 (January 15, 2017): 136–144, doi: 10.1016/j.biopsych .2016.07.008, Epub July 26, 2016.

21. M. A. Carskadon et al., "A Pilot Prospective Study of Sleep Patterns and DNA Methylation-Characterized Epigenetic Aging in Young Adults," *BMC Research Notes* 12, no. 583 (2019), doi: 10.1186/s13104-019-4633-1.

22. R. Massart et al., "The Genome-Wide Landscape of DNA Methylation and Hydroxymethylation in Response to Sleep Deprivation Impacts on Synaptic Plasticity Genes," *Translational Psychiatry* 4, no. 1 (January 21, 2014): e347, doi: 10.1038 /tp.2013.120; J. E. Carroll et al., "Partial Sleep Deprivation Activates the DNA Damage Response (DDR) and the Senescence-Associated Secretory Phenotype (SASP)

in Aged Adult Humans," *Brain, Behavior, and Immunity* 51 (2016): 223–229, doi: 10.1016/j.bbi.2015.08.024; E. K. Nilsson et al., "Epigenomics of Total Acute Sleep Deprivation in Relation to Genome-Wide DNA Methylation Profiles and RNA Expression," *OMICS* 20, no. 6 (2016): 334–342, doi: 10.1089/omi.2016.0041.

23. M. Spólnicka. et al., "Modified Aging of Elite Athletes Revealed by Analysis of Epigenetic Age Markers," *Aging* (Albany NY), 10, no. 2 (February 15, 2018): 241–252. doi: 10.18632/aging.101385.

24. H. Zeng et al., "Physical Activity and Breast Cancer Survival: An Epigenetic Link Through Reduced Methylation of a Tumor Suppressor Gene L3MBTL1," *Breast Cancer Research and Treatment* 133, no.1 (2012): 127–135, doi: 10.1007/s10549-011-1716-7.

25. A. J. White et al., "Recreational and Household Physical Activity at Different Time Points and DNA Global Methylation," *European Journal of Cancer* 49, no. 9 (2013): 2199–2206, doi: 10.1016/j.ejca.2013.02.013.

26. A. S. Zannas et al., "Lifetime Stress Accelerates Epigenetic Aging in an Urban, African American Cohort: Relevance of Glucocorticoid Signaling" [published correction appears in *Genome Biology* 19, no. 1 (May 23, 2018):61], *Genome Biology* 16 (December 17, 2015): 266, doi: 10.1186/s13059-015-0828-5.

27. E. J. Wolf et al., "Accelerated DNA Methylation Age: Associations with PTSD and Neural Integrity," *Psychoneuroendocrinology* 63 (2016): 155–162, doi: 10.1016/j.psyneuen.2015.09.020.

28. H. Ren et al., "Epigenetic Changes in Response to Tai Chi Practice: A Pilot Investigation of DNA Methylation Marks," *Evididence-Based Complementary and Alternative Medicine* 2012: 841810, doi: 10.1155/2012/841810.

29. R. Chaix et al., "Epigenetic Clock Analysis in Long-Term Meditators," *Psychoneuroendocrinology* 85 (2017): 210–214, doi: 10.1016/j.psyneuen.2017.08.016.

30. K. N. Harkess et al., "Preliminary Indications of the Effect of a Brief Yoga Intervention on Markers of Inflammation and DNA Methylation in Chronically Stressed Women," *Translational Psychiatry* 6, e965 (2016), doi: 10.1038/tp.2016.234.

31. S. Pavanello et al., "Exploring Epigenetic Age in Response to Intensive Relaxing Training: A Pilot Study to Slow Down Biological Age," *International Journal of Environmental Research and Public Health* 16, no. 17 (2019): 3074, doi: 10.3390/ijerph16173074.

32. S. Venditti et al., "Molecules of Silence: Effects of Meditation on Gene Expression and Epigenetics," *Frontiers in Psychology* 11 (2020): 1767, doi: 10.3389/fpsyg.2020.01767.

CHAPTER 4

1. T. Bergsma and E. Rogaeva, "DNA Methylation Clocks and Their Predictive Capacity for Aging Phenotypes and Healthspan," *Neuroscience Insights* (July 21, 2020), 15:2633105520942221, doi: 10.1177/2633105520942221.

2. J. C. Earls et al., "Multi-Omic Biological Age Estimation and Its Correlation with Wellness and Disease Phenotypes: A Longitudinal Study of 3,558 Individuals,"

Journal of Gerontology, Series A 74 (November 13, 2019 [Suppl. 1]): S52–S60, doi: 10.1093/geronaglz220.

CHAPTER 5

1. V. Vigorelli et al., "Abnormal DNA Methylation Induced by Hyperglycemia Reduces CXCR 4 Gene Expression in CD 34+ Stem Cells," *Journal of the American Heart Association* 8, no. 9 (2019): e010012, doi: 10.1161/JAHA.118.010012.

2. E. Hall et al., "The Effects of High Glucose Exposure on Global Gene Expression and DNA Methylation in Human Pancreatic Islets," *Molecular and Cellular Endocrinology* 472 (September 5, 2018): 57–67, doi: 10.1016/j.mce.2017.11.019; Dr. Charlotte Ling, "Effects of DNA Methylation on Diabetes," *Epigenetics Podcast*, April 1, 2021, www.podbean.com/ew/pb-t5v7z-ff5853.

3. J. A. Pinzón-Cortés et al., "Effect of Diabetes Status and Hyperglycemia on Global DNA Methylation and Hydroxymethylation," *Endocrine Connections* 6, no. 8 (2017): 708–725, doi: 10.1530/EC-17-0199.

4. M. C. L. Phillips et al., "Low-fat Versus Ketogenic Diet in Parkinson's Disease: A Pilot Randomized Controlled Trial," *Movement Disorders* 33, no. 8 (2018): 1306–1314, doi: 10.1002/mds.27390, Epub August 11, 2018, Erratum in: *Movement Disorders* 34, no. 1 (January 2019): 157.

5. H. B. Ruan and P. A. Crawford, "Ketone Bodies as Epigenetic Modifiers," *Current Opinion in Clinical Nutrition and Metabolic Care* 21, no. 4 (July 2018): 260-266, doi: 10.1097/MCO.0000000000000475.

6. A. Niedzwiecki et al., "Anticancer Efficacy of Polyphenols and Their Combinations," *Nutrients* 8, no. 9 (2016): 552, doi: 10.3390/nu8090552.

7. V. D. Longo and S. Panda, "Fasting, Circadian Rhythms, and Time-Restricted Feeding in Healthy Lifespan," *Cell Metabolism* 23, no. 6 (2016): 1048–1059, doi: 10.1016/j.cmet.2016.06.001; K. Kessler and O. Pivovarova-Ramich, "Meal Timing, Aging, and Metabolic Health," *International Journal of Molecular Sciences* 20, no. 8 (2019): 1911, doi: 10.3390/ijms20081911.

8. K. P. Kelly et al., "Eating Breakfast and Avoiding Late-Evening Snacking Sustains Lipid Oxidation," *PLoS Biology* 18, no. 2 (February 27, 2020): e3000622, doi: 10.1371/journal.pbio.3000622.

9. T. Bohn et al., "Mind the Gap—Deficits in Our Knowledge of Aspects Impacting the Bioavailability of Phytochemicals and Their Metabolites—A Position Paper Focusing on Carotenoids and Polyphenols," *Molecular Nutrition & Food Research* 59, no. 7 (2015): 1307–1323, doi: 10.1002/mnfr.201400745.

10. A. R. Hillman et al., "Exercise-Induced Dehydration With and Without Environmental Heat Stress Results in Increased Oxidative Stress," *Applied Physiology, Nutrition, and Metabolism* 36, no. 5 (October 2011): 698–706, doi: 10.1139/h11-080.

11. L. A. Frame, E. Costa, and S. A. Jackson, "Current Explorations of Nutrition and the Gut Microbiome: A Comprehensive Evaluation of the Review Literature," *Nutrition Reviews* 78, no. 10 (October 2020): 798–812, doi: 10.1093/nutrit /nuz106.

12. M. Rossi, A. Amaretti, and S. Raimondi, "Folate Production by Probiotic Bacteria," *Nutrients* 3, no. 12 (2011): 118–134, doi: 10.3390/nu3010118; D.-H. Yu et al.,

"Postnatal Epigenetic Regulation of Intestinal Stem Cells Requires DNA Methylation and Is Guided by the Microbiome," *Genome Biology* 16, no. 1 (2015): 211, doi: 10.1186/s13059-015-0763-5.

13. K. S. vel Szic et al., "From Inflammaging To Healthy Aging by Dietary Lifestyle Choices: Is Epigenetics the Key to Personalized Nutrition?," *Clinical Epigenetics* 7, no. 33 (2015), doi: 10.1186/s13148-015-0068-2.

14. A. Aljada et al., "Increase in Intranuclear Nuclear Factor KappaB and Decrease in Inhibitor KappaB in Mononuclear Cells After a Mixed Meal: Evidence for a Proinflammatory Effect," *American Journal of Clinical Nutrition* 79, no. 4 (2004): 682–690, doi: 10.1093/ajcn/79.4.682.

15. A. El-Osta et al., "Transient High Glucose Causes Persistent Epigenetic Changes and Altered Gene Expression During Subsequent Normoglycemia," *Journal of Experimental Medicine* 205, no. 10 (September 29, 2008): 2409–2417, doi: 10.1084/jem.20081188, Epub September 22, 2008, Erratum in *Journal of Experimental Medicine* 205, no. 11 (October 27, 2008): 2683.

16. Assam El-Osta et al., "Transient High Glucose Causes Persistent Epigenetic Changes and Altered Gene Expression During Subsequent Normoglycemia," *Journal of Experimental Medicine* 205, no. 10 (September 29, 2008): 2409–2417, doi: 10.1084/jem.20081188.

17. E. Hall et al., "The Effects of High Glucose Exposure on Global Gene Expression and DNA Methylation in Human Pancreatic Islets," *Molecular and Cellular Endocrinology* 472 (September 5, 2018): 57–67, doi: 10.1016/j.mce.2017.11.019.

18. A. Sharma et al., "Artificial Sweeteners as a Sugar Substitute: Are They Really Safe?" *Indian Journal of Pharmacology* 48, no. 3 (May-June 2016): 237–240, doi: 10.4103/0253-7613.182888.

19. J. B. Hoffman, M. C. Petriello, and B. Hennig, "Impact of Nutrition on Pollutant Toxicity: An Update with New Insights into Epigenetic Regulation," *Reviews on Environmental Health* 32, no. 1-2, (2017): 65–72, doi: 10.1515/reveh-2016-0041.

20. M. Varela-Rey et al., "Alcohol, DNA Methylation, and Cancer," *Alcohol Research* 35, no. 1 (2013): 25–35.

CHAPTER 6

1. J. A. King et al., "Incidence of Celiac Disease Is Increasing Over Time: A Systematic Review and Meta-Analysis," *American Journal of Gastroenterology* 115, no. 4 (2020): 507–525. doi: 10.14309/ajg.0000000000000523.

2. S. S. S. Boyanapalli and A. T. Kong, "'Curcumin, the King of Spices': Epigenetic Regulatory Mechanisms in the Prevention of Cancer, Neurological, and Inflammatory Diseases," *Current Pharmacology Reports* 1, no. 2 (2015): 129–139, doi: 10.1007/s40495-015-0018-x.

3. A. E. Connelly et al., "High-Rosmarinic Acid Spearmint Tea in the Management of Knee Osteoarthritis Symptoms," *Journal of Medicinal Food* 17, no. 12 (2014): 1361–1367, doi: 10.1089/jmf.2013.0189.

4. Y. Panahi et al., "Rosemary Oil vs Minoxidil 2% for the Treatment of Androgenetic Alopecia: A Randomized Comparative Trial," *Skinmed* 13, no. 1 (Jan–Feb 2015): 15–21.

5. J. Zhou et al., "Sulforaphane-Induced Epigenetic Regulation of Nrf2 Expression by DNA Methyltransferase in Human Caco-2 cells," *Oncology Letters* 18 (2019): 2639–2647, doi: 10.3892/ol.2019.10569.

6. L. Beaver et al., "Broccoli Sprouts Delay Prostate Cancer Formation and Decrease Prostate Cancer Severity with a Concurrent Decrease in HDAC3 Protein Expression in Transgenic Adenocarcinoma of the Mouse Prostate (TRAMP) Mice," *Current Developments in Nutrition* 2, no. 3 (2017), nzy002, doi: 10.1093 /cdn/nzy002.

7. US Department of Agriculture, "Dietary Guidelines for Americans 2015–2020, Eighth Edition," December 2015, https://health.gov/sites/default/ files/2019-09/2015-2020_Dietary_Guidelines.pdf.

8. H. Yang et al., "Preventive Effects of Lentinus Edodes on Homocysteinemia in Mice," *Experimental and Therapeutic Medicine* 6, no. 2 (2013): 465–468, doi: 10.3892/etm.2013.1130.

CHAPTER 7

1. E. Grazioli et al., "Physical Activity in the Prevention of Human Diseases: Role of Epigenetic Modifications," *BMC Genomics* 18 (November 14, 2017 [Suppl 8]): 802, doi: 10.1186/s12864-017-4193-5; F. Sanchis-Gomar et al., "Physical Exercise as an Epigenetic Modulator: Eustress, the 'Positive Stress' as an Effector of Gene Expression," *Journal of Strength Conditioning Research* 26, no. 12 (2012): 3469–3472, doi: 10.1519/JSC.0b013e31825bb594; I. Dimauro, M. P. Paronetto, and D. Caporossi, "Exercise, Redox Homeostasis and the Epigenetic Landscape," *Redox Biology* 35, 2020: 101477, doi: 10.1016/j.redox.2020.101477.

2. A. J. White et al., "Recreational and Household Physical Activity at Different Time Points and DNA Global Methylation," *European Journal of Cancer* 49, no. 9 (2013): 2199–2206, doi: 10.1016/j.ejca.2013.02.013.

3. M. D. Nitert et al., "Impact of an Exercise Intervention on DNA Methylation in Skeletal Muscle from First-Degree Relatives of Patients with Type 2 Diabetes," *Diabetes* 61, no. 12 (2012): 3322–3332, doi: 10.2337/db11-1653; T. Rönn et al., "A Six Months Exercise Intervention Influences the Genome-Wide DNA Methylation Pattern in Human Adipose Tissue," *PLoS Genetics* 9, no. 6 (2013): e1003572, doi: 10.1371/journal.pgen.1003572.

4. K. Nakajima et al., "Exercise Effects on Methylation of ASC Gene," *International Journal of Sports Medicine* 31, no. 9 (2010): 671–675, doi: 10.1055/s-0029 -1246140; T. Rönn et al., "A Six Months Exercise Intervention Influences the Genome-Wide DNA Methylation Pattern in Human Adipose Tissue," *PLoS Genetics* 9, no. 6 (2013): e1003572, doi: 10.1371/journal.pgen.1003572.

5. F. Gomez-Pinilla et al., "Exercise Impacts Brain-Derived Neurotrophic Factor Plasticity by Engaging Mechanisms of Epigenetic Regulation," *European Journal of Neuroscience* 33, no. 3 (2011): 383–390, doi: 10.1111/j.1460-9568.2010.07508.x; P. Z. Liu and R. Nusslock, "Exercise-Mediated Neurogenesis in the Hippocampus via BDNF," *Frontiers in Neuroscience* 12 (2018): 52, doi: 10.3389/fnins.2018.00052.

6. W. M. Brown, "Exercise-Associated DNA Methylation Change in Skeletal Muscle and the Importance of Imprinted Genes: A Bioinformatics Meta-Analysis,"

British Journal of Sports Medicine 49, no. 24 (2015): 1567–1578, doi: 10.1136/bj sports-2014-094073.

7. R. Barrès et al., "Acute Exercise Remodels Promoter Methylation in Human Skeletal Muscle," *Cell Metabolism* 15, no. 3 (March 7, 2012): 405–411, doi: 10.1016/j.cmet.2012.01.001.

8. W. M. Brown, "Exercise-Associated DNA Methylation Change in Skeletal Muscle and the Importance of Imprinted Genes: A Bioinformatics Meta-Analysis," *British Journal of Sports Medicine* 49, no. 24 (2015): 1567–1578, doi: 10.1136 /bjsports-2014-094073.

9. D. Moreau and E. Chou, "The Acute Effect of High-Intensity Exercise on Executive Function: A Meta-Analysis," *Perspectives on Psychological Science* 14, no. 5 (2019): 734–764, doi: 10.1177/1745691619850568.

10. F. Maillard, B. Pereira, and N. Boisseau, "Effect of High-Intensity Interval Training on Total, Abdominal and Visceral Fat Mass: A Meta-Analysis." *Sports Medicine* 48, no. 2 (February 2018): 269–288, doi: 10.1007/s40279-017-0807-y.

11. E. G. Trapp et al., "The Effects of High-Intensity Intermittent Exercise Training on Fat Loss and Fasting Insulin Levels of Young Women," *International Journal of Obesity* 32, no. 4 (2008): 684–691, doi: 10.1038/sj.ijo.0803781.

12. K. S. Weston, U. Wisloff, and J. S. Coombes, "High-Intensity Interval Training in Patients with Lifestyle-Induced Cardiometabolic Disease: A Systematic Review and Meta-Analysis," *British Journal of Sports Medicine* (Systematic Review & Meta-Analysis) 48, no. 16 (August 2014): 1227–1234, doi: 10.1136 /bjsports-2013-092576; V. S. Coswig et al. "Effects of High vs Moderate-Intensity Intermittent Training on Functionality, Resting Heart Rate and Blood Pressure of Elderly Women," *Journal of Translational Medicine* 18, no. 88 (2020), doi: 10.1186 /s12967-020-02261-8.

13. A. S. Zannas et al., "Lifetime Stress Accelerates Epigenetic Aging in an Urban, African American Cohort: Relevance of Glucocorticoid Signaling" [published correction appears in *Genome Biology* 19, no. 1 (May 23, 2018): 61], *Genome Biology* 16 (December 17, 2015): 266, doi: 10.1186/s13059-015-0828-5.

14. G. van Steenwyk et al., "Transgenerational Inheritance of Behavioral and Metabolic Effects of Paternal Exposure to Traumatic Stress in Early Postnatal Life: Evidence in the 4th Generation," *Environmental Epigenetics* 16, no. 4 (October 16, 2018): dvy023, doi: 10.1093/eep/dvy023.

15. Ewen Callaway, "Fearful Memories Passed Down to Mouse Descendants," *Nature* (December 1, 2013), www.scientificamerican.com/article/fearful-memories -passed-down/.

16. M. J. Meaney and M. Szyf, "Environmental Programming of Stress Responses Through DNA Methylation: Life at the Interface Between a Dynamic Environment and a Fixed Genome," *Dialogues in Clinical Neuroscience* 7, no. 2 (2005): 103–123.

17. S. R. Pilkay et al., "Maternal Trauma and Fear History Predict BDNF Methylation and Gene Expression in Newborns," *PeerJ* 8 (May 22, 2020): e8858, doi: 10.7717/peerj.8858.

18. L. Ramo-Fernández et al., "The Effects of Childhood Maltreatment on Epigenetic Regulation of Stress-Response Associated Genes: an Intergenerational Approach," *Scientific Reports*, 9, no. 983 (2019), doi: 10.1038/s41598-018 -36689-2.

19. M. A. Aristizabal et al., "Biological Embedding of Experience: A Primer on Epigenetics," *Proceedings of the National Academy of Sciences*, 117, no. 38 (September 2020): 23261–23269, doi: 10.1073/pnas.1820838116.

20. D. Mehta et al., "A Systematic Review of DNA Methylation and Gene Expression Studies in Posttraumatic Stress Disorder, Posttraumatic Growth, and Resilience," *Journal of Traumatic Stress* 33, no. 2 (April 2020): 171–180, Epub January 17, 2020, doi: 10.1002/jts.22472.

21. T. X. Fujisawa et al., "Oxytocin Receptor DNA Methylation and Alterations of Brain Volumes in Maltreated Children," *Neuropsychopharmacology* 44, no. 12 (2019): 2045–2053, doi: 10.1038/s41386-019-0414-8.

22. D. Mehta et al., "A Systematic Review of DNA Methylation and Gene Expression Studies in Posttraumatic Stress Disorder, Posttraumatic Growth, and Resilience," *Journal of Traumatic Stress* 33, no. 2 (April 2020): 171–180, Epub January 17, 2020, doi: 10.1002/jts.22472.

23. A. S. Zannas et al., "Lifetime Stress Accelerates Epigenetic Aging in an Urban, African American Cohort: Relevance of Glucocorticoid Signaling" [published correction appears in *Genome Biology* 19, no. 1 (May 23, 2018): 61], *Genome Biology* 16 (December 17, 2015): 266, doi: 10.1186/s13059-015-0828-5; E. Wolf et al., "Accelerated DNA Methylation Age: Associations w/PTSD and Neural Integrity," *Psychoneuroendocrinology* 63 (January 2016): 155–162, doi: 10.1016/j.psyneuen .2015.09.020; S. R. Moore et al., "Epigenetic Correlates of Neonatal Contact in Humans," *Development and Psychopathology* 29, no. 5 (2017): 1517–1538, doi: 10.1017/S0954579417001213; E. M. Vidrascu et al., "Effects of Early- and Mid-Life Stress on DNA Methylation of Genes Associated with Subclinical Cardiovascular Disease and Cognitive Impairment: A Systematic Review," *BMC Medical Genetics* 20, no. 39 (2019), doi: 10.1186/s12881-019-0764-4.

24. R. Chaix et al., "Differential DNA Methylation in Experienced Meditators After an Intensive Day of Mindfulness-Based Practice: Implications for Immune-Related Pathways," *Brain, Behavior, and Immunity* 84 (February 2020): 36–44, doi: 10.1016/j.bbi.2019.11.003.

25. S. Venditti et al., "Molecules of Silence: Effects of Meditation on Gene Expression and Epigenetics," *Frontiers in Psychology* 11 (2020): 1767, doi: 10.3389 /fpsyg.2020.01767.

26. R. Chaix et al., "Epigenetic Clock Analysis in Long-Term Meditators," *Psychoneuroendocrinology* 85 (2017): 210–214, doi: 10.1016/j.psyneuen.2017.08 .016.

27. S. Pavanello et al., "Exploring Epigenetic Age in Response to Intensive Relaxing Training: A Pilot Study to Slow Down Biological Age," *International Journal of Environmental Research Public Health* 16, no. 17 (2019), doi: 10.3390 /ijerph16173074.

28. "No Rest for the Aged: As People Get Older, Sleep Quantity and Quality Decline," *Cell Press*, April 5, 2017, www.eurekalert.org/pub_releases/2017-04/cp-nrf 033017.php.

29. J. J. Gooley et al., "Exposure to Room Light Before Bedtime Suppresses Melatonin Onset and Shortens Melatonin Duration in Humans," *Journal of Clinical Endocrinology and Metabolism* 96, no. 3 (March 2011): E463-72, doi: 10.1210 /jc.2010-2098.

30. American Sleep Association, "Deep Sleep: How to Get More of It," www .sleepassociation.org/about-sleep/stages-of-sleep/deep-sleep/.

31. Alzheimer's Drug Discovery Foundation, "Diphenhydramine (e.g., Benadryl)," CognitiveVitality.org, August 29, 2017, www.alzdiscovery.org/uploads/cognitive _vitality_media/Diphenhydramine-Cognitive-Vitality-For-Researchers.pdf.

32. Y. M. Lee, D. R. Jacobs Jr., and D. H. Lee, "Persistent Organic Pollutants and Type 2 Diabetes: A Critical Review of Review Articles," *Frontiers in Endocrinology* (Lausanne, Switzerland) 9 (November 27, 2018): 712, doi: 10.3389 /fendo.2018.00712.

33. Moshe Szyf, "The Implications of DNA Methylation for Toxicology: Toward Toxicomethylomics, the Toxicology of DNA Methylation," *Toxicological Sciences* 120, no. 2 (April 2011): 235–255, doi: 10.1093/toxsci/kfr024.

34. M. Manikkam et al., "Pesticide Methoxychlor Promotes the Epigenetic Transgenerational Inheritance of Adult-Onset Disease Through the Female Germline," *PLoS One* 9, no. 7 (July 24, 2014): e102091, doi: 10.1371/journal .pone.0102091.

35. G. H. Heinz et al., "Enhanced Reproduction in Mallards Fed a Low Level of Methylmercury: An Apparent Case of Hormesis," *Environmental Toxicology and Chemistry* 29, no. 3 (March 2010): 650–653, doi: 10.1002/etc.64.

36. S. Sutou, "Low-Dose Radiation from A-Bombs Elongated Lifespan and Reduced Cancer Mortality Relative to Un-Irradiated Individuals," *Genes and Environment* 40, no. 26 (2018), doi: 10.1186/s41021-018-0114-3.

37. Randy L. Jirtle, "Epigenetic Responses to Low Dose Ionizing Radiation," *Free Radical Biology and Medicine* 124 (2018): 559, doi: 10.1016/j.freeradbiomed .2018.05.014.

38. M. P. Mattson, "Hormesis Defined," *Ageing Research Review* 7, no. 1 (January 2008): 1–7, doi: 10.1016/j.arr.2007.08.007. Epub December 5, 2007.

39. D. Lamming, J. G. Wood, and D. Sinclair, "MicroReview: Small Molecules That Regulate Lifespan: Evidence for Xenohormesis," *Molecular Microbiology* 53 (2004). doi: 10.1111/j.1365-2958.2004.04209.x.

40. R. E. Hodges and D. M. Minich, "Modulation of Metabolic Detoxification Pathways Using Foods and Food-Derived Components: A Scientific Review with Clinical Application," *Journal of Nutrition and Metabolism* 2015 (2015): 760689, doi: 10.1155/2015/760689.

41. B. Hennig et al., "The Role of Nutrition in Influencing Mechanisms Involved in Environmentally Mediated Diseases," *Reviews on Environmental Health* 33, no. 1 (March 28, 2018): 87–97, doi: 10.1515/reveh-2017-0038.

42. M. Beidelschies et al., "Patient Outcomes and Costs Associated with Functional Medicine-based Care in a Shared Versus Individual Setting for Patients with Chronic Conditions: A Retrospective Cohort Study," *BMJ Open* 11 (2021): e048294. doi: 10.1136/bmjopen-2020-048294.

43. R. Huffmeijer, M. H. van Ijzendoorn, and M. J. Bakermans-Kranenburg, "Ageing and Oxytocin: A Call for Extending Human Oxytocin Research to Ageing Populations—A Mini-Review," *Gerontology* 59, no. 1 (2013): 32-39, doi: 10.1159/000341333; S.-Y. Cho et al., "Impact of Oxytocin on Skin Ageing," *British Journal of Dermatology* 181 (2019): e148-e148, doi: 10.1111/bjd.18568; C. Elabd et al., "Oxytocin Is an Age-Specific Circulating Hormone That Is Necessary for Muscle Maintenance and Regeneration," *Nature Communications* 5 (June 10, 2014): 4082, doi: 10.1038/ncomms5082; A. B. Reiss et al., "Oxytocin: Potential to Mitigate Cardiovascular Risk," *Peptides* 117 (July 2019): 170089, doi: 10.1016/j .peptides.2019.05.001.

44. C. I. Park et al., "Reduced DNA Methylation of the Oxytocin Receptor Gene Is Associated with Obsessive-Compulsive Disorder," *Clinical Epigenetics* 20, no. 1 (2020): 101, doi: 10.1186/s13148-020-00890-w.

45. A. Klockars, A. S. Levine, and P. K. Olszewski, "Central Oxytocin and Food Intake: Focus on Macronutrient-Driven Reward," *Frontiers in Endocrinology* (Lausanne, Switzerland) 6 (April 28, 2015): 65, doi: 10.3389/fendo.2015.00065.

46. C. Maud et al., "The Role of Oxytocin Receptor Gene (OXTR) DNA Methylation (DNAm) in Human Social and Emotional Functioning: A Systematic Narrative Review," *BMC Psychiatry* 18, no. 154 (2018), doi: 10.1186/s12888-018 -1740-9.

47. S. R. Moore et al., "Epigenetic Correlates of Neonatal Contact in Humans," *Development and Psychopathology* 29, no. 5 (December 2017): 1517–1538, doi: 10 .1017/S0954579417001213.

48. Ibid.

49. C. H. Zeanah et al., "Sensitive Periods," *Monographs of the Society for Research in Child Development* 76, no. 4 (December 2011): 147–162, doi: 10.1111/j.1540-5834.2011.00631.x.

50. E. Agerbo, P. B. Mortensen, and T. Munk-Olsen, "Childlessness, Parental Mortality and Psychiatric Illness: A Natural Experiment Based on In Vitro Fertility Treatment and Adoption," *Journal of Epidemiology & Community Health* 67 (2013): 374–376, doi: 10.1136/jech-2012-201387.

51. P. F. McArdle et al., "Does Having Children Extend Life Span? A Genealogical Study Of Parity and Longevity in the Amish," *Journals of Gerontology Series A: Biological Sciences and Medical Sciences* 61, no. 2 (February 2006): 190–195, doi: 10.1093/gerona/61.2.190.

52. J. Mitteldorf, "Female Fertility and Longevity," *Age* (Dordrecht, Netherlands: Online) 32, no. 1 (March 2010): 79–84, doi: 10.1007/s11357-009-9116-1.

53. M. S. Carmichael et al., "Relationships Among Cardiovascular, Muscular, and Oxytocin Responses During Human Sexual Activity," *Archives of Sexual Behavior* 23 (1994): 59–79, doi: 10.1007/BF01541618.

54. J. A. Barraza and P. J. Zak, "Empathy Toward Strangers Triggers Oxytocin Release and Subsequent Generosity," *Annals of the New York Academy of Sciences* 1167 (June 2009): 182–189, doi: 10.1111/j.1749-6632.2009.04504.x.

55. C. Grape et al., "Does Singing Promote Well-Being?: An Empirical Study of Professional and Amateur Singers During a Singing Lesson," *Integrative Physiological and Behavioral Science* 38, no. 1 (Jan-Mar 2003): 65–74, doi: 10.1007/BF02734261.

56. Michael J. Poulin and E. Alison Holman, "Helping Hands, Healthy Body? Oxytocin Receptor Gene and Prosocial Behavior Interact to Buffer the Association Between Stress and Physical Health," *Hormones and Behavior* 63, no. 3 (2013): 510–517, doi: 10.1016/j.yhbeh.2013.01.004.

57. V. Morhenn, L. E. Beavin, and P. J. Zak, "Massage Increases Oxytocin and Reduces Adrenocorticotropin Hormone in Humans," *Alternative Therapies in Health and Medicine* 18, no. 6 (Nov-Dec 2012): 11–18.

CHAPTER 8

1. H. Andersson et al., "Oral Administration of Lactobacillus plantarum 299v Reduces Cortisol Levels in Human Saliva During Examination Induced Stress: A Randomized, Double-Blind Controlled Trial," *International Journal of Microbiology* 2016 (2016): 8469018, doi: 10.1155/2016/8469018.

2. F. Watanabe et al., "Vitamin B_{12}-Containing Plant Food Sources for Vegetarians," *Nutrients* 6, no. 5 (May 5, 2014): 1861–1873, doi: 10.3390/nu6051861.

3. C. Paul and D. M. Brady, "Comparative Bioavailability and Utilization of Particular Forms of B12 Supplements with Potential to Mitigate B_{12}-Related Genetic Polymorphisms," *Integrative Medicine: A Clinician's Journal* 16, no. 1 (February 2017): 42–49.

4. F. L. Crowe et al., "Plasma Concentrations of 25-Hydroxyvitamin D in Meat Eaters, Fish Eaters, Vegetarians and Vegans: Results from the EPIC-Oxford Study," *Public Health Nutrition* 14, no. 2 (February 2011): 340–346, doi: 10.1017/S1368980010002454.

5. J. L. Harper and M. E. Conrad, "Iron Deficiency Anemia Treatment and Management," *Medscape* (September 30, 2020), https://emedicine.medscape.com/article/202333-treatment#d7.

6. I. S. Fetahu, J. Höbaus, and E. Kállay, "Vitamin D and the Epigenome," *Frontiers in Physiology* 5 (April 29, 2014): 164, doi: 10.3389/fphys.2014.00164.

7. E. Roshdy et al., "Treatment of Symptomatic Uterine Fibroids with Green Tea Extract: A Pilot Randomized Controlled Clinical Study," *International Journal of Women's Health* 5 (August 7, 2013): 477–486, doi: 10.2147/IJWH.S41021.

8. J. Hu et al., "The Safety of Green Tea and Green Tea Extract Consumption in Adults — Results of a Systematic Review," *Regulatory Toxicology and Pharmacology* 95 (June 2018): 412–433, doi: 10.1016/j.yrtph.2018.03.019.

9. A. Bielak-Zmijewska et al., "The Role of Curcumin in the Modulation of Ageing," *International Journal of Molecular Sciences* 20, no. 5 (March 12, 2019): 1239, doi: 10.3390/ijms20051239.

10. R. J. Keegan et al., "Photobiology of Vitamin D in Mushrooms and Its Bioavailability in Humans," *Dermatoendocrinology* 15, no. 1 (January 1, 2013): 165–176, doi: 10.4161/derm.23321.

11. R. Cooper et al., "Creatine Supplementation with Specific View to Exercise/Sports Performance: An Update," *Journal of the International Society of Sports Nutrition*, 9, no.1 (July 20, 2012): 33, doi:10.1186/1550-2783-9-33.

12. Y. Heianza et al., "Long-Term Changes in Gut Microbial Metabolite Trimethylamine N-Oxide and Coronary Heart Disease Risk," *Journal of the American College of Cardiology* 75, no. 7 (February 25, 2020): 763–772, doi: 10.1016/j.jacc.2019.11.060.

13. Y. Heianza and L. Qi, "Reply: TMAO Changes and Coronary Heart Disease Risk: Potential Impact and Study Considerations," *Journal of the American College of Cardiology* 75, no. 24 (June 23, 2020): 3102–3104, doi: 10.1016/j.jacc.2020.04.050.

14. Linus Pauling Institute, "Choline," Micronutrient Information Center, https://lpi.oregonstate.edu/mic/other-nutrients/choline#safety/; C. Roncal et al., "Trimethylamine-N-Oxide (TMAO) Predicts Cardiovascular Mortality in Peripheral Artery Disease," *Scientific Reports* 9, no. 15580 (2019), doi: 10.1038/s41598-019-52082-z.

15. R. W. Dellinger et al., "Repeat Dose NRPT (Nicotinamide Riboside and Pterostilbene) Increases NAD+ Levels in Humans Safely and Sustainably: A Randomized, Double-Blind, Placebo-Controlled Study," *NPJ Aging and Mechanisms of Disease* 3 (November 24, 2017): 17, doi: 10.1038/s41514-017-0016-9, Erratum in *NPJ Aging and Mechanisms of Disease* 4 (August 20, 2018): 8.

16. Wen Li et al., "Emerging Senolytic Agents Derived from Natural Products," *Mechanisms of Ageing and Development* 181 (2019): 1–6, doi: 10.1016/j.mad.2019.05.001.

17. M. J. Yousefzadeh et al., "Fisetin Is a Senotherapeutic That Extends Health and Lifespan," *EBioMedicine* 36 (October 2018): 18–28, doi: 10.1016/j.ebiom.2018.09.015.

18. A. Farsad-Naeimi et al., "Effect of Fisetin Supplementation on Inflammatory Factors and Matrix Metalloproteinase Enzymes in Colorectal Cancer Patients," *Food and Function* 9, no. 4 (April 25, 2018): 2025–2031, doi: 10.1039/c7fo01898c.

19. M. P. K. J. Engelen and N. E. P. Deutz, "Is ß-hydroxy β-methylbutyrate an Effective Anabolic Agent to Improve Outcome in Older Diseased Populations?," *Current Opinion in Clinical Nutrition and Metabolic Care* 21, no. 3 (May 2018): 207–213, doi: 10.1097/MCO.0000000000000459.

20. Y. Lin et al., "Luteolin, a Flavonoid with Potential for Cancer Prevention and Therapy," *Current Cancer Drug Targets* 8, no. 7 (November 2008): 634–646, doi: 10.2174/156800908786241050.

21. G. Lai et al., "Alcohol Extracts from Ganoderma lucidum Delay the Progress of Alzheimer's Disease by Regulating DNA Methylation in Rodents," *Frontiers in Pharmacology* 10 (March 26, 2019): 272, doi: 10.3389/fphar.2019.00272.

CHAPTER 9

1. G. Du Toit et al.; LEAP Study Team, "Randomized Trial of Peanut Consumption in Infants at Risk for Peanut Allergy," *New England Journal of Medicine* 372, no. 9 (February 26, 2015): 803–813, doi: 10.1056/NEJMoa1414850, Epub February 23, 2015, Erratum in: *New England Journal of Medicine* 375, no. 4 (July 28, 2016): 398; M. R. Perkin et al.; EAT Study Team, "Randomized Trial of Introduction of Allergenic Foods in Breast-Fed Infants," *New England Journal of Medicine* 374, no 18 (May 5, 2016): 1733–1743, Epub March 4, 2016, doi: 10.1056 /NEJMoa1514210.

2. I. C. Weaver et al., "Epigenetic Programming by Maternal Behavior," *Nature Neuroscience* 7, no. 8 (August 7, 2004): 847–854, doi: 10.1038/nn1276.

3. E. C. Dunn et al., "Sensitive Periods for the Effect of Childhood Adversity on DNA Methylation: Results from a Prospective, Longitudinal Study," *Biological Psychiatry* 85, no. 10 (May 15, 2019): 838–849, doi: 10.1016/j.biopsych.2018.12.023, Epub January 21, 2019, Erratum in *Biological Psychiatry* 86, no. 1 (July 1, 2019): 76.

4. K. L. Wisner et al., "Onset Timing, Thoughts of Self-harm, and Diagnoses in Postpartum Women with Screen-Positive Depression Findings," *JAMA Psychiatry* 70, no. 5 (2013): 490–498, doi: 10.1001/jamapsychiatry.2013.87.

5. M. Kimmel et al., "Oxytocin Receptor DNA Methylation in Postpartum Depression," *Psychoneuroendocrinology* 69 (July 2016): 150–160, doi: 10.1016/j.psyneuen .2016.04.008.

6. S. Bhattacharya et al., "Stress Across Generations: DNA Methylation as a Potential Mechanism Underlying Intergenerational Effects of Stress in Both Post-Traumatic Stress Disorder and Pre-Clinical Predator Stress Rodent Models," *Frontiers in Behavioral Neuroscience* 13 (2019): 113, doi: 10.3389/fnbeh.2019.00113.

7. C. Nagy and G. Turecki, "Sensitive Periods in Epigenetics: Bringing Us Closer to Complex Behavioral Phenotypes," *Epigenomics* 4, no. 4 (August 2012): 445–457, doi: 10.2217/epi.12.37.

8. D. Vågerö et al., "Paternal Grandfather's Access to Food Predicts All-Cause and Cancer Mortality in Grandsons," *Nature Communications* 9, no. 5124 (2018), doi: 10.1038/s41467-018-07617-9.

9. H. Wu et al., "Environmental Susceptibility of the Sperm Epigenome During Windows of Male Germ Cell Development," *Current Environmental Health Reports* 2, no. 4 (December 2015): 356–366, doi: 10.1007/s40572-015-0067-7.

10. A. Soubry et al., "A Paternal Environmental Legacy: Evidence for Epigenetic Inheritance Through the Male Germ Line," *Bioessays* 36, no. 4 (April 2014): 359–371, doi: 10.1002/bies.201300113.

11. L. Han et al., "Changes in DNA Methylation from Pre- to Post-Adolescence Are Associated with Pubertal Exposures," *Clinical Epigenetics* 11, no. 176 (2019), doi: 10.1186/s13148-019-0780-4.

12. D. K. Eaton et al., "Prevalence of Insufficient, Borderline, and Optimal Hours of Sleep Among High School Students—United States, 2007," *Journal of Adolescent Health* 46, no. 4 (April 2010): 399–401, doi: 10.1016/j.jadohealth.2009.10.011.

13. G. V. Skuladottir et al., "One-Night Sleep Deprivation Induces Changes in the DNA Methylation and Serum Activity Indices of Stearoyl-CoA Desaturase in Young Healthy Men," *Lipids in Health and Disease* 15, no. 1 (August 26, 2016): 137, doi: 10.1186/s12944-016-0309-1.

14. M. Amatruda et al., "Epigenetic Effects of n-3 LCPUFAs: A Role in Pediatric Metabolic Syndrome," *International Journal of Molecular Sciences* 20, no. 9 (April 29, 2019): 2118, doi: 10.3390/ijms20092118.

15. M. Varela-Rey et al., "Alcohol, DNA Methylation, and Cancer," *Alcohol Research* 35, no. 1 (2013): 25–35.

16. G. C. Williams, "Pleiotropy, Natural Selection, and the Evolution of Senescence," *Science of Aging Knowledge Environment* 2001, no. 1 (October 3, 2001): cp13, http://sageke.sciencemag.org/cgi/content/abstract/sageke.2001/1/cp13.

17. S. Bhasin et al., "Age-Related Changes in the Male Reproductive System" [Updated December 14, 2018], in K. R. Feingold et al., editors, Endotext, (South Dartmouth, MA: MDText.com, Inc., 2000–), www.ncbi.nlm.nih.gov/books /NBK278998/; American College of Obstetricians and Gynecologists, "Having a Baby After Age 35: How Aging Affects Fertility and Pregnancy," www.acog.org/wom ens-health/faqs/having-a-baby-after-age-35-how-aging-affects-fertility-and-pregnan cy#:~:text=A%20woman's%20peak%20reproductive%20years,is%20unlikely%20 for%20most%20women.

18. A. Strittmatter, U. Sunde, and D. Zegners, "Life Cycle Patterns of Cognitive Performance over the Long Run," *Proceedings of the National Academy of Sciences of the United States of America* 117, no. 4 (November 3, 2020): 27255–27261, Epub October 19, 2020, doi: 10.1073/pnas.2006653117.

19. A. Salas-Huetos et al., "Sperm DNA Methylation Changes After Short-Term Nut Supplementation in Healthy Men Consuming a Western-style Diet" [published online ahead of print], September 23, 2020, *Andrology* 2020, doi: 10.1111/ andr.12911.

20. R. Schrott et al., "Sperm DNA Methylation Altered by THC and Nicotine: Vulnerability of Neurodevelopmental Genes with Bivalent Chromatin," *Scientific Reports* 10, no. 1 (September 29, 2020): 16022, doi: 10.1038/s41598-020-72783-0.

21. M. Ben Maamar et al., "Epigenome-Wide Association Study for Glyphosate Induced Transgenerational Sperm DNA Methylation and Histone Retention Epigenetic Biomarkers for Disease," *Epigenetics* (December 9, 2020): 1–18, doi: 10.1080/15592294.2020.1853319.

22. R. Elango and R. O. Ball, "Protein and Amino Acid Requirements During Pregnancy," *Advances in Nutrition* 7, no. 4 (July 15, 2016): 839S-44S, doi: 10.3945 /an.115.011817.

23. L. P. Stone et al., "Customized Nutritional Enhancement for Pregnant Women Appears to Lower Incidence of Certain Common Maternal and Neonatal Complications: An Observational Study," *Global Advances in Health and Medicine* 3, no. 6 (November 2014): 50–55, doi: 10.7453/gahmj.2014.053.

24. Centers for Disease Control and Prevention, "Folic Acid," www.cdc.gov /ncbddd/folicacid/about.html.

25. National Institutes of Health, Office of Dietary Supplements, "Folate: Fact Sheet for Consumers," https://ods.od.nih.gov/factsheets/Folate-Consumer/#h8.

26. E. Keating et al., "Excess Perigestational Folic Acid Exposure Induces Metabolic Dysfunction in Post-natal Life," *Journal of Endocrinology* 224, no. 3 (March 2015): 245–259, doi: 10.1530/JOE-14-0448.

27. D. C. Dolinoy et al., "Maternal Genistein Alters Coat Color and Protects Avy Mouse Offspring from Obesity by Modifying the Fetal Epigenome," *Environmental Health Perspectives* 114, no. 4 (April 2006): 567–572, doi: 10.1289/ehp .8700.

28. American College of Obstetricians and Gynecologists, "Nutrition During Pregnancy," www.acog.org/womens-health/faqs/nutrition-during-pregnancy.

29. L. P. Stone et al., "Customized Nutritional Enhancement for Pregnant Women Appears to Lower Incidence of Certain Common Maternal and Neonatal Complications: An Observational Study," *Global Advances in Health and Medicine* 3, no. 6 (November 2014): 50–55, doi: 10.7453/gahmj.2014.053.

30. M. E. Levine et al., "Menopause Accelerates Biological Aging," *Proceedings of the National Academy of Sciences of the United States of America* 113, no. 33 (August 16, 2016): 9327–9332, Epub July 25, 2016, doi: 10.1073/pnas.1604558113.

31. C. L. Kuo et al., "Biological Aging Predicts Vulnerability to COVID-19 Severity in UK Biobank Participants," *Journals of Gerontology Series A: Biological Sciences and Medical Sciences* (March 4, 2021): glab060, Epub ahead of print, doi: 10.1093/gerona/glab060.

CHAPTER 10

1. Kirsty J. Flower et al., "DNA Methylation Profiling to Assess Pathogenicity of BRCA1 Unclassified Variants in Breast Cancer," *Epigenetics* 10, no. 12 (2015): 1121–1132, doi: 10.1080/15592294.2015.1111504.

2. M. C. King et al., "Breast and Ovarian Cancer Risks Due to Inherited Mutations in BRCA1 and BRCA2," *Science* 2003 302, no. 5645 (October 24, 2003): 643–646, doi: 10.1126/science.1088759.

3. Ibid.

4. R. L. Baldwin et al., "BRCA1 Promoter Region Hypermethylation in Ovarian Carcinoma: A Population-Based Study," *Cancer Research* 60, no. 19 (October 1, 2000): 5329–5333.

5. N. Al-Moghrabi et al., "Methylation of BRCA1 and MGMT Genes in White Blood Cells Are Transmitted from Mothers to Daughters," *Clinical Epigenetics* 10, no. 99 (2018), doi: 10.1186/s13148-018-0529-5.

6. G. A. Millot et al. on behalf of ENIGMA Consortium Functional Assay Working Group, "A Guide for Functional Analysis of BRCA1 Variants of Uncertain Significance." *Human Mutation* 33 no. 11 (November 2012): 1526–1537, doi: 10.1002/humu.22150, Epub July 16, 2012.

7. Ranjit Manchanda et al., "Economic Evaluation of Population-Based BRCA1/BRCA2 Mutation Testing Across Multiple Countries and Health Systems," *Cancers* (2020), doi: 10.3390/cancers12071929.

8. Kirsty J. Flower et al., "DNA Methylation Profiling to Assess Pathogenicity of BRCA1 Unclassified Variants in Breast Cancer," *Epigenetics* 10, no. 12 (2015): 1121–1132, doi: 10.1080/15592294.2015.1111504.

9. S. S. Oltra et al., "Acceleration in the DNA Methylation Age in Breast Cancer Tumours from Very Young Women," *Scientific Reports* 9, no. 14991 (2019), doi: 10.1038/s41598-019-51457-6.

10. A. J. Papoutsis et al., "BRCA-1 Promoter Hypermethylation and Silencing Induced by the Aromatic Hydrocarbon Receptor-Ligand TCDD Are Prevented by Resveratrol in MCF-7 Cells," *Journal of Nutritional Biochemistry* 23, no. 10 (October 2012): 1324–1332, doi: 10.1016/j.jnutbio.2011.08.001; A. J. Papoutsis et al., "Resveratrol Prevents Epigenetic Silencing of BRCA-1 by the Aromatic Hydrocarbon Receptor in Human Breast Cancer Cells," *Journal of Nutrition* 140, no. 9 (September 2010): 1607–1614, doi: 10.3945/jn.110.123422.

11. P. Selvakumar et al., "Flavonoids and Other Polyphenols Act as Epigenetic Modifiers in Breast Cancer," *Nutrients* 12, no. 3 (March 13, 2020): 761, doi: 10.3390/nu12030761.

12. R. Bosviel et al., "Epigenetic Modulation of BRCA1 and BRCA2 Gene Expression by Equol in Breast Cancer Cell Lines," *British Journal of Nutrition* 108, no. 7 (2012): 1187–1193, doi: 10.1017/S000711451100657X.

13. B. Mayo, L. Vázquez, and A. B. Flórez, "Equol: A Bacterial Metabolite from the Daidzein Isoflavone and Its Presumed Beneficial Health Effects," *Nutrients* 11, no. 9 (September 16, 2019): 2231, doi: 10.3390/nu11092231.

14. S. Kundur et al., "Synergistic Anticancer Action of Quercetin and Curcumin Against Triple-Negative Breast Cancer Cell Lines," *Journal of Cellular Physiology* 234, no. 7 (July 2019): 11103–11118, doi: 10.1002/jcp.27761.

15. N. Petrucelli, M. B. Daly, and T. Pal, "BRCA1- and BRCA2-Associated Hereditary Breast and Ovarian Cancer," September 4, 1998 [updated December 15, 2016], in M. P. Adam et al., editors, *GeneReviews* (Seattle, WA: University of Washington, 1993–2020) www.ncbi.nlm.nih.gov/books/NBK1247/.

16. G. Luo et al., "Pancreatic Cancer: BRCA Mutation and Personalized Treatment," *Expert Review of Anticancer Therapy* 15, no. 10 (2015): 1223–1231, doi: 10.1586/14737140.2015.1086271; J. Mijnes et al., "Promoter Methylation of DNA Damage Repair (DDR) Genes in Human Tumor Entities: RBBP8/CtIP Is Almost Exclusively Methylated in Bladder Cancer," *Clinical Epigenetics* 10 (February 6, 2018): 15, doi: 10.1186/s13148-018-0447-6; S. M. Shalaby et al., "Promoter Methylation and Expression of DNA Repair Genes MGMT and ERCC1 in Tissue and Blood of Rectal Cancer Patients," *Gene* 644 (February 20, 2018): 66–73, doi: 10.1016/j.gene.2017.10.056; I. Arora, M. Sharma, and T. O. Tollefsbol, "Combinatorial Epigenetics Impact of Polyphenols and Phytochemicals in Cancer Prevention and Therapy," *International Journal of Molecular Sciences* 20, no. 18 (September 14, 2019): 4567, doi: 10.3390/ijms20184567; A. Wojtczyk-Miaskowska et al., "Gene Expression, DNA Methylation and Prognostic Significance of DNA Repair Genes in Human Bladder Cancer," *Cellular Physiology and Biochemistry* 42 (2017): 2404–2417, doi: 10.1159/000480182; V. Shilpa et al., "BRCA1 Promoter

Hypermethylation and Protein Expression in Ovarian Carcinoma—An Indian Study," *Tumor Biology* 35 (2014): 4277–4284, doi: 10.1007/s13277-013-1558-5; A. J. Papoutsis et al., "BRCA-1 Promoter Hypermethylation and Silencing Induced by the Aromatic Hydrocarbon Receptor-Ligand TCDD Are Prevented by Resveratrol in MCF-7 Cells," *Journal of Nutritional Biochemistry* 23, no. 10 (October 2012): 1324–1332, doi: 10.1016/j.jnutbio.2011.08.001; P. Selvakumar et al., "Flavonoids and Other Polyphenols Act as Epigenetic Modifiers in Breast Cancer," *Nutrients* 12, no. 3 (March 13, 2020): 761, doi: 10.3390/nu12030761.

17. M. Imran et al., "Kaempferol: A Key Emphasis to Its Anticancer Potential," *Molecules* 24, no. 12 (June 19, 2019): 2277, doi: 10.3390/molecules24122277.

18. L. J. Fu et al., "The Effects of Lycopene on the Methylation of the GSTP1 Promoter and Global Methylation in Prostatic Cancer Cell Lines PC3 and LNCaP," *International Journal of Endocrinology* 2014 (2014): 620165, doi: 10.1155/2014/620165; C. Fang et al., "Aberrant GSTP1 Promoter Methylation Is Associated with Increased Risk and Advanced Stage of Breast Cancer: A Meta-Analysis of 19 Case-Control Studies," *BMC Cancer* 15, no. 920 (2015), doi: 10.1186/s12885-015-1926-1; J. Cui et al., "GSTP1 and Cancer: Expression, Methylation, Polymorphisms and Signaling (Review)," *International Journal of Oncology* 56, no. 4 (2020): 867–878, doi: 10.3892/ijo.2020.4979.

19. N. Mukherjee, A. P. Kumar, and R. Ghosh, "DNA Methylation and Flavonoids in Genitourinary Cancers," *Current Pharmacology Reports* 1, no. 2 (April 1, 2015): 112–120, doi: 10.1007/s40495-014-0004-8.

20. K. Yari and Z. Rahimi, "Promoter Methylation Status of the Retinoic Acid Receptor-Beta 2 Gene in Breast Cancer Patients: A Case Control Study and Systematic Review," *Breast Care* (Basel, Switzerland) 14, no. 2 (April 2019): 117–123, doi: 10.1159/000489874.

21. R. Chen et al. "Association Between MGMT Promoter Methylation and Risk of Breast and Gynecologic Cancers: A Systematic Review and Meta-Analysis," *Scientific Reports* 7, no. 1 (October 6, 2017): 12783, doi: 10.1038/s41598-017-13208-3; I. Arora, M. Sharma, and T. O. Tollefsbol, "Combinatorial Epigenetics Impact of Polyphenols and Phytochemicals in Cancer Prevention and Therapy," *International Journal of Molecular Sciences* 20, no. 18 (September 14, 2019): 4567, doi: 10.3390/ijms20184567.

22. U. Smrdel et al., "Long-Term Survival in Glioblastoma: Methyl Guanine Methyl Transferase (MGMT) Promoter Methylation as Independent Favourable Prognostic Factor," *Radiology and Oncology* 50, no. 4 (November 10, 2016): 394–401, doi: 10.1515/raon-2015-0041.

23. G. Tezcan et al., "Olea europaea Leaf Extract Improves the Efficacy of Temozolomide Therapy by Inducing MGMT Methylation and Reducing P53 Expression in Glioblastoma," *Nutrition and Cancer* 69, no. 6 (Aug-Sep 2017): 873–880, doi: 10.1080/01635581.2017.1339810.

24. M. Beetch et al., "Dietary Antioxidants Remodel DNA Methylation Patterns in Chronic Disease," *British Journal of Pharmacology* 177, no. 6 (March 2020): 1382–1408, doi: 10.1111/bph.14888; E. Collignon et al., "Immunity Drives TET1

Regulation in Cancer Through NF-κB," *Science Advances* 4, no. 6 (June 20, 2018): eaap7309, doi: 10.1126/sciadv.aap7309.

25. C. Busch et al., "Epigenetic Activities of Flavonoids in the Prevention and Treatment of Cancer," *Clinical Epigenetics* 7, no. 1 (July 10, 2015): 64, doi: 10.1186/s13148-015-0095-z.

26. C. Li et al., "OPCML Is Frequently Methylated in Human Colorectal Cancer and Its Restored Expression Reverses EMT via Downregulation of Smad Signaling," *American Journal of Cancer Research* 5, no. 5 (April 15, 2015): 1635–1648; Y. Cui et al., "OPCML Is a Broad Tumor Suppressor for Multiple Carcinomas and Lymphomas with Frequently Epigenetic Inactivation," *PLoS One* 3, no. 8 (August 20, 2008): e2990, doi: 10.1371/journal.pone.0002990, erratum in *PLoS One* 3, no.9 (2008), doi: 10.1371/annotation/f394b95b-c731-41a3-b0dc-be25fb6a227c.

27. A. Torkamani, N. E. Wineinger, and E. J. Topol, "The Personal and Clinical Utility of Polygenic Risk Scores," *Nature Reviews Genetics* 19, (2018): 581–590, doi: 10.1038/s41576-018-0018-x.

28. C. Sae-Lee et al., "Dietary Intervention Modifies DNA Methylation Age Assessed by the Epigenetic Clock," *Molecular Nutrition and Food Research* 62 (2018): 1–7, doi: 10.1002/mnfr.201800092.

CHAPTER 11

1. K. Loria, "A Rogue Doctor Saved a Potential Miracle Drug by Storing Samples in His Home After Being Told to Throw Them Away," *Business Insider*, February 20, 2015, www.businessinsider.com/suren-sehgal-saved-rapamycin-anti-aging-drug-2015-2.

2. M. Easter, "This Obscure, Potentially Dangerous Drug Could Stop Aging," *Men's Health*, July 19, 2019, www.menshealth.com/health/a28440858/anti-aging -rapamycin.

3. M. V. Blagosklonny, "Fasting and Rapamycin: Diabetes Versus Benevolent Glucose Intolerance," *Cell Death and Disease* 10, 607 (2019), doi: 10.1038 /s41419-019-1822-8.

4. Rapamune (Sirolimus) tablets label, www.accessdata.fda.gov/drugsatfda _docs/label/2010/021110s058lbl.pdf.

5. A. A. Soukas, H. Hao, and L. Wu, "Metformin as Anti-Aging Therapy: Is It for Everyone?," *Trends in Endocrinology & Metabolism* 30, no. 10 (October 2019): 745–755, doi: 10.1016/j.tem.2019.07.015.

6. A. Protti et al., "Metformin Overdose Causes Platelet Mitochondrial Dysfunction in Humans," *Critical Care* (London, England) 1 (2012): R180, doi: 10.1186 /cc1166.

7. A. R. Konopka et al., "Metformin Inhibits Mitochondrial Adaptations to Aerobic Exercise Training in Older Adults," *Aging Cell* 18, no. 1 (February 2019): e12880, doi: 10.1111/acel.12880.

8. Ibid.

9. National Institute on Aging, "Adverse Cardiovascular Events Reported in Testosterone Trial in Older Men," June 30, 2010, www.nih.gov/news-events /news-releases/adverse-cardiovascular-events-reported-testosterone-trial-older-men.

10. P. E. Norman et al., "Cohort Profile: The Health In Men Study (HIMS)," *International Journal of Epidemiology* 38, no. 1 (February 2009): 48–52, doi: 10.1093 /ije/dyn041.

11. Y. Li et al., "Reprogramming Somatic Cells to Potency: A Fresh Look at Yamanaka's Model," *Cell Cycle* 12, no. 23 (2013): 3594–3598, doi: 10.4161/cc .26952.

12. Y. Lu et al., "Reprogramming to Recover Youthful Epigenetic Information and Restore Vision," *Nature* 588, no. 7836 (February 2009): 124–129, doi: 10.1038 /s41586-020-2975-4.

13. Harvard Medical School, "Scientists Reverse the Aging Clock: Restore Age-Related Vision Loss Through Epigenetic Reprogramming," December 2, 2020, https://scitechdaily.com/scientists-reverse-the-aging-clock-restore-age-related -vision-loss-through-epigenetic-reprogramming/.

14. S. Horvath et al., "Reversing Age: Dual Species Measurement of Epigenetic Age with a Single Clock," bioRxiv (preprint), (May 8, 2020), doi: 10.1101/2020.05.07.082917.

15. L. Gong et al., "Cancer Cell Reprogramming: A Promising Therapy Converting Malignancy to Benignity," *Cancer Communications* (London, England) 39 no. 1 (2019): 48, doi: 10.1186/s40880-019-0393-5.

16. M. Müller et al., "The Role of Pluripotency Factors to Drive Stemness in Gastrointestinal Cancer," *Stem Cell Research* 16, no. 2 (March 2016): 349–357, doi: 10.1016/j.scr.2016.02.005.

17. The Royal Swedish Academy of Sciences, "The Nobel Prize in Chemistry, 2020," October 7, 2020, www.nobelprize.org/prizes/chemistry/2020/press-release/.

18. Associated Press, "Lab Tests Show Risks of Using CRISPR Gene Editing on Embryos," October 29, 2020, www.statnews.com/2020/10/29/lab-tests-show-risks -of-using-crispr-gene-editing-on-embryos/.

19. Natalie Kolfer, "Why Were Scientists Silent over Gene-edited Babies?," *Nature*, February 26, 2019, www.nature.com/articles/d41586-019-00662-4.

20. Wallace Ravven, "Could Gene Editing Enable Us to Reverse Some of the Ravages of Aging?," Stanford Engineering, March 6, 2020, engineering .stanford.edu/magazine/article/could-gene-editing-enable-us-reverse-some-ravages -aging.

21. W. Wang et al., "A Genome-Wide CRISPR-Based Screen Identifies KAT7 as a Driver of Cellular Senescence," *Science Translational Medicine* 13, no. 575 (January 2021): eabd2655, doi: 10.1126/scitranslmed.abd2655.

22. J. D. Gillmore et al., "CRISPR-Cas9 In Vivo Gene Editing for Transthyretin Amyloidosis," *New England Journal of Medicine* 385 no. 6 (August 5, 2021): 493–502, doi: 10.1056/NEJMoa2107454.

23. S. Horvath et al., "Reversing Age: Dual Species Measurement of Epigenetic Age with a Single Clock," bioRxiv (preprint), (May 8, 2020), doi: 10.1101 /2020.05.07.082917.

24. Kira Peikoff, "Anti-Aging Pioneer Aubrey de Grey: 'People in Middle Age Now Have a Fair Chance,'" Leaps.org, January 31, 2018, https://leaps.org/anti-aging -pioneer-aubrey-de-grey-people-middle-age-now-fair-chance/particle-11.

THE RECIPES

1. G. Cardwell et al., "A Review of Mushrooms as a Potential Source of Dietary Vitamin D," *Nutrients* 10, no. 10 (October 13, 2018): 1498, doi: 10.3390/nu10101498.

NUTRIENT REFERENCE

1. B. W. Bolling, D. L. McKay, and J. B. Blumberg, "The Phytochemical Composition and Antioxidant Actions of Tree Nut," *Asia Pacific Journal of Clinical Nutrition* 19 no. 1 (2010): 117–123;

N. Brown, J. A. John, and F. Shahidi, "Polyphenol Composition and Antioxidant Potential of Mint Leaves," *Food Production, Processing, and Nutrition* 1, no. 1 (2019), doi: 10.1186/s43014-019-0001-8;

C. Busch et al., "Epigenetic Activities of Flavonoids in the Prevention and Treatment of Cancer," *Clinical Epigenetics* 7, no. 1 (2015): 64, doi: 10.1186/s13148-015-0095-z;

J. Cotas et al., "Seaweed Phenolics: From Extraction to Applications," *Marine Drugs* 18, no. 8 (2020): 384, doi: 10.3390/md18080384;

D. Y. Seo et al., "Ursolic Acid in Health and Disease," *Korean Journal of Physiology & Pharmacology* 22, no. 3 (2018): 235. doi: 10.4196/kjpp.2018.22.3.235;

Q. Dong et al., "Comparative Study on Phenolic Compounds, Triterpenoids, and Antioxidant Activity of *Ganoderma lucidum* Affected by Different Drying Methods," *Journal of Food Measurement and Characterization* 13 (2019): 3198–3205, doi: 10.1007/s11694-019-00242-0;

US Department of Agriculture, "FoodData Central," https://fdc.nal.usda.gov/;

M. J. Feeney et al., "Mushrooms and Health Summit Proceedings," *Journal of Nutrition* 144, no. 7 (2014): 1128S–1136S, doi: 10.3945/jn.114.190728;

M. Górecki and E. Hallmann, "The Antioxidant Content of Coffee and Its In Vitro Activity as an Effect of Its Production Method and Roasting and Brewing Time," *Antioxidants* (Basel, Switzerland) 9, no. 4 (2020): 308, doi: 10.3390/antiox9040308;

X. Han et al., "Dietary Polyphenols and Their Biological Significance," *International Journal of Molecular Sciences* 8, no. 9 (2007): 950–988, doi: 10.3390/i8090950;

D. Guo, et al., "Phenolics Content and Antioxidant Activity of Tartary Buckwheat from Different Locations." *Molecules*, 16, no. 12 (2011): 9850–9867. doi: 10.3390/molecules16129850;

D. G. Hayward, J. W. Wong, and H. Y. Park, "Determinations for Pesticides on Black, Green, Oolong, and White Teas by Gas Chromatography Triple-Quadrupole Mass Spectrometry," *Journal of Agricultural and Food Chemistry* 63, no. 37 (2015): 8116–8124, doi: 10.1021/acs.jafc.5b02860;

T. A. Hore, "Modulating Epigenetic Memory Through Vitamins and TET: Implications for Regenerative Medicine and Cancer Treatment," *Epigenomics* 9, no. 6 (2017), doi: 10.2217/epi-2017-0021;

C. A. Houghton, R. G. Fassett, and J. S. Coombes, "Sulforaphane and Other Nutrigenomic Nrf2 Activators: Can the Clinician's Expectation Be Matched by the Reality?," *Oxidative Medicine and Cellular Longevity* (2016), 7857186: doi: 10.1155/2016/7857186;

Phenol-Explorer: Database on Polyphenol Content in Foods, http://phenol -explorer.eu/;

D. B. Haytowitz, X. Wu, and S. Bagwat, "USDA Databsae for the Flavonoid Content of Selected Foods, Release 3.3," Nutrient Data Laboratory, Agricultural Research Service, US Department of Agriculture, March 2018, www.ars.usda.gov /ARSUserFiles/80400535/Data/Flav/Flav3.3.pdf;

X. Y. Huang et al., "Variation of Major Minerals and Trace Elements in Seeds of Tartary Buckwheat (Fagopyrum tataricum Gaertn.)," *Genetic Resources and Crop Evolution* 61 (2014): 567–577;

S. Ikeda et al., "Nutritional Characteristics of Minerals in Tartary Buckwheat," *Fagopyrum* 21 (2004): 79–84;

J. M. Calderon-Montano et al., "A Review on the Dietary Flavonoid Kaempferol," *Mini-Reviews in Medicinal Chemistry* 11 (2011): 298, doi: 10.2174/138955711795305335;

S. J. Kim et al., "Identification of Anthocyanins in the Sprouts of Buckwheat," *Journal of Agricultural and Food Chemistry* 55, no. 15 (2007): 6314–6318; doi: 10.1021/jf0704716;

Y. B. Kim et al., "Characterization of Genes for a Putative Hydroxycinnamoyl-coenzyme A Quinate Transferase and p-coumarate 3'-hydroxylase and Chlorogenic Acid Accumulation in Tartary Buckwheat," *Journal of Agricultural and Food Chemistry* 61, no. 17 (2013): 4120–4126, doi: 10.1021/jf4000659;

H. E. Khoo et al., "Anthocyanidins and Anthocyanins: Colored Pigments as Food, Pharmaceutical Ingredients, and the Potential Health Benefits," *Food & Nutrition Research* 61, no.1 (2017): 1361779, doi: 10.1080/16546628.2017 .1361779;

L. Machu et al., "Phenolic Content and Antioxidant Capacity in Algal Food Products," *Molecules* (Basel, Switzerland) 20, no.1 (2015): 1118–1133, doi: 10.3390 /molecules20011118;

S. Maina et al., "Human, Animal and Plant Health Benefits of Glucosinolates and Strategies for Enhanced Bioactivity: A Systematic Review," *Molecules* (Basel, Switzerland) 25, no. 16 (2020), doi: 10.3390/molecules25163682;

D. McCormack and D. McFadden, "A Review of Pterostilbene Antioxidant Activity and Disease Modification," *Oxidative Medicine and Cellular Longevity* (2013): 575482, doi: 10.1155/2013/575482;

B. Mahayothee at al., "Phenolic Compounds, Antioxidant Activity, and Medium Chain Fatty Acids Profiles of Coconut Water and Meat at Different Maturity Stages," *International Journal of Food Properties*, 19, no. 9 (2016): 2041–2051, doi: 10.1080/10942912.2015.1099042;

K. H. Miean and S. Mohamed, "Flavonoid (Myricetin, Quercetin, Kaempferol, Luteolin, and Apigenin) Content of Edible Tropical Plants," *Journal of Agricultural and Food Chemistry* 49, no. 6 (June 2001): 3106–3112, doi: 10.1021/jf000892m;

L. Němcová et al., "Determination of Resveratrol in Grains, Hulls and Leaves of Common and Tartary Buckwheat by HPLC with Electrochemical Detection at

Carbon Paste Electrode," *Food Chemistry* 126, no. 1 (2011): 374–378, doi: 10.1016/j .foodchem.2010.10.108;

"Dietary Supplement Fact Sheets," National Institutes of Health, https://ods .od.nih.gov/factsheets/;

H. C. Pal, R. L. Pearlman, and F. Afaq, "Fisetin and Its Role in Chronic Diseases," *Advances in Experimental Medicine and Biology* 928 (2016): 213–244, doi: 10.1007/978-3-319-41334-1_10;

S. Paul et al., "Dietary Intake of Pterostilbene, a Constituent of Blueberry, Inhibits the Beta-Catenin/p65 Downstream Signaling Pathway and Colon Carcinogenesis in Rats," *Carcinogenesis* 31, no. 7 (2010): 1272–1278, doi: 10.1093/carcin /bgq004;

P. Qin et al., "Nutritional Composition and Flavonoids Content of Flour from Different Buckwheat Cultivars," *International Journal of Food Science & Technology* 45, no. 5 (2010): 951–958, doi: 10.1111/j.1365-2621.2010.02231.x;

P. Qin et al., "Changes in Phytochemical Compositions, Antioxidant and α-glucosidase Inhibitory Activities During the Processing of Tartary Buckwheat Tea," *Food Research International* 50, no. 2 (2013): 562–567; doi: 10.1016/j.foodres .2011.03.028;

S. C. Ren and J. T. Sun, "Changes in Phenolic Content, Phenylalanine Ammonia-lyase (PAL) Activity, and Antioxidant Capacity of Two Buckwheat Sprouts in Relation to Germination," *Journal of Functional Foods* 7 (2014): 298–304, doi: 10.1016/j.jff.2014.01.031;

S. C. Rha et al., "Antioxidative, Anti-Inflammatory, and Anticancer Effects of Purified Flavonol Glycosides and Aglycones in Green Tea," *Antioxidants* 8, no. 8 (2019): 278, doi: 10.3390/antiox8080278;

A. M. Rimando et al., "Resveratrol, Pterostilbene, and Piceatannol in Vaccinium Berries," *Journal of Agricultural and Food Chemistry* 52, no. 15 (July 2004): 4713–4719, doi: 10.1021/jf040095e;

K. Szarc vel Szic et al., "Nature or Nurture: Let Food Be Your Epigenetic Medicine in Chronic Inflammatory Disorders," *Biochemical Pharmacology* 80, no. 12 (December 15, 2010): 1816–1832, Epub August 3, 2010, doi: 10.1016/j.bcp.2010.07.029;

C. A. Thomson, E. Ho, and M. B. Strom, "Chemopreventive Properties of 3,3'-Diindolylmethane in Breast Cancer: Evidence from Experimental and Human Studies," *Nutrition Review* 74, no. 7 (2016): 432–443, doi: 10.1093/nutrit/nuw010;

T. Watanabe, M. Kioka, and A. Fukushima, "Biotin Content Table of Select Foods and Biotin Intake in Japanese," *International Journal of Analytical Bio -Science* 2, no. 4 (2014): 109–125;

Z. Yiming et al., "Evolution of Nutrient Ingredients in Tartary Buckwheat Seeds During Germination," *Food Chemistry* 186 (November 1, 2015): 244–248, doi: 10.1016/j.foodchem.2015.03.115;

F. Zhang et al., "Oleanolic Acid and Ursolic Acid in Commercial Dried Fruits," *Food Science and Technology Research* 19, no. 1 (2013): 113–116, doi: 10.3136/fstr.19.113;

X. Zhou et al., "Relationships Between Antioxidant Compounds and Antioxidant Activities of Tartary Buckwheat During Germination," *Journal of Food Science and Technology* 52, no. 4 (2015): 2458–2463, doi: 10.1007/s13197-014-1290-1;

S. Baghwat, D. B. Haytowitz, and J. M. Holden, "USDA Database for the Flavonoid Content of Selected Foods," Release 3, Nutrient Data Laboratory, Beltsville Human Nutrition Research Center, Agricultural Research Service, US Department of Agriculture, September 2011, www.ars.usda.gov/ARSUserFiles /80400525/Data/Flav/Flav_R03.pdf;

C. Ozuna and M.F. León-Galván, "Cucurbitaceae Seed Protein Hydrolysates as a Potential Source of Bioactive Peptides with Functional Properties," *BioMed Research International*, 2017 (2017): 2121878, doi: 10.1155/2017/2121878;

National Institutes of Health Office of Dietary Supplements, "Iron: Fact Sheet for Health Professionals," updated March 30, 2021, https://ods.od.nih.gove /factsheets/Iron-HealthProfessional/.

2. T. A. Hore et al., "Retinol and Ascorbate Drive Erasure of Epigenetic Memory and Enhance Reprogramming to Naive Pluripotency by Complementary Mechanisms," *Proceedings of the National Academy of Sciences of the United States of America* 113 (2016): 12202–12207, doi: 10.1073/pnas.1608679113.

3. L. Chen et al., "Effects of Vitamin D_3 Supplementation on Epigenetic Aging in Overweight and Obese African Americans with Suboptimal Vitamin D Status: A Randomized Clinical Trial," *Journals of Gerontology Series A: Biological Sciences and Medical Sciences* 74, no. 1 (January 1, 2019): 91–98, doi: 10.1093/gerona/gly223.

4. G. Rizzo and A. S. Laganà, "The Link between Homocysteine and Omega-3 Polyunsaturated Fatty Acid: Critical Appraisal and Future Directions," *Biomolecules* 10, no. 2 (February 2, 2020): 219, doi: 10.3390/biom10020219.

INDEX

RECIPE INDEX